Spinal Manual Therapy

An Introduction to
Soft Tissue Mobilization,
Spinal Manipulation,
Therapeutic and
Home Exercises

Spinal Manual Therapy

An Introduction to Soft Tissue Mobilization, Spinal Manipulation, Therapeutic and Home Exercises

Howard W. Makofsky, PT, DHSc, OCS
Assistant Professor, New York Institute of Technology
Old Westbury, New York

Adjunct Professor, Touro College School of Health Sciences
Bay Shore and New York, New York

Clinical Assistant Professor, University at Stony Brook
Stony Brook, New York

Codirector, TMJ Center, Southside Institute for Physical Therapy
Bay Shore, New York

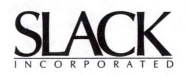

SLACK
INCORPORATED

An innovative information, education, and management company
6900 Grove Road • Thorofare, NJ 08086

Makofsky, Howard W., 1955-
  Spinal manual therapy : an introduction to soft tissue mobilization,
spinal manipulation, therapeutic and home exercises / Howard W.
Makofsky.
     p. ; cm.
  Includes bibliographical references and index.
  ISBN 1-55642-569-4 (alk. paper)
  1. Spinal adjustment.
  [DNLM: 1. Manipulation, Spinal--methods. 2. Musculoskeletal
Manipulations--methods. 3. Pelvis. 4. Temporomandibular Joint. WB 535
M235s 2003] I. Title.
RZ265.S64M355 2003
615.8'2--dc21
                              2003004761

Printed in the United States of America.

Published by: SLACK Incorporated
                         6900 Grove Road
                         Thorofare, NJ 08086 USA
                         Telephone: 856-848-1000
                         Fax: 856-853-5991
                         www.slackbooks.com

Last digit is print number: 10 9 8 7 6 5 4 3 2 1

Dedication

To my wife, Frances (Nak), whose faith and love of the Scriptures inspire and
strengthen me

To my children, Katherine, Margaret, Russell, and Daniel, who are the pride and
joy of my life

To my parents, Mildred Makofsky and the late Abe Makofsky, and to Margaret
and Dr. Christopher Willis,
for their guidance and love

To my brother and sister, Bob and Sharon, and close relatives, your enduring support and concern are a great blessing

To Christ, my King!

In memory of Jeffrey J. Ellis, PT, manual therapist par excellence, who went home
to be with his Lord on May 18, 2001.

"Fantasy abandoned by reason produces monsters,
but when united to it, is the mother of all art."
Francisco Goya

Contents

Acknowledgments

King Solomon once said, "There is nothing new under the sun. Is there anything of which it may be said, 'See, this is new?' It has already been in ancient times before us." This is especially true when dealing with the healing art of manual therapy. To this end, I cannot help but acknowledge those who have helped to lay the foundation upon which the rest of us have been building. Some of the "all-stars" who have helped to establish many of the principles found in this text and whom I have had the privilege of learning from firsthand include S. Paris, C. Steele, M. Bookhout, E. Stiles, P. Greenman, J. Bourdillion, F. Mitchell Jr, P. Kimberly, L. Rex, J. Mennell, M. Rocabado, S. Kraus, O. Grimsby, F. Kaltenborn, C. Patla, S. Burkhart, R. Bowling, R. Woodman, B. Biondi, A. DiMaggio, R. Sofer, J. Ellis, J. Mannheimer, M. Dorfman, A. Grodin, G. Johnson, T. Sexton, P. Loubert, B. Miller, S. Cooper, L. Goldfarb, A. Warmerdam, D. Plante, M. Dunn, M. Helland, G. Willner, B. Libin, J. Kahn, R. Sprague, and P. Fabian.

In any large-scale effort, there are those individuals without whom success could not have been possible. I want to express my gratitude to my wife, Frances, for her support and love from the beginning; to my sons, Russell and Daniel, for their help with photography; and a heartfelt thank you to my brother-in-law and photographer, Bill Willis, who gave self-lessly of his time and expertise. Thanks to Dorothea and Paula for their assistance and expertise at a crucial juncture early in the project and to Ed Klein for a great job with various illustrations.

Sincere thanks to John Bond, Amy McShane, Lauren Plummer, April Billick, and the whole team at SLACK Incorporated for making this book a reality, especially Carrie Kotlar, acquisitions editor, who patiently guided me through the entire publication process. Appreciation is expressed to friends and colleagues at the New York Institute of Technology (thanks Bill for showing me the "undo typing" function on my tool bar!), Touro College, and the Southside Institute for Physical Therapy. Special thanks to the library staff at NYCOM and Touro College for their assistance with articles, books, etc; to Serenity Photo for their patience and hard work; and to Neil Solina for helping with last minute pictures on such short notice.

There are several colleagues who gave me inspiration and encouragement along the way and to them I'd like to say thanks as well. They are L. Goldstein, P. Douris, W. Werner, K. Friel, V. Southard, K. Hewson, R. McKenna, L. Morrone, P. Gambardella, K. Cerrone, T. Ingenito, J. Benanti, P. McQuade, B. Davis, J. Megna, D. Dougherty, R. Streb, W. DeTurk, P. Szabo, J. Magel, N. Machnik, R. Spagnoli, R. Fernandez, F. Corio, S. Jacobson, R. Shapiro, J. Macaluso, I. Flattau, K. Correia, D. O'Brien, R. Lov, D. Porter, C. Foster, R. Mattfeld, R. Anziano, L. Schonbrun, A. Kosiba, M. Nolan, B. Finnerty, D. Diamond, B. August, J. Weisberg, L. Mancini, K. Sheehan, C. Hall, J. Handrakis, C. Mereday, B. Silvestri, S. Waldman, F. Bowman, and J. Schleichkorn.

Appreciation is also expressed to the undergraduate/graduate physical therapy students at the New York Institute of Technology, Touro College, and the University at Stony Brook, as well as the practicing physical therapists whom I have had the privilege of instructing over the past 17 years. You thought I was the teacher, when all the time you were teaching me!

About the Author

Howard W. Makofsky, PT, DHSc, OCS is an assistant professor of physical therapy at the New York Institute of Technology, Old Westbury, NY, an adjunct professor of physical therapy at the Touro College School of Health Sciences, Bay Shore and New York, NY, and a clinical assistant professor of physical therapy at the University at Stony Brook, Stony Brook, NY. Dr. Makofsky holds a BSc degree in Physiology from McGill University, a BS in Physical Therapy and an MS in Health Science from the University at Stony Brook, and a Doctor of Health Science from the University of St. Augustine for Health Sciences.

Dr. Makofsky is an APTA board certified orthopaedic clinical specialist with 24 years of clinical experience in the management of neuromusculoskeletal impairment of the vertebral column, temporomandibular joint, pelvic girdle and extremity joints. From 1985 through 1995, Dr. Makofsky was the chief therapist at the Southside Institute for Physical Therapy in Bay Shore, NY where he developed the TMJ and Headache Centers, based upon his experience from 1982 through 1985, with the Facial Pain Clinic at the Braintree Rehabilitation Center in Braintree, MA.

Dr. Makofsky has published numerous articles in both the physical therapy and dental literature and is currently on the editorial board of the Journal of Craniomandibular Practice and the Journal of Manual & Manipulative Therapy. Dr. Makofsky maintains a small private practice in Mastic Beach, NY with emphasis on manipulative therapy and therapeutic exercise for painful conditions of the spine, pelvis, TMJ, and extremity joints.

Howard and his wife Frances reside on eastern Long Island with their sons Russell and Daniel. Their two daughters, Katherine and Margaret, attend university in Montreal, Quebec. The highlight of Dr. Makofsky's career was participating in a medical mission's trip to La Calera, Chile in 1993 with Healthcare Ministries.

Preface

The field of manual physical therapy experienced unprecedented growth at the end of the 20th century with an unparalleled proliferation of journal articles, textbooks, CD-ROMS, course offerings, and web sites. Today's manual physical therapy instructors are well-equipped with a plethora of basic science and clinical resource material with which to educate students at all levels of experience, from the novice to the advanced practitioner. Though manual therapy instructors have access to many excellent publications on the topic, there are few books that are suitable as textbooks in an introductory college course on spinal manual therapy. Among these few, there is still the need for a user-friendly, *Guide to Physical Therapist Practice*-compatible approach to the basic examination and intervention of spinal impairment utilizing myofascial, articular, and exercise therapies.

The purpose of this textbook is to provide manual therapy instructors with a reference text on the spine, pelvis, and temporomandibular joint that covers all the clinical aspects of an introduction to spinal manual therapy. It is not intended, however, to provide the basic science component of such a course, but is geared toward the clinical application of spinal manual therapy and is intended for use during the lab portion of the course. It will also have utility on clinical rotations in spinal manual therapy and upon entry into the field as a new graduate.

Section I establishes the basic principles upon which the remainder of the book is based. It presents the essential concepts of an eclectic approach that attempts to integrate the major schools of thought in manual therapy education today. These principles are based upon the art and science of practice and are consistent with the conceptual models of disablement and functional limitations. These foundational principles will serve as a compass as we navigate our way through this material. As a matter of clarification, this text is consistent with the 2001 edition of the *Guide to Physical Therapist Practice* and the American Academy of Orthopedic Manual Physical Therapists, and uses the terms *manipulation* and *mobilization* interchangeably.

Through the remaining sections of the book, the student is presented with a comprehensive approach to manual therapy that includes all aspects of physical therapy examination, diagnosis, and intervention, with emphasis on soft tissue mobilization, spinal manipulative therapy, and therapeutic and home exercises. The scapulothoracic region is addressed first because of its importance to both the upper and lower half of the body. In my opinion, it, like the hip region, is where the manipulation of joint and soft tissue impairment is most needed. The approach taught in this book is not based in theory, but upon my own clinical and academic experience in manual physical therapy over the past 24 years of practice.

The reader will note that there are no specific manual techniques of examination and intervention for either upper cervical or sacral dysfunction. Because of the mechanical complexity of these regions, they are best covered in textbooks on advanced spinal manual therapy. The basic treatment techniques and therapeutic/home exercises covered in this text are more than adequate for the majority of patients with impairment of these areas.

The goal of this introductory textbook is "to make the complex simple." It is my hope that those who work through this material find this to be the case.

Howard W. Makofsky, PT, DHSc, OCS

Foreword

Manual therapy is finally receiving the attention that it most certainly deserves in the curriculum of physical therapy education. The debate continues as to whether the practice of manual therapy is a science or an art. This book is written in an attempt to address this question from both perspectives, presenting evaluation and treatment strategies with the supporting scientific rationale, when known, for their use.

There are few books currently available that present more than one approach to the evaluation and treatment of spinal dysfunction. This author emphasizes an eclectic approach and covers "all the basics" that a physical therapist needs to thoroughly evaluate and treat the vast majority of patients presenting with spinal pain/dysfunction.

The author's intent is for this book to be used as a reference text for physical therapy students who are being introduced to spinal manual therapy. It helps to bridge the gap between classroom instruction and the actual application of various manual therapy approaches. The case presentations at the end of the book help to foster the clinical decision-making process our students so urgently need to develop, particularly if we, as a profession, are to be recognized as frontline practitioners.

Mark R. Bookhout, PT, MS

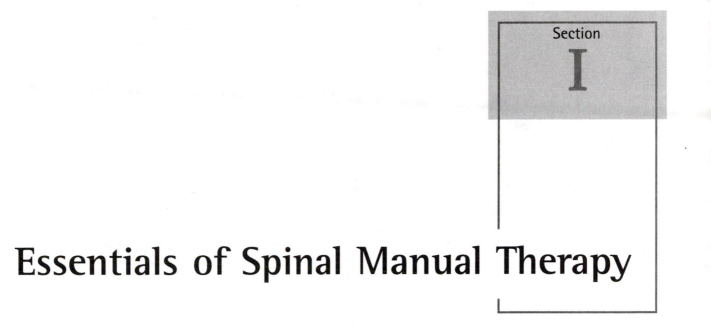

Section

I

Essentials of Spinal Manual Therapy

Vertebral Motion Dynamics

The Vertebral Motion Segment

The basic unit of spinal motion is the vertebral motion segment. It consists of two connecting vertebrae—the superior and the inferior—and all related anatomic structures, including the intervertebral disc, two apophyseal joints, and various soft tissues. An example of a vertebral motion segment is the third cervical vertebra (C3) situated above the fourth cervical vertebra (C4). The nomenclature used to describe this union is the C3,4 motion segment. Other examples are T8,9 (thoracic spine) and L3,4 (lumbar spine). A junction or transitional segment is an area where one region of the spine is joined to a different region. Examples are the cervicothoracic, the thoracolumbar, and the lumbosacral junctions. The cervicothoracic junction is synonymous with C7,T1; the thoracolumbar junction with T12,L1; and the lumbosacral junction with L5,S1.

Physiologic Motion

Each of the 24 vertebrae (7 cervical, 12 thoracic, and 5 lumbar) have the ability to move in four planes of reference. These motions include forward bending or flexion, backward bending or extension, side bending or lateral flexion to the right and left, and rotation to the right and left.

Motion Axes

Each of these four spinal motions can be considered rotations about an orthogonal axis (Figure 1-1). Forward and backward bending are rotations about the X or horizontal axis, side bending is a rotation about the Z or antero-posterior axis, and axial rotation occurs about the Y or vertical axis. The thumb, index, and middle fingers of one hand can be used to assist in recalling these three axes of spinal motion. The thumb pointing to the ceiling represents the Y or vertical axis, the middle finger flexed to 90 degrees at the metacarpophalangeal joint represents the X axis, and the index finger at a right angle to the middle finger, directed anteriorly, represents the Z axis (Figure 1-2).

Rule of Superior Motion

When manual therapists describe segmental motion, it is understood that the superior vertebra is mentioned first. For example, side bending right at the T5,6 motion segment suggests that the fifth thoracic vertebra (T5) is side bending right on T6. Most often this will be documented as T5,6 side bending right. However, some clinicians may describe this in short form as T5 side bending right. When only one vertebral level is noted, it denotes that segment's motion not under the level above but rather over the level below. Consequently, T5 side bending right refers to its motion relative to T6; L4 rotation left is motion relative to L5. This is the case whether spinal motion is initiated from above down or from below up. For example, trunk rotation that is initiated by rotating the lower extremities and pelvis to the right and proceeding up to and including T8 is still described as T7,8 rotation left by virtue of the fact that T7 is left rotated relative to T8.

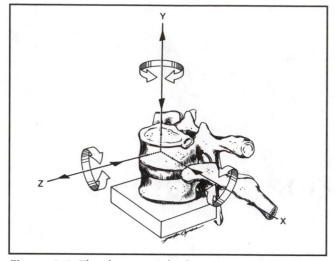

Figure 1-1. The three vertebral motion axes (reprinted with permission from Lee D. Biomechanics of the thorax: a clinical model of in vitro function. *J Man & Manip Ther*. 1993;1(1):14).

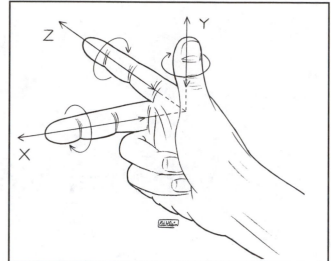

Figure 1-2. Manual illustration of the three cardinal axes. (Illustration by Ed Klein)

Rule of Vertebral Body Motion

A vertebra's motion is always described by the direction of vertebral body motion and not spinous process movement. Consequently, a passive movement of the T11 spinous process to the left, which induces vertebral rotation to the right, is described as T11,12 rotation right because of the direction of vertebral body motion.

Fryette's Rules of Spinal Motion

Rule 1

When one or more motion segments are positioned in neutral (ie, loose-packed) with the apophyseal joints "idling," side bending and rotation are coupled to opposite sides (Figure 1-3). For example, in a neutral lordosis, side bending to the left from L1 through L5 is associated with Y-axis rotation to the right. Rule 1 is referred to as neutral or type 1 spinal mechanics. Neutral mechanics occur in all vertebral segments except from C2 through C7, where there is no true neutral position of the apophyseal joints.

Rule 2

When a spinal motion segment is positioned in either flexion or extension such that the apophyseal joints are in apposition (ie, engaged), side bending to one side is coupled with Y-axis rotation to the same side (Figure 1-4). For example, side bending to the right at T7,8 from a position of trunk flexion is associated with T7 rotation right. Rule 2 is referred to as non-neutral or type 2 spinal mechanics. Non-neutral mechanics occur in all vertebral segments

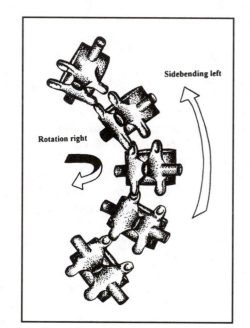

Figure 1-3. Type 1 spinal mechanics (reprinted from Gibbons P, Tehan P. *Manipulation of the Spine, Thorax, and Pelvis: An Osteopathic Perspective*. Edinburgh: Churchill Livingstone; 2000, by permission of the publisher Churchill Livingstone).

except in the upper cervical spine (occipitoatlantal and atlantoaxial joints) where only neutral mechanics prevail. At the L5,S1 motion segment, studies[1] have demonstrated that non-neutral mechanics predominate regardless of trunk position (ie, neutral, flexion, or extension).

It is now believed that the upper thoracic region from T1 through T4 tends to follow the lower cervical spine in type 2 mechanics. It is also believed that the thoracic region from T5 through T12 follows type 2 mechanics, when Y-axis rotation precedes Z-axis side bending.[2]

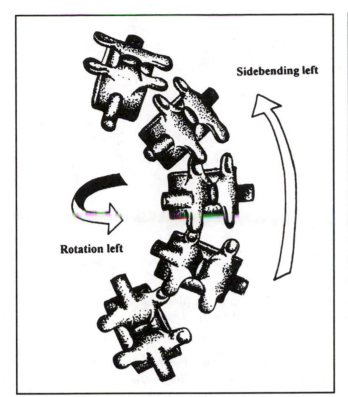

Figure 1-4. Type 2 spinal mechanics (reprinted from Gibbons P, Tehan P. *Manipulation of the Spine, Thorax, and Pelvis: An Osteopathic Perspective.* Edinburgh: Churchill Livingstone; 2000, by permission of the publisher Churchill Livingstone).

A final exception to Fryette's rules or "laws" involves the lumbar spine from L1 through L4. It is now believed that these segments demonstrate type 1 mechanics, not type 2 in which the motion occurs from an extended position of the lumbar spine.[1]

Rule 3

When motion is introduced in one plane, the available motion in the remaining planes is reduced. For example, rotation of the head-neck is greater in an upright posture than it is in a slumped posture. Likewise, trunk side bending is greater in a neutral position of the spine than in a flexed or extended position of the spine.

The converse of this also applies (ie, if motion is increased in one plane, it will also be increased in the other planes as well). For example, if lumbar spine side bending is increased through manipulative therapy, then the other motions of flexion, extension, and rotation will increase as well.

Type 1 and 2 Impairment

Restricted spinal motion involving three or more segments in a neutral position of the trunk is referred to as type 1 or neutral impairment (ie, dysfunction).

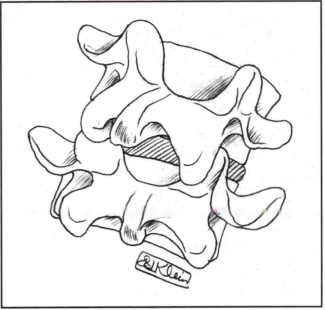

Figure 1-5. Facet opening of L5,S1 on the left. (Illustration by Ed Klein)

For example, in a neutral trunk position a restriction in left side bending from T9 through T12 is associated with a restriction at the same levels in right rotation. This is also referred to as a type 1 rotoscoliosis, and its position can often be identified on an anteroposterior spinal radiograph.

Restricted spinal motion of one segment in a non-neutral position is referred to as type 2 or non-neutral impairment. For example, T3,4 is said to be FRS (flexed, rotated, and side bent) right when it is limited in the opposite directions (ie, extension, rotation, and side bending to the left). Conversely, L4,5 is said to be ERS (extended, rotated, and side bent) left when it is limited in flexion, rotation, and side bending to the right. These one-segment motion impairments may not be easily seen on a spinal radiograph, but can be readily diagnosed through osteopathic segmental motion analysis.[2]

Apophyseal Joint Kinematics

Facet Opening

The term *facet opening* refers to the anterior and superior glide of the inferior articular process of the superior vertebra on the superior articular process of the vertebra below. For example, the L5,S1 facets are said to open bilaterally in lumbar flexion; open on the left during flexion, side bending, and rotation to the right (Figure 1-5); or open on the right during flexion, side bending, and rotation to the left.

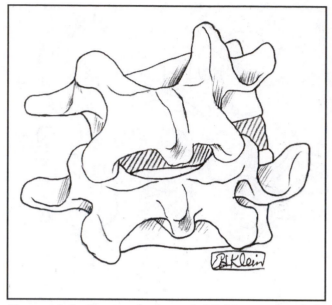

Figure 1-6. Facet closing of L5,S1 on the left. (Illustration by Ed Klein)

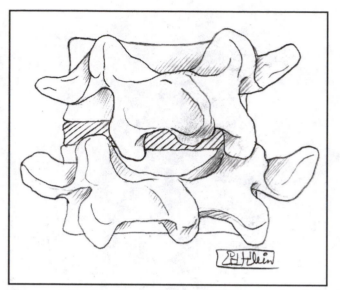

Figure 1-7. Facet gapping of L5,S1 on the left. (Illustration by Ed Klein)

Facet Closing

The term *facet closing* refers to the posterior and inferior glide of the inferior articular process of the superior vertebra on the superior articular process of the vertebra below. For example, the L5,S1 facets are said to close bilaterally in lumbar extension; close on the left during extension, side bending, and rotation to the left (Figure 1-6); or close on the right during extension, side bending, and rotation to the right.

Facet Gapping

The term *facet gapping* refers to the separation or distraction of the joint surfaces in a perpendicular direction. If the L5,S1 facet were to gap on the left, this implies that the inferior articular process of L5 separates away from the superior articular process of S1. Gapping in the facets generally occurs in the thoracic and lumbar spines in response to neutral rotation on the ipsilateral side (Figure 1-7). On the contralateral side, the facets approximate each other as they are compressed together.

Roll-Gliding

According to Kaltenborn,[3] the vertebral motion segment, not unlike the extremity joints, moves in a roll-gliding fashion. Except for the occipital condyles, which are convex surfaces moving on the concave surfaces of the atlas, the remainder of the motion segments of the spine behave as a concave surface moving on a convex one. This suggests that the roll of the superior component will glide in the same direction on the inferior component below. We have previously described the X, Y, and Z motion axes, but

only with regard to rotation. However, to appreciate how a rigid body moves in space (ie, the helical axis of motion), we need to consider not only rotation (roll) about a given axis, but also the translation that occurs along a different axis (see Figure 1-1). For example, forward bending of the T7,8 motion segment involves anterior rotation (roll) of T7 about an X axis as well as anterior translation (glide) of T7 along the Z axis. Backward bending of T7,8 involves X axis posterior rotation and Z axis posterior translation. For side bending motion about a Z axis, there is vertebral translation in the same direction along the X axis. The roll-gliding that occurs with Y axis rotation is dependent upon the vertebral segment involved. At the atlantoaxial segment, axial rotation about the Y axis is associated with a craniocaudal translation along the same Y axis such that there is a slight loss of height as the extreme of rotation is reached. The vertical height is then restored when the head is rotated to neutral. Consequently, each vertebral motion segment has a total of six degrees of freedom—three for rotation and three for translation.

Based upon this review of spinal mechanics, it can be said that motion of the superior component of the motion segment demonstrates both rotation and translation in the same direction. If we accept the premise that the superior and inferior components of the motion segment have relative motions that are out of phase with each other, then it can also be said that the superior component of the segment will roll in one direction while the inferior component will glide in the opposite direction. For example, backward bending of T5,6 involves a backward roll of T5 about the X axis with an anterior glide of T6 along the Z axis. This is not unlike an extremity joint in which a concave surface moves upon a convex one as at the trapezium-scaphoid joint in the midcarpal region of the wrist. Just as wrist extension involves a posterior roll of the trapezium with

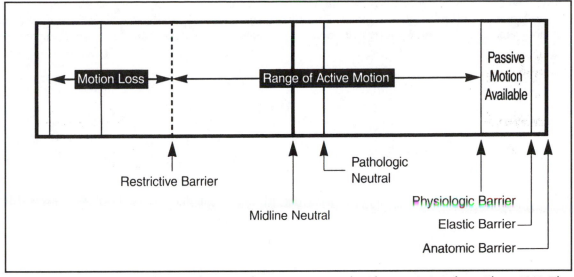

Figure 1-8. Normal and abnormal motion barriers (reprinted with permission from Flynn TW. *The Thoracic Spine and Rib Cage: Musculoskeletal Evaluation and Treatment.* Boston, Mass: Butterworth-Heinemann; 1996).

concurrent anterior gliding of the scaphoid, likewise T6 "dives" underneath the extending T5 as one would do at the beach in the presence of a formidable wave. Consequently, a manipulation of T6 in a posteroanterior direction will improve backward bending range at the T5,6 segment. Since translation is a mechanically simpler movement to perform manually, therapists routinely manipulate the inferior component of a segment to achieve improvement in range. It is also common to perform a combination of roll-gliding in the spine with a simultaneous roll of the superior component while gliding the inferior component in the opposite direction. A second example involves the motion of side bending. Side bending left at L4,5 involves a Z axis roll to the left of L4 and a glide of L5 along the X axis to the right. Consequently, a translational manipulation of L5 to the right under L4 or a manipulative combination of an L4 roll in left side bending with a concurrent glide of L5 to the right can be utilized to enhance the motion of left side bending at L4,5. Another commonly used term for rotation or roll is *overturning*; another term for translation or glide is *slide*.

Motion Barriers

There are three normal and one abnormal barriers to joint motion (Figure 1-8).

Physiologic Barrier

The end of an active, voluntary effort in a normal joint is the physiologic barrier for that motion. Every movement in the body has an associated physiologic barrier.

Elastic Barrier

The elastic barrier is the point at which the soft tissue slack is taken up during a passive movement in a normal joint.

Anatomic Barrier

The anatomic barrier is the absolute end-point in the passive range of motion in a normal joint beyond which tissue injury occurs.

Restrictive Barrier

The premature motion loss in an impaired joint is known as the restrictive barrier. It may represent a restriction at any point in the overall range of motion of a joint. It is associated with an abnormal end-feel (ie, hard or nonyielding versus resilient and supple). Restrictive barriers have multiple causes (ie, muscle splinting, capsular fibrosis, internal derangement, myofascial tightness, etc) and are responsible for causing either a major motion loss when 50% or more of the range is restricted or a minor motion loss involving less than 50% of the range of motion in a specific direction.

It is important to understand that the restrictive barrier presents as a range of restriction rather than as a definitive end-point. This restricted "range" spans from the initial sense of tension, which osteopathic physicians refer to as the "feather edge," to the end-range of the restriction in which all the "slack" has been taken up. The feather edge is the point used for localization purposes in osteopathic muscle energy technique, whereas the end-range is challenged during certain articular manipulative procedures.

The restrictive barrier is an impairment that results from tissue pathology and can lead to functional limitation and disability if not given the appropriate intervention. The goal of manual therapy is to diagnose and correct these impairments so that the associated functional limitation and disability are minimized or ideally eliminated.

McKenzie's Three Syndromes

Postural Syndrome

According to McKenzie,[4] patients with postural syndrome are usually under 30 years of age and, by definition, are devoid of restrictive barriers. These patients develop symptoms that appear locally and usually adjacent to the spine. The pain is provoked by mechanical deformation of normal, healthy tissue when spinal segments are subjected to static loading over prolonged periods of time. The resulting pain disappears when the structure under load is released from tension.

The pain from postural syndrome is not induced by movement and is never referred to a distant site. Because there is no associated inflammation, it is never constant. Examination of these patients fails to reveal impairment because there is no underlying tissue pathology. The only consistent finding is pain provocation with static loading at end-range. Simply put, postural pain develops gradually when normal tissues are overstretched.

The most useful intervention is to correct the faulty alignment wherever it is found (ie, sitting, standing, lying, walking, etc). This may also involve an ergonomic assessment of furniture, mattresses, pillows, etc, as well as an analysis of the patient's conditions at the worksite.

The long-term complication of postural syndrome is that it can eventually cause pathologic changes in the soft tissues with resultant impairment. However, this will not likely occur with proper instruction in correct posture, ergonomic intervention, and proper body mechanics.

Dysfunction Syndrome

An uncorrected postural problem will cause pathologic changes over time. For example, a 35-year-old computer operator who spends 8 hours per day in a forward head position will eventually develop adaptive shortening of the occipital extensor muscles. Likewise, the 40-year-old truck driver who spends 10 hours per day in a slumped sitting posture will eventually discover an inability to assume a normal lumbar lordosis in standing because of adaptive shortening of the trunk flexors.

As per the Nagi Functional Limitations Model,[5] these adaptive changes in connective tissue (ie, adhesions, depletion of hyaluronic acid, etc) represent pathophysiologic events that cause such macroscopic tissue impairment as restricted joint mobility, muscle weakness, and the faulty alignment that is often associated with imbalance in the musculoskeletal system. If the patient does not correct his or her impairment with the proper interventions, he or she can go on to develop functional limitations and disability, which can adversely affect performance at work, home, etc.

A distinguishing feature of the patient with dysfunction syndrome includes painful symptoms that tend to arise at the end of range rather than during movement. This patient has intermittent pain similar to the postural patient, but differs in that his or her soft tissues are abnormally tight. The symptoms are usually adjacent to the spine and are never referred distally except in the case of an adherent nerve root. Simply stated, the pain of dysfunction syndrome is produced immediately when shortened tissues are overstretched.

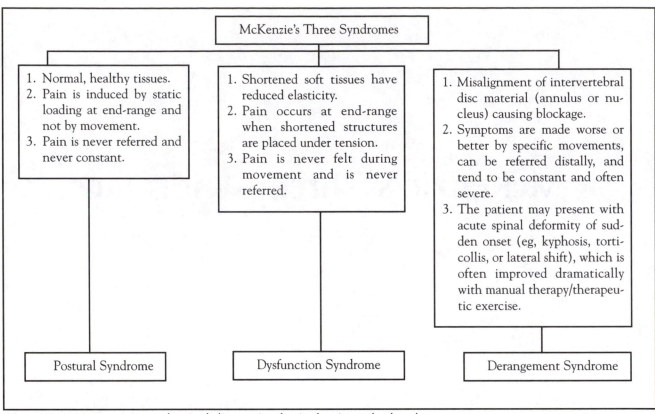

Figure 2-1. McKenzie's mechanical diagnosis of spinal pain and related symptoms.

As with postural syndrome, dysfunction syndrome also has a long-term complication. If untreated with the appropriate intervention (ie, manipulative therapy), it can cause more destructive pathology and result in the last of McKenzie's three syndromes, namely derangement syndrome. However, in some cases a traumatic event in the absence of preexisting dysfunction is enough to cause derangement of the intervertebral disc.

Derangement Syndrome

Characteristics of this syndrome can include neurologic signs and symptoms, pain during movement, acute deformity (eg, torticollis, lumbar kyphosis, lateral shift phenomenon), and pain that is severe and disabling. Patients with derangement syndrome often have a history of poor posture and progressive stiffness. It is believed that the lack of motion-based nutrition in conjunction with off-center loading on the intervertebral disc causes the displacement of disc material. The young are more likely to have a nuclear displacement, while those over the age of 50 tend to develop annular lesions. With the onset of degenerative disc disease, patients may develop segmental instability, which requires stabilization training of the hypermobile segment(s) in conjunction with manual therapy of the stiff, hypomobile segments above and/or below.

Patients with derangement syndrome (primarily occurring in the cervical and lumbar spine) often describe their neck and/or back as being "out." It is imperative that these patients be correctly diagnosed lest they be deprived of the correct intervention. The deranged disc requires an approach that is quite different from dysfunction syndrome and will not respond unless managed appropriately. The goals of intervention are as follows:

1. The derangement must be properly reduced.

2. The reduction must be stabilized.

3. Once the derangement is stable, lost function must be recovered.

4. The prevention of recurrence of the derangement must be emphasized.

The classification of spinal impairment into one of McKenzie's three syndromes (Figure 2-1) is just the beginning of establishing the correct intervention. There are further subclassifications of both the dysfunction and derangement syndromes. These are made during the evaluation process and are necessary in establishing the correct diagnosis. Though the theory behind McKenzie's approach[4] can and should be presented in every textbook on spinal manual therapy, it is not until the therapist attends a McKenzie workshop that a true understanding of this unique problem-based approach to spinal patients takes place.

Principles of Manual Examination, Diagnosis, and Intervention

Somatic Impairment

When asked about the manipulable lesion, osteopathic physicians for years described the "osteopathic lesion." This lesion has been replaced with the term *somatic dysfunction* over the past 20 years. With the advent of the *Guide to Physical Therapist Practice* and the sweeping changes that are occurring within physical therapy, it seems more appropriate that the term *dysfunction* be replaced by *impairment*. The term *somatic impairment* will be used to describe an impairment of function in the neuromusculoskeletal system that is mechanical in nature. It is a term to be contrasted with systemic disease,[6] requiring the expertise of a physician for diagnosis and management. Whereas disease is within the realm of medicine and surgery, physical or somatic impairment is within the realm of physical therapy. It develops as a result of tissue pathology, but the pathology is of a mechanical nature and can be traced to nonsystemic causes, including macrotrauma, cumulative microtrauma, immobilization, etc.

As per McKenzie's classification, it is useful to subclassify somatic impairment as either a dysfunction or a derangement. As stated previously, these syndromes, though both are somatically based, behave quite differently. Whereas dysfunction is related to adaptive shortening of tissue, a derangement involves displacement of an intrajoint structure (ie, meniscus, intervertebral disc, etc). Both are amenable to manual therapy, but in severe cases a nonreducing derangement may require the skills of a surgeon to correct the problem.

Schafer and Faye[7] subclassify dysfunction as either class I, II, or III and refer to them as fixations. Class I fixations are muscular in nature, class II fixations are related to the shortening of ligaments, and class III fixations represent true articular hypomobility. This classification system is based upon motion palpation and helps to determine the type of manual therapy that is utilized.

Stiles[8] emphasizes the area of greatest restriction (AGR) in his attempt to prioritize manipulative management. It is based upon the premise that areas of major hypomobility in the body are the "engines" that drive the entire system into an inefficient state in which impairment develops and symptoms result. Whereas a symptom-oriented approach to therapy addresses secondary and compensatory areas of impairment, a manually-oriented approach seeks to locate the AGR, even though it is usually asymptomatic and often found some distance away from the patient's complaint. It is the author's opinion that the AGR is most often found in the thoracic cage and hips. Most of the neck, shoulder, and low back pain that present clinically would be better managed by identifying and treating the AGR rather than applying "fake, shake, and bake" therapy to the symptomatic areas of hypermobile compensation.

Joint mobility is evaluated with regard to the quality of motion, the quantity of motion, and the end-feel. Normal joints demonstrate smooth, friction-free, and interference-free movement and have a healthy degree of "play" at the end-range. In contrast, pathologic joints demonstrate friction, joint sounds, and deviations from normal motion. They may feel blocked, restricted, or abnormally loose at the end-range and have either limited or excessive gliding motions. Most approaches to manual therapy utilize the 0 to 6 scale for grading joint mobility where 0 = ankylosed, 1 = markedly hypomobile, 2 = slightly hypomobile, 3 = normal, 4 = slightly hypermobile, 5 = markedly hypermobile, and 6 = unstable.[9]

The CHARTS Method of Manual Examination

The ART method of physical examination has been the mainstay of the osteopathic diagnosis of somatic dysfunction for several years.[+] This diagnostic triad identifies three key components of a somatic dysfunction. They are as follows: A stands for *asymmetry* of related parts of the musculoskeletal system; R stands for *range of motion* of a joint, several joints, or region of the musculoskeletal system; and T stands for *tissue texture abnormality* of the soft tissues of the musculoskeletal system (eg, skin, fascia, muscle, ligament, capsule). It is believed that a true somatic dysfunction demonstrates all three components of the triad. For example, spasm of the right levator scapulae muscle will be associated with the following findings: A—elevation of the right scapula, R—restricted cervical spine side bending left, and T—increased tone and tenderness of the right levator scapulae.

In the late 1980s, physical therapists at Southside Hospital in Bay Shore, NY, under the direction of Jeffrey Ellis,[10] elaborated on the ART diagnostic triad by adding C for chief complaint, H for histories (eg, family, psychosocial, past medical, a description of the presenting problem, pharmacologic), and S for special tests (eg, neurologic, orthopaedic, vascular, gait, functional capacity, radiologic and lab results). This resulted in the acronym CHARTS, which has gained widespread acceptance within the field of orthopaedic physical therapy as an extremely useful tool in the examination and evaluation of patients presenting with somatic impairment.

An efficient way of collecting information about the patient's chief complaint is to use the o, p, q, r, s, t method. This consists of several questions, including the following:

➡ Onset—Did the problem have a sudden or an insidious onset?

➡ Pain—What makes it better or worse?

➡ Quality—What is the nature of the symptoms? (The adjectives used to describe the pain are quite helpful in diagnosing the problem. Words such as burning, shooting, and piercing suggest pain of neurologic origin; words such as deep, aching, and vague suggest pain of somatic origin; the words throbbing and pulsing suggest pain of vascular origin.)

➡ Radiating—How far down the extremity do the symptoms travel? The symptoms from a dysfunction do not generally travel past the elbow or knee whereas the referred symptoms of a derangement can.

➡ Severity—How intense (mild to severe) is the chief complaint? An analogue or a 0 to 10 scale is useful in determining pain intensity.

➡ Timing—Is the chief complaint constant, intermittent, or occasional?

Though it is not the role of the therapist to manage symptoms of systemic origin, it is certainly the therapist's responsibility to recognize them so that the appropriate medical/surgical referral can be made. To this end the student of manual therapy is encouraged to develop basic competency in the process of differential diagnosis in physical therapy.[6]

Direct versus Indirect Technique

Osteopathic manipulative therapy (OMT) can be divided into two approaches.[2] Therapy that engages the motion barrier directly is referred to as direct technique. Examples include non-thrust joint manipulation, muscle energy, high-velocity thrust, myofascial release, and direct fascial technique. Manipulative therapy, which moves away from the motion barrier in the direction of "ease" in the tissues, comprises those techniques that are known as indirect. Examples include strain/counterstrain, functional, facilitated positional release, integrated neuromuscular inhibition, and induration technique.

The effective manipulator is skilled in both approaches and knows when "to go direct and when to go indirect." In general, direct techniques are applied to tissues that demonstrate contracture (ie, thick, fibrotic, and shortened tissues), whereas indirect techniques are more suited for states of contraction (ie, hypertonic, inflamed, and hyperalgesic). The author subscribes to the phrase "a time to hold and a time to scold" as related to child rearing. As a child at times needs comfort but at others requires discipline, so too the soft tissues need an indirect approach that will settle them down when inflamed. However, when stubbornly tight, they must be challenged with a direct technique that will release, elongate, and correct the underlying impairment. Because of the gentle nature of indirect techniques, they can be safely and effectively utilized in acute conditions in which direct techniques would be contraindicated. Therapists who have difficulty with "right brain" activities that require less analysis and more creative thought may have difficulty with the feeling-oriented indirect methods. However, the skills necessary to master these techniques can be learned by even the most "left-brained" among us!

Sequencing Therapeutic Interventions

When it comes to managing somatic impairment, we must consider whether we are dealing with tissue dysfunction or internal joint derangement. As mentioned previously, the approach to derangement involves the following:

➡ Reduction of the derangement
➡ Maintenance of the reduction for healing to occur
➡ Recovery of function
➡ Prevention of recurrence

To assist us with the sequencing of interventions in the management of a symptomatic dysfunction patient, we will use a case study approach. Our patient is a 32-year-old female attorney. The patient is married to an accountant and has two children ages 3 years and 9 months. The patient was involved in a rear-end motor vehicle accident 6 weeks before presenting in the physical therapist's office for treatment. Ms. Jones reports chronic daily headaches as well as neck pain and stiffness. She is taking naproxen and Flexeril (Merck, West Point, Pa) and is wearing a cervical collar. The examination reveals moderate forward head posture; symmetrical limitation in neck rotation and side bending, moderate in nature; muscle hypertonus of the levator scapulae and suboccipital muscles, bilaterally; and moderate limitation of jaw opening with tenderness and tightness of the temporalis muscles, bilaterally. Neurologic examination for sensation, deep tendon reflexes, and muscle strength is normal.

The evaluation of Ms. Jones places her in practice pattern 4B in the *Guide to Physical Therapist Practice*,[5] which consists of soft tissue injuries of the cervical spine and temporomandibular joint involving pain, poor posture, and myalgia. The ICD-9 CM codes used for billing purposes are 723.1, 781.92, and 524.6. As per the *Guide*, the expected number of visits for this episode of care is 6 to 20.

The topic of sequencing intervention becomes relevant when considering how one proceeds with the management of Ms. Jones' symptoms and many impairments. The recommended sequence of dealing with what appears to be a symptomatic dysfunction will now be covered in detail.

1. Reduce the patient's reactivity to a more tolerable level. By reactivity, we are referring to the irritability of the symptomatic area.[9] High levels of reactivity are present when pain precedes stiffness in the impaired range of motion. Low levels of reactivity are present when stiffness precedes pain; moderate levels are present when pain and stiffness simultaneously limit motion. Tissue reactivity is based upon the inflammatory process and correlates well with it. When high levels of tissue reactivity are present, direct techniques are contraindicated. Instead, indirect manipulative techniques in conjunction with cryotherapy and electrotherapeutic modalities should be employed for the purpose of reducing pain, inflammation, and reflex-induced muscle splinting.

2. Restore impaired myofascial extensibility. Once the tissues can be moved without provoking pain and muscle splinting, it is time to commence connective tissue techniques, including myofascial release and direct fascial technique.[11] The soft tissues function as "guy wires," and the bony skeleton cannot assume optimal alignment and functional mobility without normal extensibility within the myofascial system. It is the author's belief that musculoskeletal motion loss within the spine and extremities is more often a problem of myofascial extensibility than true articular dysfunction or derangement. If, however, joint dysfunction is present, there is almost always an associated loss of myofascial extensibility. As a general rule, the connective tissue component should always be treated first. The reasons for this are that the unnecessary repeated manipulation of a joint predisposes that joint to hypermobility and joint manipulation in the presence of unresolved myofascial dysfunction is often met with failure. This has been the experience of those who thrust joints without attending to the tightness in the "guy wires."

   At this point, it is necessary to discuss the work of Janda[12] from Czechoslovakia. Based upon years of clinical experience, Janda believes that there are two groups of muscles in the body: 1) those prone to becoming hypertonic, facilitated, and tight, and 2) those prone to becoming hypotonic, inhibited, and weak. Janda calls the former postural muscles and the latter phasics. It is the postural muscles, such as the upper trapezius, levator scapulae, and sternocleidomastoid, that require soft tissue mobilization and stretching; this work must be done prior to articular manipulation as previously discussed. The phasic muscles will require strengthening and will be dealt with later in the correct sequence.

3. Achieve normal joint mobility through the use of manipulative therapy. Once the reactivity is reduced to a low level and the myofascial soft tissues have regained lost extensibility, it is now necessary to use manual therapy to normalize joint motion. The term *joint manipulation* in this book is defined as, "A manual therapy technique comprising a continuum of skilled passive movements to a joint that is applied at varying speeds and amplitudes, including but not limited to a small amplitude/high velocity therapeutic movement" consistent with APTA/*Guide* terminology.[5] Consequently, the terms *manipulation* and *mobilization* will be used inter-

changeably in the chapters to follow and may certainly apply to the myofascial tissues as well as capsuloligamentous structures. Though the term *manual therapy* is synonymous with manipulation, it embodies not only the art of manipulative therapy, but also the scientific foundation upon which the art is based. As the quote by Goya on the dedication page of this book states, we certainly need both!

Now that we have defined our terms, it is important to inject some philosophy and ask what is the purpose and ultimate goal for the use of manipulation? Is it to reposition a bone that has become subluxed? Is it to cure systemic disease? No, it is much simpler than that. In the author's view, the purpose of manipulation—be it of a synovial joint of the spine or extremities or of the myofascial soft tissues—is simply to restore the normal joint play or accessory movements of a joint so that the physiologic/osteokinematic motion of the joint system can be returned to normal. When asked the same question, a panel of experts on the topic[13] stated the following: "The goal of manipulation is to restore maximal pain-free movement of the musculoskeletal system within postural balance." We have discussed the movement perspective in great detail; now we will proceed in our discussion of the importance of postural balance.

4. Attain orthostatic posture. McConnell[14] defines ideal posture as "optimal alignment with symmetrical loading of body parts." This is helpful, but we need something more specific. Johnson and Saliba[15] use the term *efficient state* and define it as "A state where each body segment distributes weight, absorbs shock, has full available range of motion and independent control of movement to meet the functional needs of both stability and mobility." Buckminster Fuller, an early 20th-century architect, discussed balance from a structural perspective.[16] He coined the term *tensegrity*, which is derived from the words tension and integrity. Whether in an edifice or in the human body, tensegrity refers to the optimal three-dimensional balance between compression and tension. Perhaps the tensegrity model captures the true essence of "postural balance" and is really what manipulative therapy aims to achieve! In theory, the terms postural balance, optimal alignment, efficient state, and tensegrity make sense. However, on a clinical level, it is important to define their parameters. To assist us further in this regard, we refer to the work of FM Alexander.[17]

The Alexander Technique is a "means whereby" each person can be taught the optimal use of his or her body. It involves a mind-body interaction in which we consciously inhibit inefficient movements to allow the body to generate movement and align-ment that is efficient, pain-free, and aesthetic. Because optimal alignment and postural balance are among some of the benefits of Alexander's work, it behooves us to review the four concepts of good use:

a. Allow your neck to release so that your head can balance forward and up.

b. Allow your torso to release into length and width.

c. Allow your legs to release away from your pelvis.

d. Allow your shoulders to release out to the sides.

When the transition is made from imbalance to balance, from malalignment to alignment, and from inefficient to efficient, we then see the improvement in symptoms that we seek for our patients. To operate in a clinical environment in which patients are treated more like "cattle" than the unique and wonderful creations that they truly are should be unacceptable. We can and should do better!

Achieving postural balance is not possible without the requisite work in reducing reactivity, restoring myofascial extensibility, and achieving normal joint mobility. The final step in the intervention sequence is to strengthen the weak phasic muscles.

5. Sensorimotor training and muscle strengthening procedures. At a well-attended manual therapy conference in 1985 in Boston, Mass, Sandy Burkhart made the statement, "In addition to being 'carpenters,' manual therapists need to be 'electricians' as well." That insightful comment represented a turning point in manual therapy practice, where the emphasis had always been on restoring the mechanics of the joint. With the Institute of Physical Art's integration of neurologic and orthopaedic practice into a series of seminars on "functional orthopaedics," as well as an explosive interest in "body work" (ie, Feldenkrais, Alexander, Hanna, Pilates, etc), manual therapists were suddenly interested in not only "fixing the hardware" but in "reprogramming the software." This new emphasis in manual therapy was good news for patients, as they were now able to maintain the improvement in joint mechanics by "retraining" the muscles of the body to move these more mobile structures in more efficient ways.

As discussed previously, the specific muscles that require sensorimotor reeducation and/or strengthening work are the phasics that become hypotonic, inhibited, and weak over time. Examples of such muscles include the deep neck and occipital flexors, the lower trapezius, the lower abdominals, and the gluteal muscles. One of the reasons why muscle strengthening should be performed after manual therapy is because of the reflexogenic effects of the articular mechanoreceptors on muscle tone. This neurophysiologic principle was first reported by Wyke[18] and later developed clinically by Warmerdam.[19] Because one of these effects is inhibitory in nature, it makes sense to "mobilize before strengthening" in order to remove this "neural inhibition" on the phasic muscles that are prone to developing weakness. The specific joint-muscle relationships involved will be covered at various points in this textbook.

With the understanding that orthopaedic patients could benefit from neurologic techniques came the realization that neurologic patients could likewise benefit from orthopaedic/manual therapy techniques. This represented significant progress in the physical therapy profession, and it is the patient who is the beneficiary in this process of integration.

Body Holism and Adaptive Potential

Sir William Osler,[8] the famous McGill physician, is quoted as saying, "It is more important to know the patient who has a disease than the disease that has the patient." This approach to patient care recognizes that the body functions as a whole, well-integrated unit. The basic components of the individual represent the "triad of health" and include physical structure, biochemical processes, and the mental/spiritual state.[20] When all three components are integrated and functioning normally, the individual is healthy and functional. However, when there is an imbalance in one or more areas, this represents "dis-ease," impairment, and/or disability.

When considering a "holistic" rather than a "localistic" approach to the patient, it is necessary to consider every factor that represents a source of potential "dis-ease" or imbalance to the patient. These include macrotrauma, cumulative microtrauma, psychological distress, nutritional deficiencies, infection, environmental and ergonomic influences, etc. It is always in the best interest of the patient to address as many of these "stressors" as possible. Commenting on the role of chronic overuse (ie, cumulative microtrauma), Sahrmann[21,22] states, "Musculoskeletal problems are seldom caused by isolated precipitating events, but are a consequence of habitual imbalances in the movement system."

The term that represents an individual's ability to cope with these negative influences is *adaptive potential*. In health, a person's adaptive potential is high; in states of impairment and/or disability adaptive potential is low. The advantage of approaching the patient from a perspective of body holism is that intervention, whether it is physical, psychological, nutritional, etc, has the desired effect of restoring adaptive potential. This is turn raises the patient's tolerance, and the result is improved overall health and wellness.

Stiles[8] discusses the clinical "equation": Host + Disease = Illness. In this equation, the host represents adaptive potential; when it is compromised the patient suffers, but when it is improved the patient benefits. As manual therapists, we may not have control over various disease states, but we can "fortify the host." We do this by managing his or her somatic impairment and by referring him or her, when necessary, to other health care providers who can assist them with the other health-limiting factors with which they deal.

Contraindications to Spinal Manual Therapy

The following conditions are contraindications to the use of direct joint manipulative technique (ie, low/high velocity manipulation/mobilization, muscle energy, etc):

➡ Acute arthritis of any type
➡ Rheumatoid arthritis
➡ Acute ankylosing spondylitis
➡ Hypermobility/instability, including patients with generalized hypermobility as in Ehlers-Danlos syndrome
➡ Calvé-Perthes disease
➡ Fracture
➡ Ligamentous rupture
➡ Malignancy (primary or secondary)
➡ Osteomalacia
➡ Paget's disease
➡ Severe osteoporosis
➡ Osteomyelitis
➡ Tuberculosis
➡ Disc prolapse with serious neurologic impairment (including cauda equina syndrome)
➡ Evidence of involvement of more than two adjacent nerve roots in the lumbar spine
➡ Lower limb neurologic symptoms due to cervical or thoracic spine involvement
➡ Painful movement in all directions
➡ Infectious disease
➡ Depleted general health
➡ Patient intolerance
➡ Inability of the patient to relax
➡ Rubbery end-feel of the joint
➡ Undiagnosed pain

➡ Protective joint muscle spasm

➡ Segments adjacent to the level being manipulated that are too irritable or hypermobile to tolerate the stress of proper positioning prior to or during the manipulation

In the event that any of these conditions are undiagnosed but present, the astute clinician is still protected providing he or she recognizes the level of reactivity in the pathologic tissues and acts accordingly. Regarding the use of indirect techniques, with the exception of frank disease, they may be effectively utilized in cases of high tissue reactivity because of their gentle nature. However, for the inexperienced novice the above list should serve as contraindications to all manual techniques.

There are two axioms in medicine that are extremely useful in uncertain times of clinical practice. They are:

1. Do no harm!

2. When in doubt, don't!

To further assist in distinguishing pain of different origins, the reader is referred to Figure 3-1. It is helpful to remember that although technology has its place in physical therapy, as in medicine, there is no substitute for a good history and physical examination of the patient!

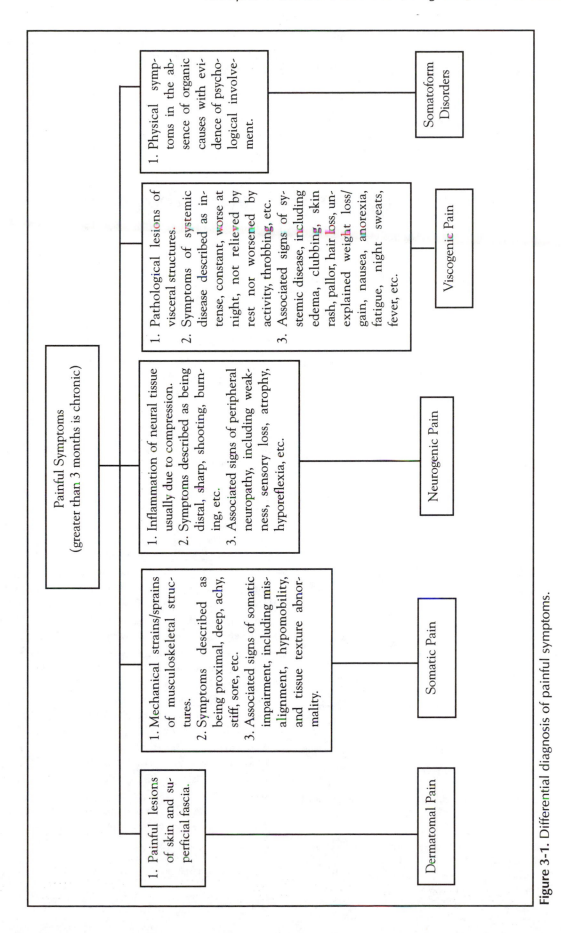

Figure 3-1. Differential diagnosis of painful symptoms.

References and Bibliography

References

1. Gibbons P, Tehan P. *Manipulation of the Spine, Thorax and Pelvis: An Osteopathic Perspective.* Edinburgh: Churchill Livingstone; 2000.

2. Greenman PE. *Principles of Manual Medicine.* 2nd ed. Philadelphia, Pa: Lippincott Williams & Wilkins; 1996.

3. Kaltenborn FM. *The Spine: Basic Evaluation and Mobilization Techniques.* Minneapolis, Minn: OPTP; 1993.

4. McKenzie RA. *The Cervical and Thoracic Spine: Mechanical Diagnosis and Therapy.* Walkanae, New Zealand: Spinal Publications; 1990.

5. Guide to physical therapist practice. 2nd ed. *Phys Ther.* 2001;81(1):1-768.

6. Goodman CC, Snyder TE. *Differential Diagnosis in Physical Therapy.* 3rd ed. Philadelphia, Pa: WB Saunders; 2000.

7. Schafer RC, Faye LJ. *Motion Palpation and Chiropractic Technique: Principles of Dynamic Chiropractic.* 2nd ed. Huntington Beach, Calif: The Motion Palpation Institute; 1989.

8. Stiles EG. Clinical presentations and examples: an osteopathic perspective. In: Flynn TW, ed. *The Thoracic Spine and Rib Cage: Musculoskeletal Evaluation and Treatment.* Boston, Mass: Butterworth-Heinemann; 1996.

9. Paris SV, Loubert PV. *FCO: Foundations of Clinical Orthopaedics, Seminar Manual.* St. Augustine, Fla: Institute Press; 1999.

10. Ellis JJ, Johnson GS. Myofascial considerations in somatic dysfunction of the thorax. In: Flynn TW, ed. *The Thoracic Spine and Rib Cage: Musculoskeletal Evaluation and Treatment.* Boston, Mass: Butterworth-Heinemann, 1996.

11. Andrade CK, Clifford P. *Outcome-Based Massage.* Philadelphia, Pa: Lippincott, Williams & Wilkins; 2001.

12. Janda V. Pain in the locomotor system—a broad approach. In: Glasgow EF, Twomey LT, Scull ER, Kleynhans AM, Idczak RM, eds. *Aspects of Manipulative Therapy.* Melbourne: Churchill Livingstone; 1985.

13. Dvorak J, Dvorak V, Schneider W, eds. *Manual Medicine.* Heidelberg: Springer-Verlag; 1985.

14. McConnell J. *McConnell Institute: The McConnell Approach to the Problem Shoulder.* Course Manual; 1994.

15. Johnson GS, Saliba VL. *Functional Orthopedics I: Soft Tissue Mobilization, PNF, and Joint Mobilization.* Steamboat Springs, Colo: IPA Course Notes; 2001.

16. Orient JM. *Sapira's Art & Science of Bedside Diagnosis.* 2nd ed. Philadelphia, Pa: Lippincott Williams & Wilkins; 2000.

17. Caplan D. *Back Trouble: A New Approach to Prevention and Recovery.* Gainesville, Fla: Triad Publishing; 1987.

18. Wyke BD. Articular neurology and manipulative therapy. In: Glasgow EF, Twomey LT, Scull ER, Kleynhans AM, Idczak RM, eds. *Aspects of Manipulative Therapy.* Melbourne: Churchill Livingstone; 1985.

19. Warmerdam A. *Manual Therapy: Improve Muscle and Joint Functioning.* Wantagh, NY: Pine Publications; 1999.

20. Valentine T, Valentine C. *Applied Kinesiology.* Rochester, Vt: Healing Arts Press; 1987.

21. Sahrmann SA. *The Movement System Balance Theory: Relationship to Musculoskeletal Pain Syndromes.* Course Notes; 1990.

22. Sahrmann SA. *Diagnosis and Treatment of Movement Impairment Syndromes.* St. Louis, Mo: Mosby-Year Book; 2002.

Bibliography

Bland JH. Pain in the head and neck: where does it come from? *J Craniomandib Pract*. 1989;7(3):167.169.

Chaitow L. *Positional Release Techniques*. 2nd ed. Edinburgh: Churchill Livingstone; 2002.

DiGiovanna EL, Schiowitz S, eds. *An Osteopathic Approach to Diagnosis and Treatment*. Philadelphia, Pa: Lippincott-Raven; 1997.

Donatelli R, Wooden MJ. *Orthopaedic Physical Therapy*. 3rd ed. New York, NY: Churchill Livingstone; 2001.

Grant R, ed. *Physical Therapy of the Cervical and Thoracic Spine*. 3rd ed. New York, NY: Churchill Livingstone; 2002.

Hanna T. *Somatics*. New York, NY: Addison-Wesley Publishing; 1988.

Lewit K. *Manipulative Therapy in Rehabilitation of the Locomotor System*. Oxford: Butterworth-Heinemann; 1993.

McGill SM, Cholewicki J. Biomechanical basis for stability: an explanation to enhance clinical utility. *J Orthop Sports Phys Ther*. 2001;31:96-100.

McGonigle T, Matley KW. Soft tissue treatment and muscle stretching. *Journal of Manual & Manipulative Therapy*. 1994;2: 55-62.

Mennell JM. *Joint Pain*. Boston, Mass: Little, Brown and Co; 1964.

Nordin M, Frankel VH. *Basic Biomechanics of the Musculoskeletal System*. Philadelphia, Pa: Lippincott Williams & Wilkins; 2001.

Panjabi MM, White AA. *Biomechanics in the Musculoskeletal System*. New York, NY: Churchill Livingstone; 2001.

Petty NJ, Moore AP. *Neuromusculoskeletal Examination and Assessment*. Edinburgh: Churchill Livingstone; 1998.

Warwick R, Williams P, eds. *Gray's Anatomy*. 36th ed. Philadelphia, Pa: WB Saunders; 1980.

Scapulothoracic Region

Examination and Evaluation of the Scapulothoracic Region

Posture

Consistent with the CHARTS methodology, the evaluation of postural alignment is performed following the interview in which the chief complaint (C) and history (H) are recorded. This component of the examination consists of a detailed inspection for the presence of asymmetry (A). In the scapulothoracic region, this will be accomplished by analyzing posture in three ways. The patient will be observed from the side (ie, lateral view), back (ie, posterior view), and front (ie, anterior view). The purpose of the postural assessment is to identify areas of potential impairment. For instance, a patient who demonstrates exaggeration of the thoracic kyphosis is likely to develop a restriction in backward bending over time as adaptive shortening of anterior structures occurs. However, one should not assume that impairment of mobility exists based upon posture alone. Recall that it is the combined ART triad that signals somatic dysfunction (ie, impairment).

The standing lateral view of the scapulothoracic region enables the therapist to inspect the following structures for faulty alignment (Figure 4-1):

1. Scapular position in the horizontal plane (normal, protracted or abducted, retracted or adducted).

2. Scapular position in the sagittal plane (a common misalignment is an anterior scapular tilt; the superior or aspect of the scapula drops anterior/inferior as the inferior angle is displaced posterior/superior).

3. Sternal angle or manubriosternal junction (it should have a slight upward inclination but is often in a downward or depressed position).

4. Humeral head position.[1] No more than one-third of the humeral head should be anterior to the acromion. Alexander teachers place the humeral head at the midpoint of the trunk, halfway between the sternum in the front and the root of the scapular spine posteriorly.[2] Anterior displacement of the humeral head suggests anterior glenohumeral joint hypermobility and/or posterior glenohumeral capsular tightness.

5. Thoracic kyphosis (normal, increased, decreased). The upper (T1 to T4), mid (T5 to T8), and lower (T9 to T12) thoracic regions should be assessed separately. Flattening of the curve represents an extended position, whereas an accentuated kyphosis represents a flexed position of the spine.

A common postural problem seen in many patients, young and old alike, is a combination of scapular protraction and sternal depression with an increased mid/lower thoracic kyphosis. Prior to assuming that an increased thoracic kyphosis has a postural or functional basis, structural causes, such as Scheuermann's disease or adolescent kyphosis, ankylosing spondylitis, tuberculous spondylitis, osteoporosis, or fracture-dislocation, must be ruled out first.[3]

There are structural deformities of the chest wall[4] that may have significance in the evaluation of the pulmonary patient (eg, Harrison's sulcus, pigeon breast, and pectus excavatum) but are not of major consequence in the

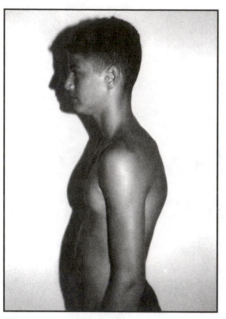

Figure 4-1.

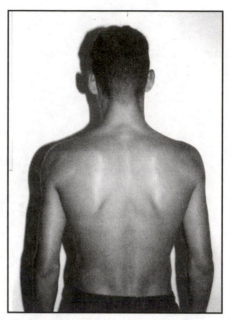

Figure 4-2.

patient with somatic impairment. However, the presence of the barrel chest deformity, although a sign of emphysema, represents a typical pattern of expiratory rib restriction that may derive some benefit from manual therapy.

The standing posterior view of the scapulothoracic region allows us to detect the following positional relationships (Figure 4-2):

1. Scapular position in the frontal plane (the scapulae should be symmetrical and almost parallel to the spine; note elevation and upward or downward rotation).

2. Scapular position in the sagittal plane (note an anterior tilt with inferior angle prominence, which is confirmed in supine with anterior displacement of the coracoid process versus the contralateral side).

3. Scapular position about the vertical Y axis (external and internal rotation). Excessive internal scapular rotation about a vertical axis results in posterior displacement of the vertebral border (ie, "winging" of the scapula).

4. Rotoscoliosis of the upper, mid, and lower thoracic spine.

5. Posterior rib prominence.

6. Contour of the neck-shoulder line.

7. Waist angle acuity.

8. Position of the upper extremities (eg, neutral, internally/externally rotated).

Common clinical findings related to misalignments/asymmetries in the posterior view include the following:

1. Elevation with downward rotation of the scapula secondary to a combination of levator scapulae and latissimus dorsi tightness (shoulders that are above the T1 level suggest scapular elevation).

2. Anterior tilting or "tipping" of the scapula related to a combination of pectoralis minor tightness and/or weakness of the lower scapular stabilizers (ie, serratus anterior, rhomboids, middle and lower trapezius).

3. "Winging" of the vertebral border of the scapula secondary to either excessive scapular internal rotation or serratus anterior weakness (this weakness of serratus anterior is often associated with flattening and restricted flexion in the midthoracic region).

4. Posterior rib prominence on the convex side of a mid/lower side bending curve related to type 1 or neutral mechanics.

5. "Gothic" shoulders or straightening of the neck-shoulder line secondary to levator scapulae and upper trapezius tightness.

6. Internally rotated upper extremities secondary to tightness of the latissimus dorsi.

In addition to the above functional misalignments/asymmetries, the therapist should be cognizant of the structural/pathological deviations in form that affect the scapulothoracic region. Examples include Klippel-Feil syndrome, which can cause bilateral scapular elevation, and Sprengel's deformity, another congenital deformity that is associated with an abnormally small/high scapula and poor development on the affected side.[3]

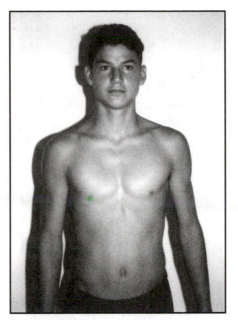

Figure 4-3.

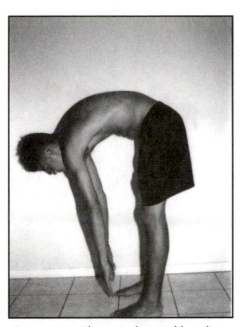

Figure 4-4a. Thoracic forward bending.

The final anterior view in stance (Figure 4-3) provides an analysis of these relationships:

1. Clavicular alignment (the distal end of the clavicle should ideally be horizontal or only slightly elevated relative to the proximal end at the sternoclavicular joint; the clavicles should be symmetrical).

2. The linea alba should be straight up and down.

3. In males, symmetry of nipple height is assessed.

4. The anterior aspect of the rib cage is observed for asymmetry.

Common anterior view asymmetries/misalignments include the following:

➡ Bilateral clavicular angulation in which the distal end of the clavicles are superior to the proximal attachment. This is a response to protraction of the scapulae, which is enhanced when the scapulae are also elevated. A unilateral angulation of the clavicle is seen when the shoulder girdle is elevated on the ipsilateral side.

➡ Asymmetric linea alba and nipple height consistent with the side-bending component of a rotoscoliosis.

➡ Anterior rib cage prominence on the concave side of a rotoscoliosis (the rotational component of the curve forces the ribs forward on the concave side and backward on the convex side of the curve).

In the final analysis there are four abnormal postural patterns in the scapulothoracic region that are routinely encountered in clinical practice. They are as follows:

1. Scapular protraction/elevation associated with an increased mid/lower thoracic kyphosis, sternal depression, and angulated clavicles.

2. Scapular protraction/depression associated with an increased mid/lower thoracic kyphosis, sternal depression, and angulated clavicles.

3. Scapular "winging" associated with flattening of the thoracic kyphosis.

4. Thoracic spine rotoscoliosis associated with an anterior rib prominence on the concave side of the curve and posterior rib prominence on the convex side of the curve. The shoulder girdle will tend to be higher on the convex side of the curve and the waist angle sharper on the concave side.

According to Kendall,[5] we must remember that hand dominance plays a role in spinal asymmetry such that an individual who is right hand dominant would be expected to carry his or her right shoulder slightly lower and the right hip slightly higher as a normal variation. It is when the low shoulder is found on the nondominant side that our index of suspicion is raised.

Active Movements

Now that C, H, and A have been completed, we can move onto R, which begins with an assessment of active range of motion. The examination of active thoracic movements consists of an analysis of six motions (Figures 4-4a to 4-4f). They are forward bending (ie, flexion), backward bending (ie, extension), side bending (ie, lateral flexion) to the left and right, and rotation to the left and right.

This part of the examination, as with the postural assessment, is performed while the patient stands. There is highly important information to be gleaned from the observa-

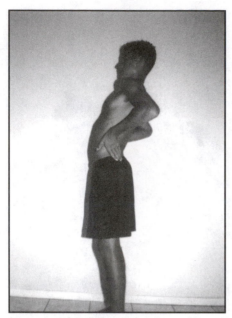

Figure 4-4b. Thoracic backward bending.

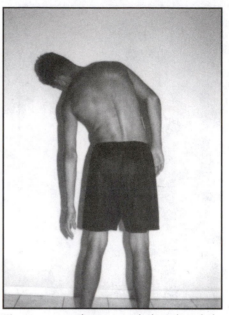

Figure 4-4c. Thoracic side bending left.

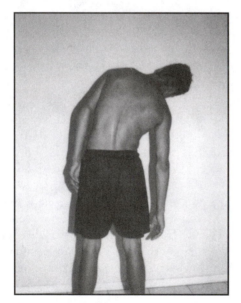

Figure 4-4d. Thoracic side bending right.

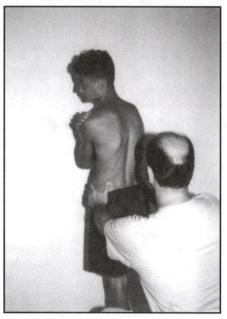

Figure 4-4e. Thoracic rotation left.

tion of active spinal motion. The following are a summary of points of which to take note:

1. The patient should stand in a comfortable and relaxed position in as close to the neutral position as possible.

2. Motion should start from the head and proceed to the neck and spine.

3. Though the quantity of movement is important and can certainly be measured with various devices, it is the quality of motion that is most important to the

manual therapist. For example, a patient may appear to have normal spinal flexion in that he or she can easily touch the floor. However, on closer inspection it is noted that it is the hamstrings that are flexible, whereas the lumbar spine shows limitation of motion. The assessment of an active movement's quality requires skill in observation, which becomes better with practice. Optimal human motion is described as effortless, efficient, and smooth. It is without interference, restriction, or hypermobility. Whether the curve is anteroposterior as in forward and backward

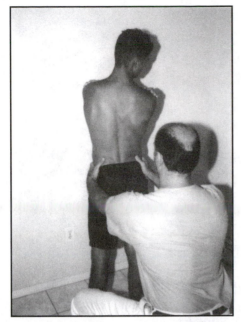

Figure 4-4f. Thoracic rotation right.

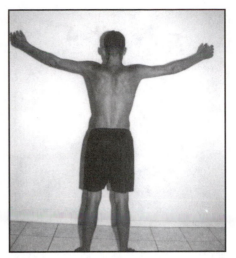

Figure 4-5.

bending or mediolateral as in side bending, it should be a well-contoured and unbroken curve. Impaired movement is characterized by flat or straight lines that may cause effort and even pain. Motion loss in one area of the spine will cause another area to compensate and this is represented by "pivot" points or "fulcrums." It is these areas of compensation that tend toward hypermobility and become symptomatic, while the areas of hypomobility remain stiff but asymptomatic. The "mission" of the manual therapist is to locate these stiff segments and to then decide which is the area of greatest restriction. It is with this "culprit" lesion that we commence manipulative intervention.

4. By means of a comparison between pain and tissue stiffness, the therapist is able to determine the tissue's level of reactivity. This determination will serve as a guide in our choice of intervention later (ie, high reactivity will require indirect treatment methods and the use of pain-relieving modalities, whereas low reactivity responds better to direct techniques, as discussed in Chapter 3).

5. Whenever possible, a correlation between positional asymmetry and impaired mobility should be established. This correlation, in conjunction with tissue texture abnormality, provides the basis for diagnosing somatic impairment. For example, a correlation between an increased thoracic kyphosis from T5 to T10 and restricted backward bending in the same region has more clinical significance for the manual therapist than either one by itself.

The final aspect of active motion testing in the scapulothoracic region involves an assessment of scapular upward rotation. This is accomplished by having the patient abduct both upper extremities while the therapist observes scapular rotation from a posterior view (Figure 4-5). A normal response is to observe upward rotation of the scapulae through a range of 60 degrees beginning at approximately 30 degrees of shoulder abduction. A common abnormal pattern associated with shoulder impingement syndrome is a restriction of scapular upward rotation on the side of the impingement secondary to tight downward rotators of the scapula (ie, levator scapulae, latissimus dorsi, etc). When the levator scapulae is at fault, an associated elevation or "hiking up" of the "shawl area" will occur with abduction. This is often a compensation for weakness of the shoulder abductors. In the presence of serratus anterior weakness, the inferior angle of the scapula fails to reach the midaxillary line of the trunk secondary to inadequate protraction on the affected side.

The relationship between subacromial impingement and incomplete scapular upward rotation has to do with inadequate clearance of the suprahumeral tissues under the coracoacromial arch. It is therefore crucial that these scapulothoracic influences be appreciated when managing patients with shoulder impairments. McConnell[1] also underscores the importance of thoracic spine mobility, in general, when addressing shoulder impairment, especially the movement of extension in the mid/lower thoracic region.

Passive Accessory Intervertebral Movements

There are two accessory or joint play motions in the thoracic spine that provide important information. They are posteroanterior (PA) and transverse pressures on the spinous

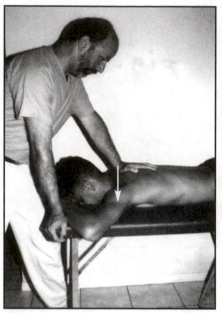

Figure 4-6.

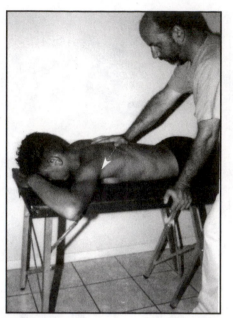

Figure 4-7.

processes. PA pressure on a thoracic spinous process (SP) induces extension, and transverse pressure on the side of the SP induces rotation. The purpose of performing passive accessory intervertebral movements (PAIVMs) is to identify motion restrictions in the 12 motion segments of the thoracic spine. When applying these manual forces, the therapist is reminded to "use as little force as possible, but as much force as necessary." There are generally three components of the accessory assessment. They are the quantity of the accessory motion, the quality of the accessory motion, and the end-feel imparted to the therapist's manual contact at the end of the available range of movement. In addition, the assessment of tissue reactivity at the dysfunctional segment(s) will help to guide the intervention to follow.

The PA central accessory movement examination is classified as a "spring" test, as it involves a small amplitude impulse over the spinous process. The therapist has the option of assessing superior vertebral motion with posterior rotation (ie, roll) or inferior vertebral motion with an anterior translation (ie, glide), because both forces induce spinal extension. However, considering that translations are easier to control and require less effort than rotations, the PA spring test is performed on the SP of the inferior vertebra.

The PA central spring test for the assessment of thoracic extension is performed as follows:

1. The patient is prone, lying with proper support provided. It is important that the thoracic spine be placed in a neutral position during testing.

2. The table height should be adjusted so that the therapist's middle finger reaches the top of the table when the therapist is standing.

3. T1 to T4 is best assessed with the therapist standing at the head of the table with the spinous process placed between the thenar and hypothenar eminence (Figure 4-6).

4. T5 to T12 is best assessed at the side of the table with the spinous process placed in the palmar groove between the thenar and hypothenar contacts and the fingers directed cranially (Figure 4-7). The therapist's other hand can be placed out of the way as illustrated, or juxtaposed inferiorly with the ulnar border placed against the heel of the active hand. The therapist must demonstrate proper body mechanics at all times (ie, neutral pelvis; optimal head, neck, and spinal alignment; etc).

5. Because the PA force induces an anterior translation of the inferior vertebrae of the motion segment, a PA central spring over T5 is an assessment of backward bending at T4,5. Therefore, an assessment of T12,L1 backward bending involves a PA central spring of L1 under T12.

6. Due to the progressive inferior angulation of the spinous processes in the thoracic spine from cranial to caudal, the therapist must incorporate a superiorly directed force below T4. A helpful landmark is to perform the PA spring anteriorly/superiorly toward the sternal angle. This will ensure that the translational motion occurs in the plane of the apophyseal joints.

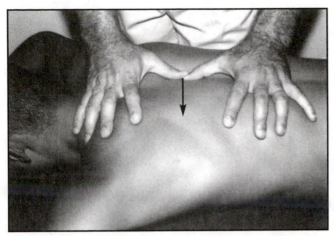

Figure 4-8.

has been used effectively. It consists of two to three sets of rapid transverse pressure oscillations for 30 to 60 seconds each in the pain-free range. The segment is essentially "bombarded" with proprioceptive afferent input, which helps to "downregulate" its neural facilitation and decrease painful symptoms.

Passive Physiologic Intervertebral Movements

This series of passive movements is a means of evaluating physiologic motion in the spine as it normally occurs during active motion. The therapist induces movement with one hand and assesses with the other. As with PAIVMs, the quantity, quality, and end-feel are assessed at each motion segment. The examination includes the motions of forward and backward bending, side bending right and left, and rotation right and left.

Upper Thoracic Spine (T1 to T4)

With the patient in the sitting position, the therapist uses the head-neck region to induce the desired physiologic motions. While this is performed with one hand, the thumb or middle finger of the other hand is assessing intervertebral motion between the spinous processes (interspinous space or simply interspace) of T1,2; T2,3; T3,4; and T4,5. For the evaluation of side bending, the palpating contact is on the ipsilateral side of the movement; for rotation, the contact is on the contralateral side of the interspinous space (Figures 4-9a to 4-9d).

The most challenging of the six motions in the upper thoracic region is definitely backward bending. In order to achieve upper thoracic extension, the therapist must induce upper cervical flexion, which will recruit lower cervical and then upper thoracic extension. If only the patient's head is extended, then the extension is confined to the craniovertebral region which is unacceptable.

Mid/Lower Thoracic Spine (T5 to T12)

As with the upper thoracic spine, T5 to T12 is assessed at the interspinous space with a palpating finger (usually the thumb or middle finger), while physiologic motion is induced through the trunk with the other hand. The patient's and therapist's positions change from one movement to the next, as illustrated, but the principles remain the same as for the upper thoracic region. Some clinicians perform these passive physiologic intervertebral movements (PPIVMs) in the sitting and recumbent positions, but a sitting examination alone is sufficient for now (Figures 4-10a to 4-10d).

7. The 0 to 6 mobility scale, described in Chapter 3, is used to document the quantity of motion at each segment. In addition, the quality of the spring through the range and the end-feel for extension at the end of range should also be reported.

8. The area of greatest restriction is identified when somatic impairment is present.

A few surface landmarks are helpful in identifying the various spinal levels. The root of the scapular spine is at the level of the T3 spinous process, and the inferior angle of the scapula is at the level of the T7 spinous process. The most reliable method, however, is to locate the spinous process of C7 (vertebra prominens) and count down from there. The location of the cervical landmarks, including C7, will be covered in a subsequent chapter on the cervical spine.

The transverse pressure test for the assessment of segmental rotation is performed as follows:

1. The patient, lying prone, is again positioned in a comfortable, neutral posture with the table at the correct height for the therapist.

2. To assess rotation right from T1 to T12 the therapist stands on the patient's right side and slowly displaces the spinous process from right to left. This is accomplished by placing the passive thumb directly over the lateral aspect of the spinous process, which is reinforced by the active thumb. The movement for this procedure is not through the thumbs but through the upper extremities. If thumb contact is uncomfortable, the therapist can use a thenar eminence contact instead (Figure 4-8).

3. As with the PA central spring test, the therapist assesses the quantity and quality of the accessory range as well as the end-feel. If impairment is present, the area of greatest restriction as well as the level of reactivity must be determined. In the presence of "segmental facilitation" with local hyperalgesia, hypertonicity, and increased sympathetic activity,[6] a technique known as "chasing the pain"

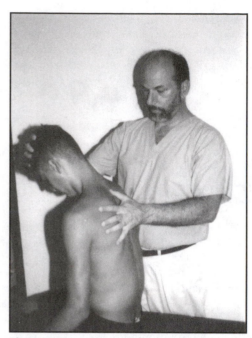

Figure 4-9a. Assessing forward bending at T2,3.

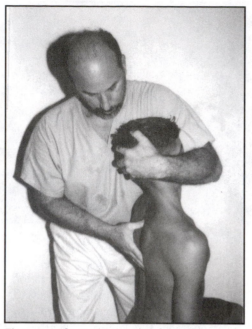

Figure 4-9b. Assessing backward bending at T3,4.

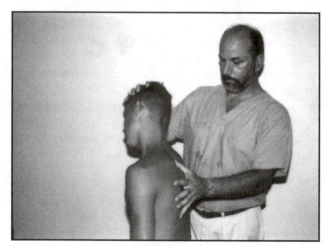

Figure 4-9c. Assessing side bending right at T3,4.

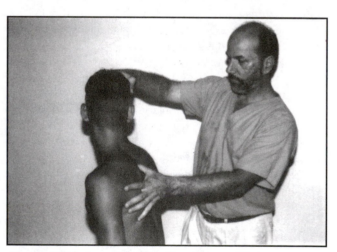

Figure 4-9d. Assessing rotation right at T3,4.

Soft Tissue Palpation

The examination of the scapulothoracic region now progresses to the evaluation of tissue texture abnormality (T). There are three markers for soft tissue impairment that are worth noting. They are tenderness, tightness, and tone. Establishing a baseline measure for the amount of pressure used when assessing tenderness is important during this aspect of the examination. Otherwise, false positive and negative errors are likely. In this regard, the therapist presses on the patient's anterior thigh with a light but firm pressure that should not be perceived by the patient as tender. If it is, then either the pressure is too strong or the other thigh should be used instead. It is this same nontender pres-

sure that is used to assess the tissues of the scapulothoracic region. In addition to the presence of tenderness, the examiner is also evaluating the patient for tightness and increased muscle tone (ie, the type associated with reflex-induced splinting or guarding as compared with neurogenic spasticity).

The entire anterior chest wall should be assessed. Structures to be examined include the following:

➡ Sternoclavicular joints

➡ Costosternal joints

➡ Costochondral junctions

➡ Xyphoid process

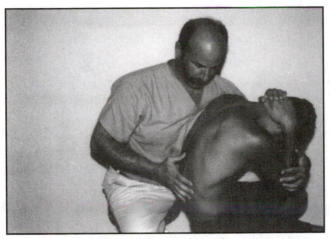

Figure 4-10a. Assessing forward bending at T9,10.

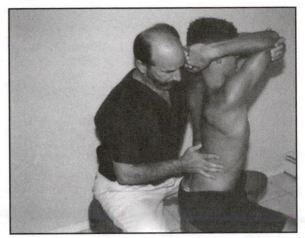

Figure 4-10b. Assessing backward bending at T9,10.

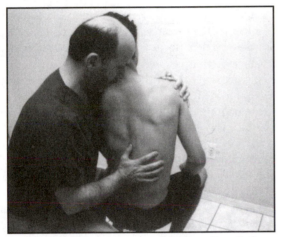

Figure 4-10c. Assessing side bending left at T9,10.

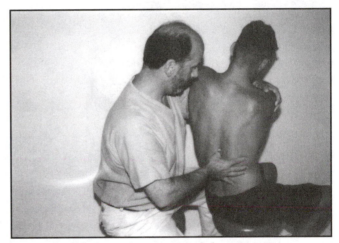

Figure 4-10d. Assessing rotation left at T10,11.

➠ Skin and superficial fascia

➠ Rectus abdominis

➠ Pectoral muscles and fascias, including the clavipectoral fascia

➠ Subclavius muscles

➠ Intercostal muscles

➠ Coracoclavicular ligament (conoid and trapezoid components)

The posterior aspect of the scapulothoracic region is examined next. Structures to be examined from superficial to deep include:

➠ Skin and superficial fascia

➠ Trapezius muscle (upper, mid, and lower fibers)

➠ Rhomboid major and minor, levator scapulae at the superior angle of the scapulae, supra/infraspinatus, teres major/minor, and latissimus dorsi

➠ Erector spinae (spinalis, longissimus, and iliocostalis at the rib angle)

➠ Transversospinales (semispinalis, multifidus, rotatores) in the medial groove of longissimus

➠ Costotransverse joints at the lateral edge of the longissimus thoracis muscle

In addition to the inspection for tenderness, tightness, and tone, the myofascial tissues of the scapulothoracic region and costal cage can also be examined for taut bands, trigger/tender points, swelling, nodules, extensibility, and length.

Special Tests

The final category in the CHARTS process is special tests (S). It is here that all neurologic, vascular, integumentary, cardiopulmonary, and additional orthopaedic procedures are performed. In the context of a basic scapulothoracic examination, the following special tests should be performed at this time:

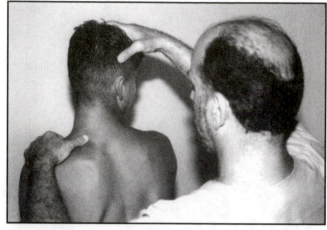

Figure 4-11.

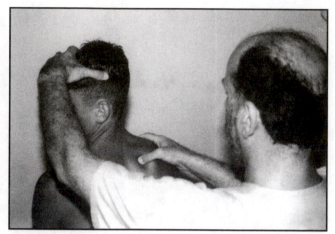

Figure 4-12.

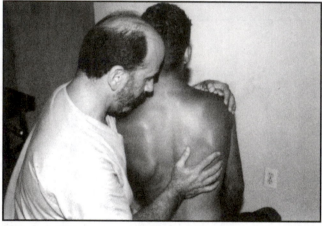

Figure 4-13.

1. Sensation in the related dermatomes.

2. Manual muscle testing with special attention given to the phasic muscles (ie, rhomboids, mid and lower trapezius, and the serratus anterior).

3. Inspection for cool/moist areas of skin consistent with localized sympathetic activation as seen in segmental facilitation[6] and T4 syndrome.[7]

4. Passive accessory rib mobility. The therapist has the option of performing this mobility test under R, but the author prefers to separate it from the spinal exam and place it under S instead.

The first rib is tested separately from the other ribs. The first rib is found at the "summit" of the shawl area, halfway between the clavicle, anteriorly, and spine of the scapula, posteriorly. With the patient seated the therapist passively right rotates the head-neck to the end of range with the right hand. With the left hand positioned over the left upper trapezius, the therapist's left thumb applies a PA pressure to the first left rib just lateral to the costotransverse joint. The motion is assessed for quantity, quality, and end-feel and compared to the other side by simply reversing the maneuver for the first right rib (Figure 4-11).

The remaining ribs (2 to 12) are also assessed in sitting. For ribs 2, 3, and 4, the head-neck can be used. The therapist passively rotates the patient's head-neck to the left until motion is perceived at the desired rib tubercle on the right. At this point, the therapist performs a PA spring test with the right thumb just lateral to the costotransverse joint (Figure 4-12). The quantity, quality, and end-feel are evaluated, and the test is repeated on the left side for comparison.

For ribs 5 to 12 the seated patient's right hand is placed on his or her left shoulder. The therapist reaches across the anterior chest wall and places his or her hand on the patient's right shoulder while placing the right thumb or thenar contact against the medial aspect of the rib angle to be assessed. With the left hand the therapist rotates the patient to the left until motion is perceived at the desired rib angle on the right. At this point in the mobility exam, the therapist displaces each of the rib angles 5 to 12 sequentially in a transverse manner to the right (Figure 4-13). The exam is repeated on the left side by simply reversing the maneuver, and a comparison is made.

Localization to the desired level is crucial with all the above passive accessory rib mobility tests. Osteopathic physicians use the term *feather edge* to describe when motion first arrives at the desired level. This concept applies to all manual procedures, whether they are for examination or intervention purposes.

Connective Tissue Techniques for the Scapulothoracic Region (Myofascial Release, Direct Fascial Technique, and Friction)

Thoracic Inlet Release

The thoracic inlet is the cephalic opening of the thoracic cage through which the esophagus, trachea, and the major vessels of the neck and upper limb traverse. Mechanically, it is important because of its soft tissue influence on the sternum, ribs, clavicles, thoracic spine, scapulae, and upper extremities. Systemically, it is important because of its relationship to the major lymphatic ducts in the anterior chest wall, as well as its role in pulmonary function and neural activity (particularly of the brachial plexus). The borders of the thoracic inlet are the manubrium and the medial aspect of clavicles and first ribs, anteriorly; the vertebral body of T1, posteriorly. Because of its complex fascial network and the influence of postural factors (ie, forward head/rounded shoulders), the thoracic inlet is an area that is prone to developing somatic impairment. For this reason, it is the first of the soft tissue areas that is addressed in the management of patients with scapulothoracic impairment.

The thoracic inlet responds well to both direct and indirect treatment methods using a "three-dimensional" approach. In the presence of highly reactive tissues or when working with anxious patients, the indirect approach is preferred. However, when there is adaptive shortening with low tissue reactivity, direct technique is the treatment of choice. An extremely useful way of employing either method is with a palpation technique developed by Peter Fabian, PT known as the "4 Ms" procedure. In order of application, the first M stands for *mold*, the second for *meld*, the third for *monitor*, and the fourth for *move*.

With the patient positioned comfortably in supine and the therapist sitting at the head of the table, the therapist places one hand lightly over the sternal angle with the fingers and thumb spread over the upper ribs and sternoclavicular joints. The other hand is placed under the patient's upper thoracic region encompassing the cervicothoracic junction (Figure 5-1). Molding is the process of conforming one's hands to the patient's unique anatomic structure (ie, "anatomy to anatomy"). Melding is the process of "tuning in" to the tissues being palpated and involves the appreciation of contour, texture, tone, moisture, temperature, etc. It is a deeper form of palpation that involves sensitivity to function (ie, "physiology to physiology"). Monitoring separates a direct from an indirect technique. During the performance of an indirect approach, the therapist is sensing what osteopathic physicians refer to as "inherent tissue motion" or the "preferred tissue pattern." Inherent tissue motion or rhythm is a compilation of all the ongoing physiologic motions in the body that affect the neuromusculoskeletal system and produce fine movements. These include cardiovascular, respiratory, neuroreflexive, and craniosacral movements, all occurring simultaneously.[8] The therapist is simply monitoring these "micromovements" and noticing their combined direction, amplitude, and velocity.

The two-hand palpation style enables the therapist to appreciate motion in three dimensions. This theoretically enlarges the receptive field of motion to all tissues between the therapist's hands due to the contiguity of myofascial structures. Monitoring tissue status in a direct technique is quite different. Here, the therapist performs a shearing

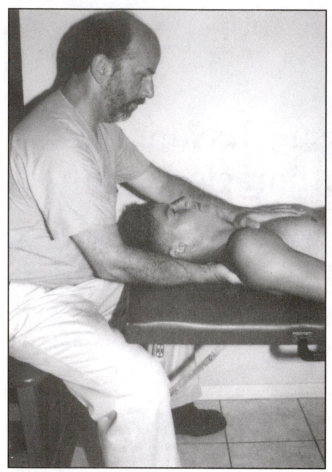

Figure 5-1.

motion with the top hand in a multidirectional manner. However, the hand is not allowed to move over the tissues, but rather "drags" the soft tissues with it until a barrier is reached. Ellis[9] developed the "shear-clock" method of assessing superficial tissue motion. It involves tissue shear in six planes corresponding to the 12 hours of a clock (eg, 12 to 6, 1 to 7, 2 to 8, 3 to 9, 4 to 10, and 5 to 11). The therapist should not apply massage lotion or lubricant for this assessment lest motion over the skin occurs. The purpose of the "shear-clock" assessment is to identify restrictive motion barriers in the thoracic inlet and chest wall tissues that require myofascial mobilization.

Moving is the final step in the 4 Ms procedure. To perform an indirect myofascial release technique, the therapist follows "ease" in the tissues. This induces neuromuscular relaxation and symptom reduction. The therapist is merely taking the tissues where they are most comfortable and thus enabling them to "unwind." A useful analogy is to consider a stick floating on a stream as it meanders through the forest. Just as the stick follows the stream's current, the therapist follows the "current" of inherent tissue motion.

Applying a slight degree of manual compression to the thoracic inlet will facilitate inherent tissue motion and enhance the efficacy of the indirect myofascial release.

Direct myofascial release techniques can be likened to a fullback on the football field. Unlike the halfback, who is quick and agile, looking for the openings on the field (ie, indirect approach), the fullback is strong and formidable, looking to run directly at anyone who dares to get in his way! So it is with direct technique. It is a means of "releasing" myofascial restrictions in the presence of contracture. It is used when stiffness is dominant and the tissue reactivity is low. The author routinely performs this "three-dimensional" thoracic inlet release in the sitting position as well.

Anterior Chest Wall Fascial Techniques

The next group of soft tissue procedures are referred to as direct fascial techniques. These soft tissue mobilizations[10] have several physiologic effects, including enhanced circulation (eg, arterial, venous, and lymphatic), increased production of glycosaminoglycans, loosening of connective tissue adhesions, and viscoelastic elongation (ie, "creep"). Direct fascial techniques utilize a variety of manual contacts (eg, thumbs, palms, knuckles, forearms, finger pads, elbows) and apply them to intermuscular septa, musculotendinous junctions, tenoperiosteal junctions, postsurgical and posttraumatic scar tissue, fascial attachments, etc. Some of the names given to these techniques include "strumming," "sculpting," rolfing, connective tissue massage, myofascial manipulation, "ironing," deep tissue massage, soft tissue mobilization, etc.

There are several principles that guide the use of these effective soft tissue procedures, including the following:

1. Commence each technique with the soft tissues in a loose or slackened state.

2. Apply manual contacts in a direction perpendicular to muscle, tendon, and collagenous fiber orientation whenever possible.

3. Combine all techniques with gentle oscillations, which are better received by the body than static pressure.

4. Progress each technique into tissue length to accomplish full range of motion of the treated structures.

5. The therapist must use a small amount of lubricant when employing these techniques (Note: The author recommends Deep Prep II [Smith & Nephew, Germantown, Wisc]).

6. The contraindications listed in Chapter 3 apply to these direct treatment procedures as well.

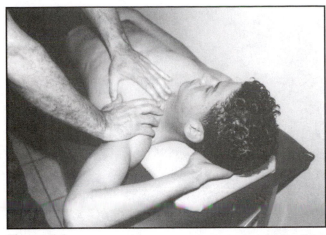

Figure 5-2.

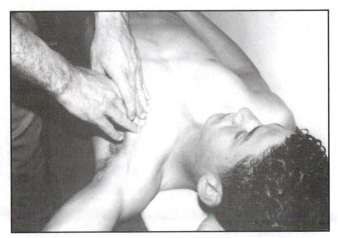

Figure 5-3.

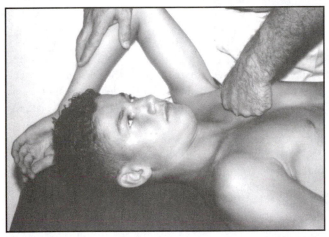

Figure 5-4.

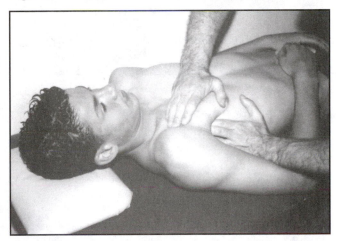

Figure 5-5.

The first two techniques illustrated are referred to as "muscle play" and "strumming." Muscle play (Figure 5-2) stretches the myofascial tissues of the anterior chest wall over the costal cage, whereas strumming (Figure 5-3) identifies and treats localized regions of dysfunction, including taut bands. The muscle play contact consists of a "triangle" formed by the two thumbs and index fingers; strumming is accomplished by joining the third, fourth, and fifth fingers of both hands with the index fingers crossed on top and the thumbs out of the way.

The "steamroller" leads with the thumb and is followed by the proximal phalanges of the second through fifth fingers (Figure 5-4). In patients with high pain tolerance, the proximal interphalangeal (PIP) joints may follow the thumb for deeper tissue penetration. The steamroller is used to accomplish deep tissue massage under the clavicle and between the ribs.

The pectoralis major/minor fascial technique is a more aggressive maneuver that requires a willing patient who is able to tolerate some degree of discomfort. The therapist probes between the two pectoral muscles with one hand while drawing the major over the probing hand with the other. Once "in" the fascial plane between the muscles, the therapist "scours" the area for tight and thickened tissue and then attempts to "free and soften" through direct digital pressure with oscillations. Applying digital pressure in the expiratory phase of breathing allows for greater penetration (Figure 5-5).

The final combined direct fascial/myofascial release technique is one of the author's favorites. With the patient in the side lying position, the therapist carefully wedges his or her body between the patient's abducted/externally rotated upper limb and the patient's trunk (Figure 5-6). Care must be taken to not cause impingement of the glenohumeral joint. The patient's only discomfort should be a stretching sensation across the anterior chest wall. In this position of pectoral elongation, the therapist's hands are free to perform muscle play, strumming, steamrolling, myofascial release (ie, manual stretching of myofascial tissues), postisometric stretching (ie, hold-relax), etc.

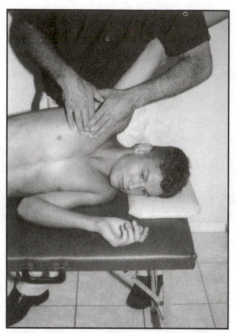

Figure 5-6.

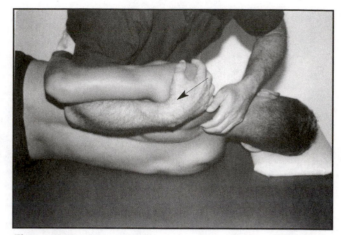

Figure 5-7.

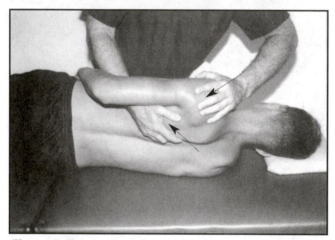

Figure 5-8.

Scapular Fascial Techniques

Once the anterior and lateral structures of the chest wall are rendered more supple and mobile, the therapist can proceed to the myofascial attachments of the scapulae. The most common restrictions in scapular motion seen clinically are depression, retraction, upward rotation, and posterior tilting (ie, superior aspect of the scapula moves posterior and inferior as the inferior angle moves anterior and superior). These restrictions are due to the pull of tight postural muscles in conjunction with weakness of the lower scapular stabilizers. Consequently, the soft tissue component of these impairments must be managed in order to enable the scapulae to assume a neutral position on the costal cage.

To accomplish this, the direct fascial technique known as "framing the scapula," as taught by Grodin,[10] will be employed. The patient is positioned in side lying as the therapist engages the restrictive motion barrier in scapular retraction/depression by grasping the patient's shoulder with the caudal-most hand. At the same time, the cranial-most hand performs a "raking" technique to the levator scapulae and upper trapezius muscles (Figure 5-7). As the tissues relax, the therapist takes up the slack toward increased depression, retraction, and posterior scapular tilt. (Note: The amount of each will vary from patient to patient and must therefore be managed on an individual basis.)

The second phase of "framing the scapula" involves switching hand position so that the cranial-most hand provides the motion against the barrier while the caudal-most hand performs the fascial technique (Figure 5-8). The mobilizing hand proceeds down the vertebral border of the scapula to the inferior angle, working the soft tissues, while simultaneously mobilizing the scapula into further depression, retraction, upward rotation, and posterior tilt. If possible, the therapist should consider an often "forgotten" movement of the scapula, which is rotation about the vertical Y axis through the acromioclavicular joint.[11,12] In patients with forward head/rounded shoulders posture, the scapulae tend to internally rotate as well as protract. Consequently, scapular mobilization should incorporate scapular external rotation, along with retraction, into the intervention described above. Postisometric relaxation can be added to enhance this multiplanar mobilization of the scapula. This combined myofascial/scapular mobilization enables the scapula to function normally by "extricating" it from its previously abnormal positions of elevation, protraction, downward rotation, anterior tilt, and internal rotation.

There are two additional scapular techniques that are quite useful, especially related to shoulder impairment. The first is a direct fascial technique of the subscapularis muscle (Figure 5-9). The subscapularis is often a key component in "frozen shoulder" and its treatment often produces dramatic results. The therapist adducts and internally rotates the

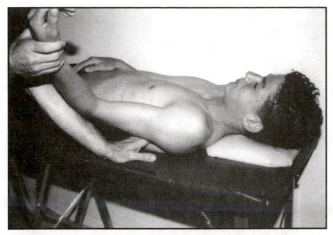

Figure 5-9.

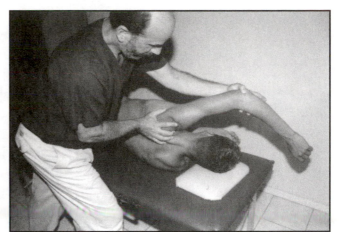

Figure 5-10.

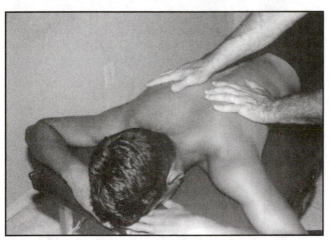

Figure 5-11.

patient's shoulder in order to gain access into the anterior surface of the scapula. Digital pressure is applied to areas of increased density in order to release, soften, and inhibit muscle tone and tightness. As softening occurs, the shoulder is abducted and externally rotated; the direct fascial technique is repeated under stretch. As with all soft tissue procedures, the application of hold-relax technique is a useful adjunctive tool in restoring myofascial length.

The second technique is of particular benefit to patients with shoulder impingement related to poor scapulohumeral rhythm. The patient is in the side lying position with the upper limb at the side. The therapist grasps the scapula with one hand and the elbow with the other (Figure 5-10). Active assisted shoulder abduction is performed while the scapula is passively upwardly rotated and depressed. This provides clearance of the suprahumeral tissues under the coracoacromial arch and also gives the patient the sensation of normal scapulohumeral rhythm. The movement is progressed to an active effort, with the patient incorporating a conscious depression of the scapula as the arm is elevated past 90 degrees. This can then be practiced in standing with the assistance of a mirror to ensure that the scapu-

la is not "hiked up" by the levator scapulae during shoulder elevation.

Superficial Posterior Tissue Release

Myofascial release of the skin, subcutaneous tissue, and superficial fascia of the posterior scapulothoracic region is indicated when the examination reveals impaired mobility (Figure 5-11). The shear-clock method described previously is an excellent tool for both the diagnosis and management of superficial tissue restriction. Once found, the therapist uses the "hold one, move one" treatment by "anchoring" the tissues with one hand and applying a sustained tensional stretch with the other in the specific direction(s) of the restriction. As viscoelastic lengthening and plastic deformation occur, the therapist will feel a "release" of tension and "follow behind" the release until a new barrier is encountered. This process continues for several minutes until the restrictions have been satisfactorily managed. Whereas indirect technique looks for "ease" in the tissues, direct myofascial release seeks tissue "bind." Following the successful "release" of the principal barrier, new areas of "bind" are sought after and "released" accordingly.

Erector Spinae Fascial Technique

The myofascial treatment of the erector spinae muscles is accomplished with a variety of techniques, including strumming and muscle play. Another useful treatment method is termed the "CPR" technique because of how it resembles the manual method used during cardiopulmonary resuscitation (Figures 5-12a and 5-12b).

The heel of the therapist's hand is placed in the medial groove of the longissimus thoracis and continues in a later-

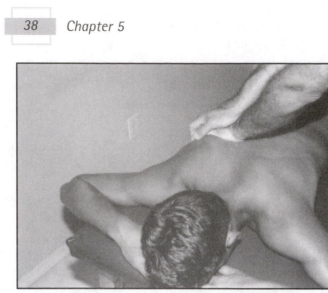

Figure 5-12a.

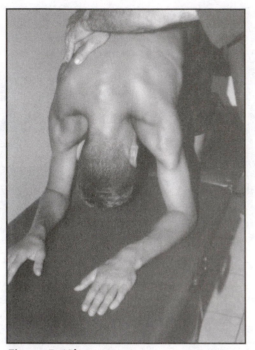

Figure 5-12b.

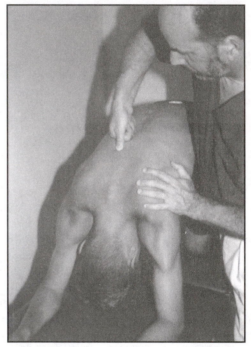

Figure 5-13a.

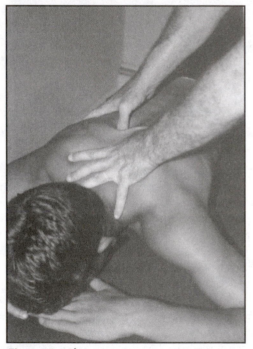

Figure 5-13b.

al direction, imparting a perpendicular stretch on all aspects of the erector spinae. A small amount of Deep Prep II is used to lessen skin friction. The therapist is encouraged to begin at the area of greatest restriction and proceed from there. Two positions are shown: prone with the muscles relaxed (Figure 5-12a) and the "scared cat" position (Figure 5-12b) with the erector spinae under stretch.

Transversospinalis Fascial Techniques and Friction

There are several techniques that address the deep spinal musculature found between the spinous and transverse

processes (ie, the medial groove of longissimus). These techniques apply manipulative contacts in a direction that is caudal or cranial and thus at an oblique angle to the fiber orientation of the semispinalis, multifidus, and rotatores. Such techniques include the "steamroller," bilateral thumb oscillations, and friction (Figures 5-13a to 5-13c).

The steamroller technique applied here is useful in detecting hypertonicity of the transversospinalis. These

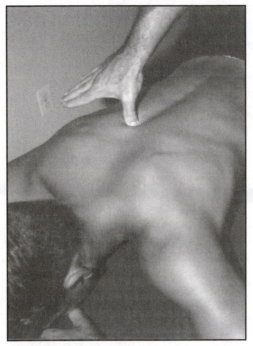

Figure 5-13c.

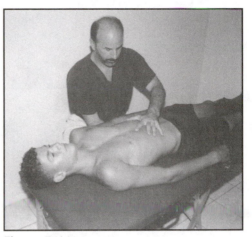

Figure 5-14.

areas of myofascial dysfunction feel like "speed bumps" or "moguls." When these areas are identified, the thumb is used to apply posteroanterior pressure in the form of myotherapy or ischemic compression,[13] as well as circular friction. Once the hypertonicity and/or myofascial trigger point is eradicated, the therapist continues with the steamroller in either a caudal or cranial direction, seeking other areas of myofascial dysfunction. As with the "CPR" technique, these too can start in prone and progress to quadruped (ie, the "scared cat" position).

Respiratory Diaphragm Release (Thoracic Outlet)

The last of the connective tissue techniques is a "three-dimensional" myofascial release of the respiratory diaphragm (Figure 5-14). The anatomic borders of the thoracic outlet (the caudal opening of the thoracic cage) consist of T12 posteriorly, the seventh through tenth costal cartilage anteriorly, and the 11th and 12th ribs laterally. The thoracic outlet is closed by the diaphragm, which separates the thoracic and abdominal cavities. As shown, this release involves both hands, with one hand placed under the thoracolumbar junction and the other hand placed over the respiratory diaphragm. As with the thoracic inlet release described earlier, the 4 Ms palpation technique is a useful way of performing either a direct or indirect technique to the diaphragm and its many attachments (ie, crural attachment to L1 to L3, lower six ribs, psoas, and quadratus lumborum muscles). Mobility of this area is important for both pulmonary and musculoskeletal physiology; it is a common area for the development of myofascial impairment. As with thoracic inlet release, the thoracic outlet can also be treated while the patient sits, where the therapist has optimal control of his or her manual contacts.

To initiate an indirect release, slight compression of the patient's abdomen, between the therapist's hands, is applied.[14] The therapist's hands are then "directed" by inherent tissue motion into a succession of myofascial "releases," which are complete when the tissues are supple and free of restriction.

Manipulation of the Thoracic Spine and Ribs

There are several components to effective manipulative technique; however, the skilled manual therapist must pay particular attention to three. They are localization, control, and balance. If the T3,4 segment is restricted in flexion, the therapist must direct the greatest force at this motion segment and not elsewhere. To ensure that the technique is efficient and effective, the therapist must have maximal control of all points of leverage leading to the restricted area. Maximal, but tension-free, control of the patient's body is also necessary for optimal balance of both the therapist and patient. When these three factors are integrated and the applied force to the impaired joint is as "gentle as possible, but as strong as necessary," the outcome is generally successful for the patient and satisfying for the therapist. A skillful manipulation—whether it be grade 1, 2, 3, 4, or 5—is characterized as graceful, gentle, and purposeful. As for the patient, he or she must be relaxed, comfortable, and confident in the therapist's ability to relieve symptoms, as well as enhance healing and wellness. The main effect of manipulation is physiologic, but enhancement through the placebo effect is of great benefit to the patient. In general, manipulation, especially on the small joints of the spine and ribs, should be of short duration (ie, 30 to 60 seconds) lest the sensitive articular tissues react adversely. It is always wise to begin gently so that the patient's response to passive motion has a chance to be accurately assessed. Both passive accessory intervertebral movements (PAIVMs) and passive physiologic intervertebral movements (PPIVMs) can be transformed into mobilization/manipulation techniques, but only PPIVMs will be used for this purpose in this text.

Thoracic Flexion

The difference between PPIVMs and manipulative technique is that PPIVMs involve the collection of data about motion, whereas spinal manipulation involves the mobilization of a restricted motion segment. The patient's and therapist's positions are identical except for the spinal contact. When performing manipulation, the spinal contact is either providing a "block" of the inferior vertebrae or is assisting the mobilization by gliding the inferior vertebra in the direction opposite the roll of the superior component.

Improving spinal flexion from T1 to T4 is shown in sitting but can easily be done in side lying as well (Figures 6-1a and 6-1b). In order to mobilize T3,4 in flexion, the therapist induces flexion of T3 through the head-neck while the thumb or thenar eminence of the other hand prevents the spinous process (SP) of T4 from moving superiorly. This is achieved by blocking it at its superior aspect. Maitland's grades,[15] excluding grade 5 (ie, manipulative thrust), are then applied in accordance with tissue reactivity. Grade 1 manipulation is a small amplitude movement performed at the beginning of the accessory range. Grade 2 is a large amplitude motion performed within the range but not reaching its limit (at the beginning of the range it is expressed as 2– and deep into the range but not at the limit it is a 2+). Grade 3 is a large amplitude movement, similar to grade 2, but from mid to end-range (3– is a gentle "nudge" at end-range, whereas 3+ is a vigorous "knock"). Grade 4 is a small amplitude movement at the end of range, which can also be described as 4+ or 4–, depending on its

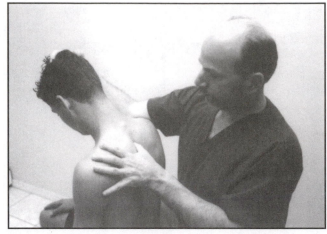

Figure 6-1a.

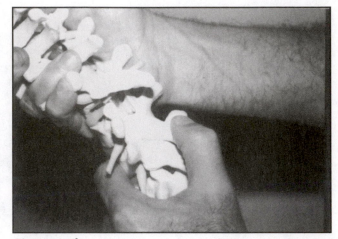

Figure 6-1b.

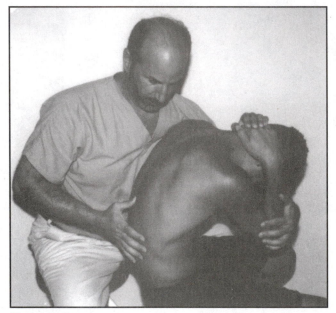

Figure 6-2a.

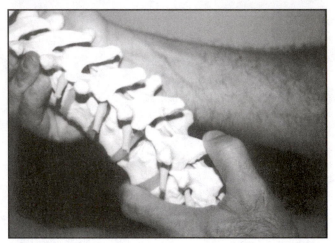

Figure 6-2b.

Clinically, the serratus anterior muscle requires normal flexion from approximately T1 to T9 in order to function optimally. Impaired mobility will weaken the serratus, while mobilization will restore it to its normal potential.

Thoracic Extension

The recovery of thoracic extension, especially from T6 to T12, is one of the most important applications of spinal manual therapy. There are many factors that contribute to this pattern of impairment, but perhaps the most common, as of late, is poor sitting posture related to spending hours at the computer.

The manipulation of extension from T1 to T4 is performed on the seated patient. To perform an extension manipulation at the T2,3 segment, the therapist lightly "cradles" the patient's head and induces extension down to T2 by gliding the head-neck dorsally (Figures 6-3a and 6-3b). Meanwhile, the other hand has the option of either preventing the T3 SP from moving inferiorly on T4 or

vigor, as described for grade 3. Grade 1 manipulation is useful when tissue reactivity is high, grade 2 and 3 manipulations are used in the presence of moderate reactivity, and grade 4 techniques are applied to low reactive, stiffness-dominant tissues. Unlike grades 1 and 2, grades 3 and 4 involve passive movements into tissue resistance against the restrictive barrier.

Flexion manipulation for the T5 to T12 region is similar to the upper thoracic spine with the obvious difference being the use of the patient's arms to induce flexion in this region of the spine (Figures 6-2a and 6-2b). All flexion manipulations can be enhanced by adding a translational component via the trunk to the inferior vertebra in an AP direction, while the superior vertebrae is flexed up and forward (ie, roll-glide).

Warmerdam[16] emphasizes the relationship between joint mobility and muscle strength (ie, the arthrokinetic reflex).

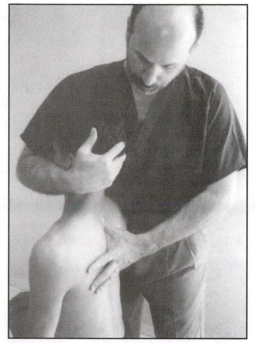

Figure 6-3a.

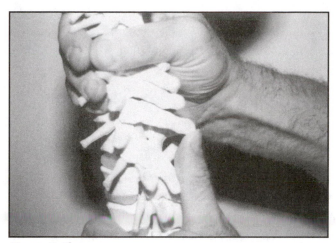

Figure 6-3b.

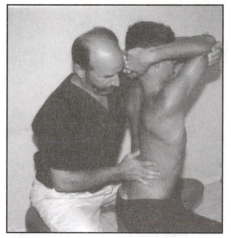

Figure 6-4b.

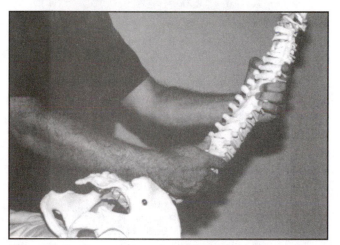

Figure 6-4a. Lower thoracic extension.

enhancing the extension mobilization by performing a PA glide on the SP of T3. Blocking the SP of T3 with either the thumb or thenar eminence at its inferior aspect is a mechanically simpler technique than performing a manipulative "roll-glide," but the latter is the treatment of choice once the requisite skill is developed. Postmenopausal women who develop a matron's or dowager's deformity may derive benefit from gentle extension work in the T1 to T4 region. The cervicothoracic region may also benefit because of its tendency to flex.

There are several ways of improving extension in the mid/lower thoracic region. Increasing extension from T6 to T12 has been shown to enhance strength of the lower trapezius muscles in normal subjects without symptoms.[17] Three methods, all in the sitting position, are illustrated in Figures 6-4a to 6-4d. In all three procedures the inferior SP is translated in an anterior direction as the superior vertebra is rotated into physiologic extension. Depending on the reactivity present, the appropriate Maitland grade is selected. To enhance the treatment's effectiveness, the patient may be asked to participate in the effort by actively extending the thoracic spine during grade 4 mobilizations. This passive/active combination technique has been referred to as "mobilization with movement" by Mulligan,[18] "functional mobilization," and "physiologically enhanced mobilization" by Ellis and Johnson.[9]

Improving mid/lower thoracic extension benefits the thoracic region but also allows for improved function of the cervical and lumbar spine as well as the shoulder girdle and upper extremity.

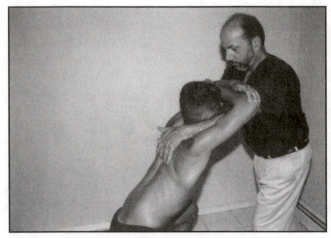

Figure 6-4c.

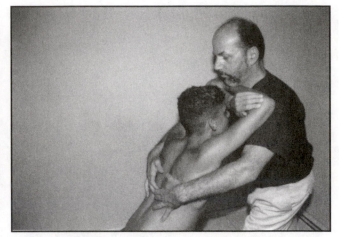

Figure 6-4d.

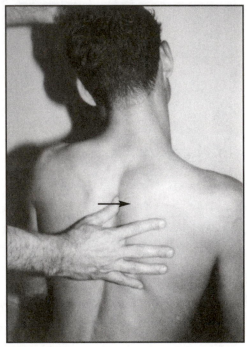

Figure 6-5a.

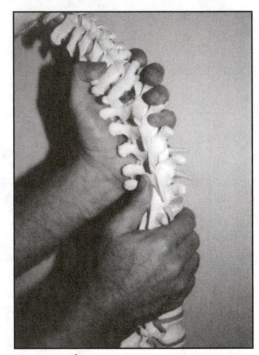

Figure 6-5b.

Thoracic Side Bending

The mobilization of thoracic side bending is first illustrated for the upper thoracic region (Figures 6-5a and 6-5b) and then for the mid/lower thoracic spine (Figures 6-6a and 6-6b). For all side-bending manipulations, the therapist can start with the traditional "hold one, move one" approach and progress to the "roll-glide" technique. For example a T4,5 side bending left maneuver with a "hold one, move one" approach involves mobilizing T4 to the left while "blocking" T5 on the left side of the SP. A "roll-glide" technique of T4,5 side bending left involves "rotating" T4 to

the left on a Z axis while simultaneously translating the T5 SP to the right with the thumb or thenar contact. Although a transverse pressure at the apex of the SP from the neutral position will normally induce vertebral rotation, when it is applied at the base of the spinous process in conjunction with a lateral bending motion, it induces enhanced side bending.

From T5 to T12, the therapist has two options. One is referred to as the "pull" technique (see Figure 6-6a), while the other is the "push" technique (see Figure 6-6b). In both procedures, the "roll-glide" manipulation is superior to the traditional "hold one, move one" approach.

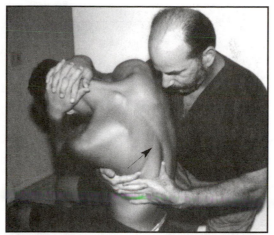

Figure 6-6a.

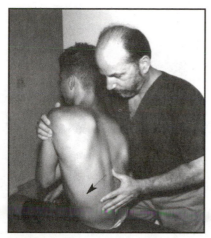

Figure 6-6b.

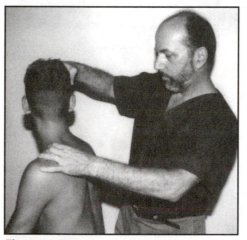

Figure 6-7a.

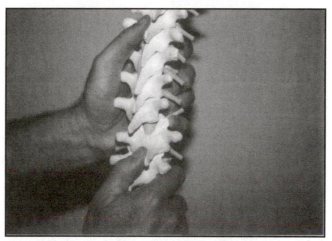

Figure 6-7b.

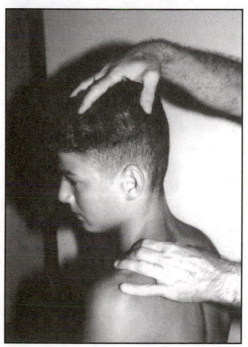

Figure 6-7c.

Thoracic Rotation

As with the other thoracic manipulations/mobilizations covered previously, the difference between PPIVMs and manipulative intervention is found in the purpose behind the technique and the slight modification in hand position. Thoracic rotation manipulation is achieved via the "hold one, move one" approach in which rotation of the superior vertebra is induced with one hand while the other hand blocks the inferior vertebra. For example, a right rotation manipulation at T2,3 involves inducing right rotation of T2 through the head-neck region as the therapist prevents T3 rotation below (Figures 6-7a and 6-7b). This "blocking" of T3 is achieved by placing the thumb or hypothenar contact against the SP of T3 on its left lateral aspect.

For rotational techniques, the concept of "pre-positioning" the segment is quite useful (Figure 6-7c). For example, prior to a T2,3 right rotation manipulation, the therapist rotates the patient's head-neck to the left. The therapist then places his or her left thumb against the spinous process of T3 on the left. The head-neck region is now rotated to

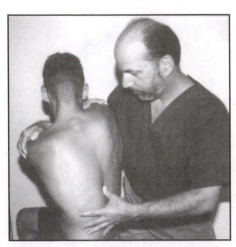

Figure 6-8a. Mobilization/manipulation of T10,11 in rotation right.

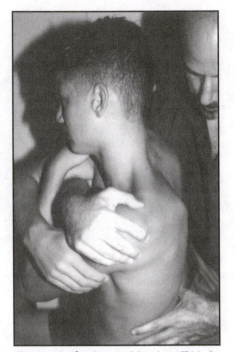

Figure 6-8b. Prepositioning T11 in left rotation for a T10,11 rotation right maneuver.

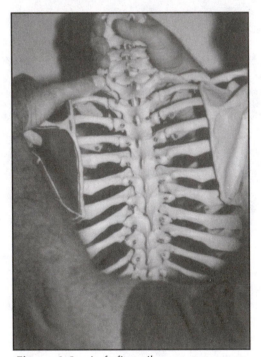

Figure 6-9a. Left first rib costotransverse joint.

the right with T3 fixed in a left rotated position. The advantage of pre-positioning is that the barrier is reached sooner and the surrounding joints are subjected to less stress. The same principles (ie, blocking, pre-positioning, etc) are applied to the T5 to T12 region; however, the trunk replaces the head-neck region as the lever arm (Figures 6-8a and 6-8b).

As emphasized earlier, all spinal manipulations, whether grade 1, 2, 3, or 4 (grade 5 thrust is not covered on the introductory level), start in the area of greatest restriction and proceed from there. The major motion losses (50% or more) are treated first; the minor motion losses (less than 50%) are treated last.

The role of the thoracic spine in the management of shoulder impairment cannot be emphasized enough. It is often the key in the treatment of chronic shoulder impingement syndromes and adhesive capsulitis.

The diagnosis and treatment of respiratory rib dysfunctions, subluxations, and torsions is beyond the scope of an introductory textbook on the topic. The objective of this section is to provide the manual therapist with one useful technique for each of the 12 ribs. These techniques in conjunction with soft tissue/spinal manipulative procedures and therapeutic exercises will ensure that patients with scapulothoracic impairment receive a basic yet comprehensive approach to their condition.

To manipulate restriction of the left first rib, the therapist rotates the patient's head-neck region to the right while palpating the left first rib just lateral to the costotransverse joint. When motion "arrives" at the first rib, a PA-graded mobilization is performed with the thumb contact (fingers are draped over the shawl area for counterbalance). With practice, both hands move simultaneously to enhance the effectiveness of the procedure. As with the spine, the choice of which grade to use depends upon the tissue reactivity present (Figures 6-9a and 6-9b).

The second, third, and fourth ribs (Figures 6-10a and 6-10b) are mobilized using the same procedure as for the first rib (ie, a graded PA pressure on the rib tubercle with simultaneous head-neck rotation).

The fifth through 12th ribs are treated as follows: to manipulate the right seventh rib by gapping its costotrans-

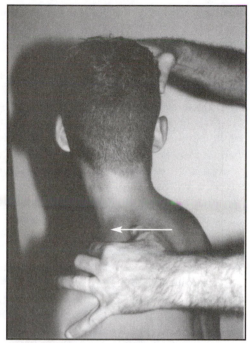

Figure 6-9b.

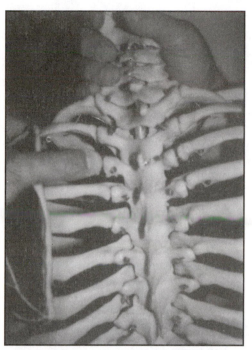

Figure 6-10a. Left third rib costotransverse joint.

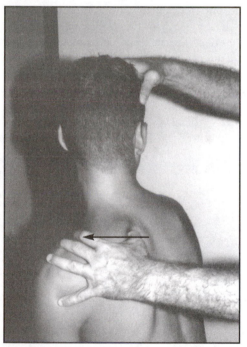

Figure 6-10b.

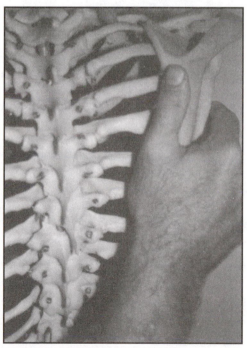

Figure 6-11a. Gapping the seventh costotransverse joint on the right.

verse joint, the patient grasps his or her right shoulder with the left hand, and the therapist reaches across the front of the patient to grasp the posterior aspect of the right shoulder (Figures 6-11a and 6-11b). The patient's trunk is then rotated to the left until motion arrives at the medial aspect of the angle of the right seventh rib (the rib angle is the most posterior aspect of the rib). The graded mobilization consists of a transverse pressure on the rib angle to the right with or without a simultaneous small amplitude rotation of the trunk to the left. The lower the rib the greater the trunk rotation. To manipulate the fifth through 12th ribs on the left, all positions and movements are reversed.

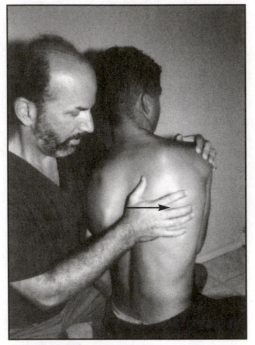

Figure 6-11b.

There are additional rib mobilizations involving the anterior costosternal joints that will not be covered in this text. Bookhout[19] has been successfully using anteroposterior (AP) mobilizations in this area of the costal cage to enhance shoulder girdle mobility in addition to managing adverse neural tension in the upper limb. The reader is encouraged to "stay tuned" to this developing area in scapulothoracic manual therapy!

Manipulation of the ribs affects the costotransverse, costovertebral, and costosternal joints as spinal manipulation affects the apophyseal joints. As with any manipulative procedure, there are both mechanical and neurological effects, but in the case of costal cage manipulation, there are beneficial effects on pulmonary function as well.

To enhance any of the manipulations described in this chapter, the therapist can add a postisometric relaxation component to the technique. This procedure, which osteopathic physicians refer to as muscle energy technique, involves the use of a patient-activated, submaximal, isometric contraction at the very beginning of the restrictive motion barrier (ie, the "feather edge"), which is in the opposite direction of the desired mobilization. Following a 6-second isometric contraction, the therapist mobilizes the affected segment until a new motion barrier is reached. This procedure is repeated three times prior to using the graded mobilizations that have been outlined above. For example, prior to applying a grade 4 extension manipulation at the T6,7 segment, the patient is asked to resist the therapist's attempt to extend for a count of 6 seconds. This activates the flexors at the T6,7 segment isometrically. According to scientific theory,[6] and in keeping with the clinical experience of those trained in these procedures, this is followed by a period of reflex inhibition in which the muscles are amenable to being stretched. The value of this technique, prior to joint mobilization, is that muscle tone is reduced, thus enhancing the efficacy of the manipulation. In the presence of neuroreflexive muscle splinting, the use of either indirect treatment methods or postisometric relaxation is indicated. However, when reactivity is low and there is more contracture than contraction, then mobilization/manipulation alone is needed.

All sitting techniques of the thoracic spine and ribs should be performed with the patient's feet in firm contact with either the floor, a chair, or a stool. Otherwise, the patient will not be secure and therefore unable to fully relax.

Therapeutic and Home Exercises for the Scapulothoracic Region

The home exercise program (HEP) is as important if not more important than the manual therapy component of the intervention process. Having said that, the HEP should never consist of merely providing a handout to the patient. The HEP should be custom-designed to address the specific needs of each patient. The patient requires individual instruction for each procedure in order to ensure its correct performance. The benefit to the patient is directly related to both the quantity and the quality of the home exercises; the time spent by the therapist facilitating the patient's independence in this process is a most worthwhile investment.

The HEP should always be presented to the patient as an exercise prescription. This involves all aspects of the exercise, including number of repetitions, sets, and seconds held. It must also include instruction in warm-up, cooldown, injury prevention, first aid for managing flare-ups, etc. For stretching procedures, the patient is advised to stop at the first feeling of tissue resistance and to hold the stretch for 30 seconds.[20,21] It is wise to escalate patients up to 30 seconds by beginning at 5 to 10 seconds and working up from there. This is then repeated three times every 2 hours if possible. For strengthening exercises, the patient is advised to avoid any and all painful muscle contractions. The patient can begin with 10 repetitions, holding each contraction for 5 to 10 seconds. Strengthening exercises are usually performed no more than three times a day because working muscles need time to rest.

It is imperative that patients understand that the HEP is not optional. If they expect results, then they must "take their medicine!"

Doorway Stretch

The doorway stretch is an excellent way to stretch the myofascial structures of the anterior chest wall (eg, pectoralis major/minor and related fascia, clavipectoral fascia). The patient should be encouraged to "explore" various aspects of the chest wall in "search" of the area of greatest tightness. The doorway stretch can be performed bilaterally (Figure 7-1a) or unilaterally (Figure 7-1b). The patient must be careful not to stress the anterior capsule of the glenohumeral joint, which in many patients is already hypermobile.

Quadruped Flexion

In order to isolate spinal flexion in the upper, mid, and lower thoracic spine, the patient is instructed to perform self-mobilization in three distinct positions. To achieve flexion from T1 to T4, the patient is placed in the "scared cat" position with the ears in line with the elbows (Figure 7-2a). To achieve flexion from T5 to T8, the patient is again placed in the "scared cat" position, but this time with the shoulders in line with the elbows (Figure 7-2b). To achieve flexion in the lower thoracic spine, T9 to T12, the patient is instructed to extend his or her arms and sit back, buttocks to heels (Figure 7-2c).

Once positioned correctly in proper alignment, the patient is instructed to "round the back" so that the thoracic kyphosis is increased. It is important that the patient

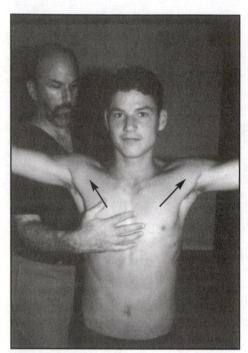

Figure 7-1a.

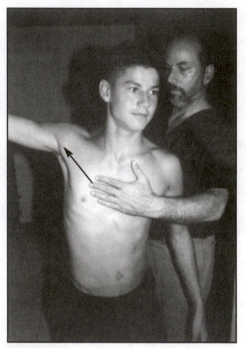

Figure 7-1b.

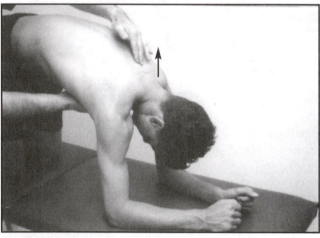

Figure 7-2a.

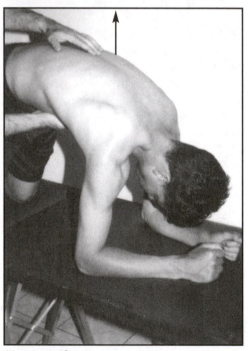

Figure 7-2b.

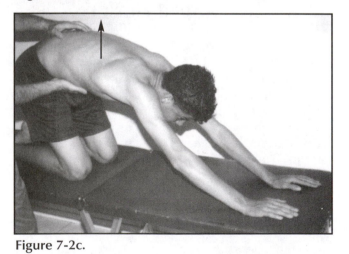

Figure 7-2c.

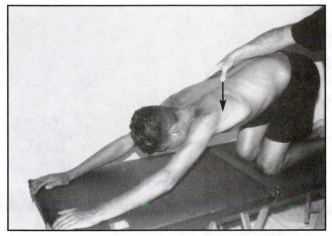

Figure 7-3a.

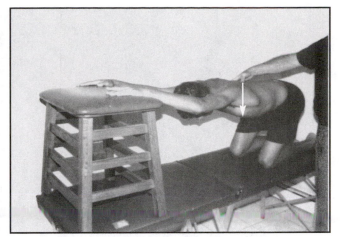

Figure 7-3b.

Quadruped Side Bending

This stretch can address tightness of the latissimus dorsi, erector spinae, quadratus lumborum, piriformis, and tensor fascia latae. It is also an excellent way to self-mobilize the thoracic and lumbar spine for increased side bending. Most patients require hands-on instruction before they attain a proper stretch. The key is to "lean" into the convex side rather than "tilt" into it (ie, the shoulders should remain level). Patients often need to be reminded not to over-stretch lest they will "pay for it" later (Figure 7-4)!

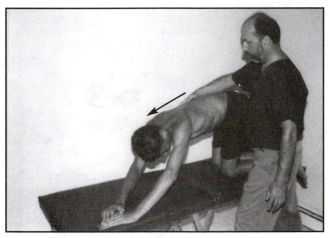

Figure 7-4.

Quadruped Rotation

The patient is advised to initiate motion with the eyes, followed by the head-neck, upper limb, and trunk. Sitting backward toward the heels reduces motion in the lower thoracic region as per Fryette's third rule. By adjusting hip position in this manner, the rotation can be biased to a given region of the thoracic spine (Figure 7-5).

understands the need to self-mobilize the region that lacks flexion. Simply flexing in an area that is already mobile is unproductive. The self-mobilization is held for 30 seconds and repeated three times every 2 hours.

Quadruped Extension

From the quadruped position, the patient's hands are placed in front of the patient to the point where thoracic extension begins to occur (Figure 7-3a). The patient must have full range of shoulder flexion in order for this stretch to be effective. The patient rocks backward with the intention of drawing the chest to the floor and flattening the thoracic kyphosis. Three repetitions of 30 seconds each are performed, with the arms placed further in front of the patient with each stretch. For those who are able to tolerate a more vigorous stretch, the patient's hands can be placed on a chair or stool as illustrated (Figure 7-3b). This also serves as an excellent stretch for the latissimus dorsi muscle.

Sensorimotor Training

Hanna[22] defined sensory-motor amnesia (SMA) as "the habituated state of memory loss of how certain muscle groups feel and how to control them." Many 20th century "body workers" (eg, Feldenkrais, Alexander, Hanna, Rolf, Pilates, Trager) contributed enormously to our understanding of mind/body connections, and physical therapists have been the conduits of much of this information into mainstream medicine.

The appreciation of neuromusculoskeletal impairment, as compared with musculoskeletal impairment alone, has greatly benefited the practice of orthopaedic physical therapy. The purpose of sensorimotor training[23] is to reduce or eliminate pain in the neuromusculoskeletal system by help-

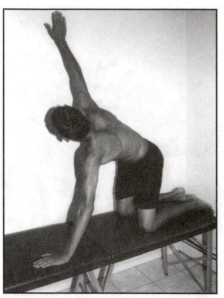

Figure 7-5.

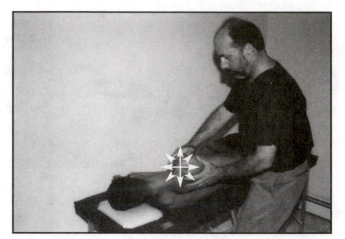

Figure 7-6.

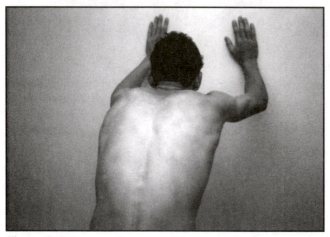

Figure 7-7.

ing the patient rediscover flexibility and ease of movement. Using an analogy from computers, manual therapy is to the "hardware" what sensorimotor training is to the "software." As mentioned earlier, it is the "electrical" connection that makes the difference between movement that is efficient and functional versus movement that is inefficient and dysfunctional.

While many options exist for the re-education of motion in the scapulothoracic region, a good place to start is with the Feldenkrais "clock" approach (Figure 7-6). In the side lying position, the patient imagines a "clock" placed upon the shoulder and upper arm. The "clock" concept can be used in a variety of ways with the motion occurring in a clockwise or counterclockwise fashion as well as in imaginary "lines" that connect opposite ends of the "clock" (ie, 12 to 6, 1 to 7, 2 to 8, 3 to 9, 4 to 10, and 5 to 11). The sequence includes passive motion, followed by active assisted, active, and resisted motion. It is crucial that all sensori-

motor training commence with passive work so that the patient can develop a "template" for what the motion should feel like. Patient guidelines for successful sensorimotor training include the following:

1. Perform the movements slowly and easily.
2. Avoid excessive effort.
3. Rest frequently.
4. Pain and discomfort should never be experienced during an exercise.

The most common movement impairment seen in the scapulothoracic region is a combination of depression and retraction. It is this "down and back" motion that will require the most work. Another useful tool for muscle re-education is rhythmic stabilization. The shoulder girdle is placed in its neutral, physiologic position. The patient then attempts to maintain this position against a variety of forces, in a variety of directions. These isometric contractions provide excellent feedback into the central nervous system for motor learning. Rhythmic stabilization is also applied with the patient in the side lying position.

Strengthening the Lower Scapular Stabilizers

The final component of the intervention process is to revisit the weak phasic muscles to ensure that their motor strength is restored to normal. Otherwise, the imbalance persists and future impairment of function is likely. According to Janda,[24] the lower scapular stabilizers consist of the serratus anterior, rhomboids, and middle/lower trapezius. Isaacs and Bookhout[25] use the "wall press" as one way of strengthening the serratus anterior. This exercise is performed in standing with the hands flat against the wall at shoulder height (Figure 7-7). From the neutral position of the spine, the patient is asked to protract the scapulae, flex the cervical spine, and tuck the pelvis under. The end-

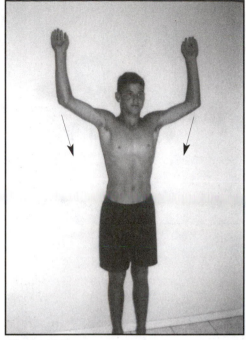

Figure 7-8a.

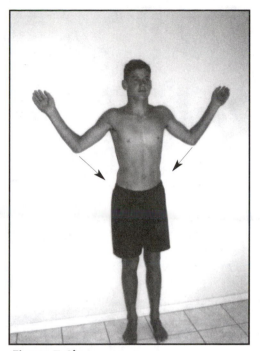

Figure 7-8b.

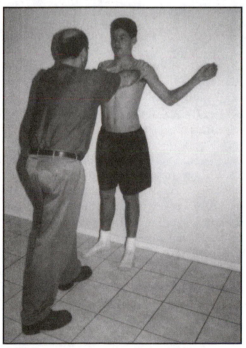

Figure 7-8c.

point of thoracic flexion is held for 5 to 10 seconds and repeated 10 times, three times per day.

There are several ways to strengthen the rhomboids and middle/lower trapezius, but one method in particular is especially effective. The patient assumes a standing position with his or her back and arms against the wall. The upper limbs should be in approximately 145 degrees of

abduction with the elbows flexed slightly (Figure 7-8a). The patient pushes back against the wall to recruit the scapular retractors and proceeds to draw the elbows down toward the low back to recruit the scapular depressors (Figure 7-8b). The combination of scapular upward rotation, retraction, and depression isolates the lower trapezius, primarily, but also facilitates the middle trapezius and rhomboids, even though the rhomboids are downward rotators of the scapulae. During this exercise the patient must be advised not to lower the upper limbs below 60 degrees of abduction lest the scapulae begin to rotate downward. Any extension of the spine should occur in the thoracic rather than the lumbar region. In fact, a slight posterior pelvic tilt is helpful in avoiding this tendency. The author finds that the addition of a bilateral, superior glide mobilization at the sternoclavicular joints in 60 degrees of abduction significantly enhances the efficacy of this strengthening maneuver (Figure 7-8c). Not illustrated but also of clinical significance is the component motion of posterior clavicular rotation, which is a requisite movement for scapular depression, retraction, and upward rotation. The next phase of the exercise is difficult but extremely effective, if performed correctly. The patient is asked to maintain the scapulae in a retracted and depressed position as the arms are slowly elevated to 145 degrees. The key to the successful execution of the return phase is that the patient must not elevate the shawl area while doing it. EMG biofeedback over the lower trapezius is a useful tool in this process of motor learning (Figure 7-9a). If the patient requires visual feedback, then performing the exercise in front of a mirror is impor-

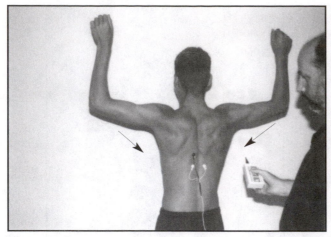

Figure 7-9a.

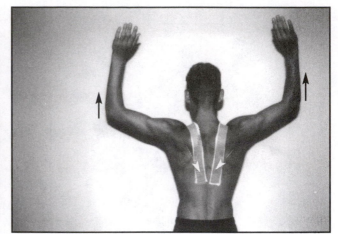

Figure 7-9b.

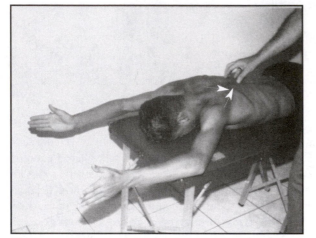

Figure 7-10a.

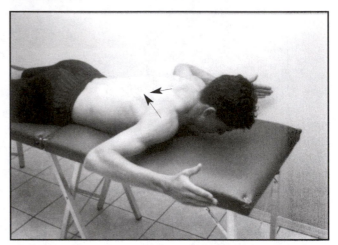

Figure 7-10b.

tant, especially during the return phase when the shawl area must remain depressed. Securing the scapulae in a position of retraction/depression (Figure 7-9b) with Leukotape P (Beiersdorf-Jobst Inc, Rutherford College, NC) is helpful in the "retraining" of scapular position, through increasing kinesthetic awareness, as well as by directly inhibiting the upper trapezius muscles.[1]

The above two-phase exercise can also be performed in the prone position as illustrated. In prone lying, care should be taken to maintain a neutral lumbopelvic region as well as a neutral craniovertebral and cervicothoracic junction by having the patient perform a chin tuck throughout the exercise (Figures 7-10a and 7-10b).

For both the standing and prone lying positions, the patient takes 5 to 10 seconds to complete each of the two phases and performs 10 repetitions of the entire up and down cycle three times per day. Some patients find the Leukotape P so helpful in facilitating a corrected position of the scapulothoracic region that they keep it on for a few days at a time. A useful Alexander movement principle regarding shoulder elevation is that motion should occur from distal to proximal (ie, fingers, wrist, elbow, and shoulder in that order). Furthermore, optimal active shoulder elevation should include the awareness of movement all the way into the sternoclavicular joint.

Lower trapezius training is a crucial component in the rehabilitation of shoulder impingement. Without normal function of the lower trapezius, the scapulae will not upwardly rotate optimally during shoulder elevation; therefore, the coracoacromial arch will fail to move away from the subacromial tissues, causing further impingement.

References and Bibliography

References

1. McConnell J. *The McConnell Approach to the Problem Shoulder.* Marina Del Rey, Calif: McConnell Institute; 1994.

2. Conable B, Conable W. *How to Learn the Alexander Technique.* Columbus, Ohio: Andover Road Press; 1992.

3. Apley AG, Solomon L. *Apley's System of Orthopaedics and Fractures.* 7th ed. Oxford: Butterworth-Heinemann; 1993.

4. Hillegrass EA, Sadowsky HS. *Essentials of Cardiopulmonary Physical Therapy.* 2nd ed. Philadelphia, Pa: WB Saunders; 2001.

5. Petty NJ, Moore AP. *Neuromusculoskeletal Examination and Assessment.* Edinburgh: Churchill Livingstone; 1998.

6. Korr IM, ed. *The Neurobiologic Mechanisms in Manipulative Therapy.* New York, NY: Plenum Press; 1978.

7. Grieve GP. Thoracic musculoskeletal problems. In: Boyling JD, Palastanga N, eds. *Grieve's Modern Manual Therapy, The Vertebral Column.* 2nd ed. Edinburgh: Churchill Livingstone; 1994.

8. Nelson KE, Sergneef N, Lipinski CM, Chapman AR, Glonek T. Cranial rhythmic impulse related to the Traube-Hering-Mayer oscillation: comparing laser-Doppler flowmetry and palpation. *J Am Osteopath Assoc.* 2001;101(3):163-173.

9. Ellis JJ, Johnson GS. Myofascial considerations in somatic dysfunction of the thorax. In: Flynn TW, ed. *The Thoracic Spine and Rib Cage: Musculoskeletal Evaluation and Treatment.* Newton, Mass: Butterworth-Heinemann; 1996.

10. Cantu RI, Grodin AJ. *Myofascial Manipulation, Theory and Clinical Application.* 2nd ed. Gaithersburg, Md: Aspen Publishers; 2001.

11. Culham E, Peat M. Functional anatomy of the shoulder complex. *J Orthop Sports Phys Ther.* 1993;18(1):342-350.

12. McQuade KJ, Smidt GL. Dynamic scapulohumeral rhythm: the effects of external resistance during elevation of the arm in the scapular plane. *J Orthop Sports Phys Ther.* 1998;27(2):125-131.

13. Simons DG, Travell JG, Simons LS. *Travell & Simons' Myofascial Pain and Dysfunction: The Trigger Point Manual. Vol 1. Upper Half of Body.* Baltimore, Md: Williams & Wilkins; 1999.

14. Manheim C. *The Myofascial Release Manual.* 3rd ed. Thorofare, NJ: SLACK Incorporated; 2001.

15. Maitland GD. *Vertebral Manipulation.* 5th ed. London: Butterworth-Heinemann; 1986.

16. Warmerdam A. *Manual Therapy: Improve Muscle and Joint Functioning.* Wantagh, NY: Pine Publications; 1999.

17. Liebler EJ, Tufano-Coors L, Douris P, et al. The effect of thoracic spine mobilization on lower trapezius strength testing. *Journal of Manual & Manipulative Therapy.* 2001;9:207-212.

18. Mulligan BR. Snags: mobilizations of the spine with active movement. In: Boyling JD, Palastanga N, eds. *Grieve's Modern Manual Therapy, The Vertebral Column.* 2nd ed. Edinburgh: Churchill Livingstone; 1994.

19. Bookhout MR. *Management of Thoracic Spine and Costal Cage Dysfunction With Manipulative Therapy, Myofascial Techniques, and Specific Exercises.* Bayshore, NY: Course Manual; 1995.

20. Bandy WD, Irion JM. The effect of time on static stretch on the flexibility of the hamstring muscles. *Phys Ther.* 1994;74:845-852.

21. Bandy WD, Irion JM, Briggler M. The effect of time and frequency of static stretching on flexibility of the hamstring muscles. *Phys Ther.* 1997;77(10):1090-1096.

22. Hanna T. *Somatics.* New York, NY: Addison-Wesley Publishing; 1988.

23. Zemach-Bersin D, Reese M. *Audiotape Program User's Guide.* Berkeley, Calif: Sensory Motor Learning Systems; 1983.

24. Janda V. Muscles and cervicogenic pain syndromes. In: Grant R, ed. *Physical Therapy of the Cervical and Thoracic Spine.* New York, NY: Churchill Livingstone; 1988.

25. Isaacs ER, Bookhout MR. *Bourdillon's Spinal Manipulation.* 6th ed. Boston, Mass: Butterworth-Heinemann; 2002.

Bibliography

Andrade CK, Clifford P. *Outcome-Based Massage.* Philadelphia, PA: Lippincott Williams & Wilkins; 2001.

Bookhout MR. Evaluation of the thoracic spine and rib cage. In: Flynn TW, ed. *The Thoracic Spine and Rib Cage.* Newton, Mass: Butterworth-Heinemann; 1996.

Cyriax J. *Textbook of Orthopaedic Medicine.* Vol 2. 9th ed. London: Bailliere Tindall; 1977.

DiGiovanna EL, Schiowitz S, eds. *An Osteopathic Approach to Diagnosis and Treatment.* 2nd ed. Philadelphia, Pa: Lippincott-Raven; 1997.

Flynn TW. *Current Concepts of Orthopedic Physical Therapy, Home Study Course 11.2.5, Thoracic Spine and Chest Wall.* Fairfax, Va: American Physical Therapy Association; 2001.

Grant R, ed. *Physical Therapy of the Cervical and Thoracic Spine.* New York, NY: Churchill-Livingstone; 2002.

Hammer WI. *Functional Soft Tissue Examination and Treatment by Manual Methods.* Gaithersburg, Md: Aspen Publishers; 1999.

Hertling D, Kessler RM. *Management of Common Musculoskeletal Disorders, Physical Therapy Principles and Methods.* 3rd ed. Philadelphia, Pa: Lippincott Williams & Wilkins; 1996.

Hendricks T. The effects of immobilization on connective tissue. *Journal of Manual & Manipulative Therapy.* 1995;3:98-103.

Kendall FP, McGreary FP, Provance PG. *Muscles: Testing and Function.* 4th ed. Baltimore, Md: Williams & Wilkins; 1993.

Knott M, Voss DE. *Proprioceptive Neuromuscular Facilitation.* 2nd ed. New York, NY: Harper & Row Publishers; 1968.

Lee D. Biomechanics of the thorax: a clinical model of in vivo function. *Journal of Manual & Manipulative Therapy.* 1993;1: 13-21.

Lee D. *The Thorax: An Integrated Approach.* White Rock, British Columbia: Diane G. Lee Physiotherapist Corp; 2003.

Lewis J, Green A, Reichard Z, Wright C. Scapular position: the validity of skin surface palpation. *Man Ther.* 2002;7(1):26-30.

Petty NJ, Bach TM, Cheek L. Accuracy of feedback during training of passive accessory intervertebral movements. *Journal of Manual & Manipulative Therapy.* 2001;9:99-108.

Roddey TS, Olson SL, Grant SE. The effect of pectoralis muscle stretching on the resting position of the scapula in persons with varying degrees of forward head/rounded shoulder posture. *Journal of Manual & Manipulative Therapy.* 2002;10(3): 124-128.

Rolf IP. *Rolfing: The Integration of Human Structures.* New York, NY: Harper & Row Publishers; 1977.

Sahrmann S. *Diagnosis and Treatment of Movement Impairment Syndromes.* St. Louis, Mo: Mosby-Year Book; 2002.

Saunders HD, Saunders R. *Evaluation, Treatment, and Prevention of Musculoskeletal Disorders, Vol. 1, Spine.* Chaska, Minn: The Saunders Group; 1995.

Stoddard A. *Manual of Osteopathic Techniques.* London: The Anchor Press; 1977.

Travell JG, Simons DG. *Myofascial Pain and Dysfunction: The Trigger Point Manual.* Baltimore, Md: Williams & Wilkins; 1983.

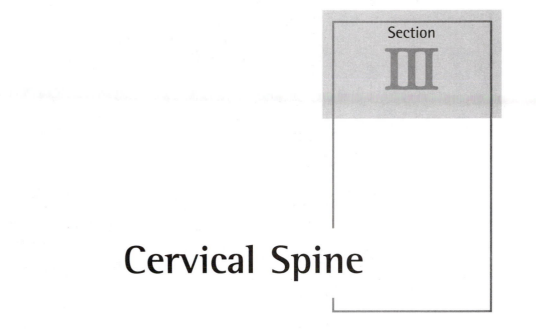

Cervical Spine

Examination and Evaluation of the Cervical Spine

Posture

For the purpose of learning the specifics of a patient's structure, a "compartmental" approach is taken in which we separate the various anatomic regions from each other (eg, scapulothoracic, cervical, lumbar, and pelvic). However, in clinical practice the entire continuum of posture from "head to toe" must be integrated. This is because of the interdependence of all body parts, which must be appreciated within a holistic paradigm.

Having said that, we come to the analysis of head and neck alignment. As in the scapulothoracic region, we will examine the standing patient from the side, back, and front. Employing the CHARTS methodology, the evaluation of posture provides much needed information on asymmetry (A). The importance of C and H was covered earlier in Chapter 3.

The standing lateral view of the cervical spine enables the therapist to inspect the following structures for faulty alignment (Figure 8-1):

1. Head and neck position in the sagittal plane. The ear lobe to acromion relationship can be assessed related to forward head posture (FHP), which can be described as minimal, moderate, or severe. A posture grid or plumb-line can be used for greater accuracy.

2. The position of the occiput. Note posterior cranial rotation (occipital extension) when present. Alexander teachers refer to this as "downward pull." The term for the preservation or recovery of the optimum dynamic relationship between the head and spine in movement and at rest is *primary control*. A recognized plane of reference for the assessment of head position is the "Frankfort plane." It suggests that a line extending from the upper margin of the external auditory meatus to the inferior aspect of the orbit should be horizontal or parallel to the ground.

3. The inferior orbit to manubrium relationship. This should ideally be a straight vertical line.

4. Rocabado[1] recommends the use of a head-neck measure that involves extending a vertical tangent from the thoracic spine from which the perpendicular distance in centimeters is recorded to the mid-cervical lordosis (Figure 8-2). A distance of 6 cm represents the optimum head-neck to back relationship.

5. Another option in measuring FHP is to use the forward head "arm" of the cervical range of motion (CROM) device (Performance Attainment Associates, Roseville, NJ).

Both the plumb-line method and the CROM device have demonstrated moderate to high intratester and intertester reliability in the evaluation of FHP.[2]

The standing posterior view (Figure 8-3) includes an assessment of the following:

1. Occipital position in the frontal plane. The ears can be used to assess for a lateral tilt of the occiput; rotation of the head is noted by observing the face on one side. A type I head tilt involves contralateral

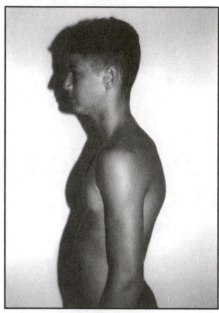

Figure 8-1.

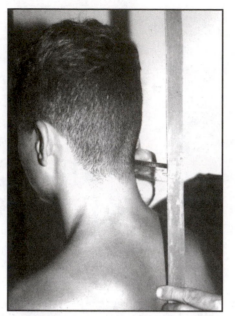

Figure 8-2.

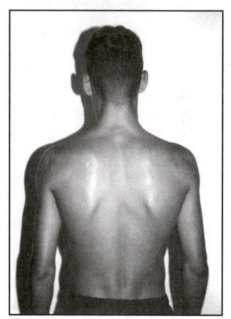

Figure 8-3.

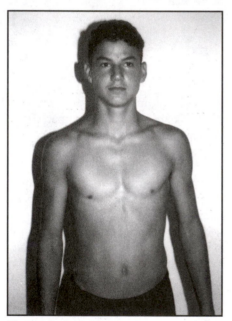

Figure 8-4.

head rotation, while a type II tilt involves ipsilateral rotation (the terms torticollis or wryneck are also used).

2. Lower neck position (C2 to C7). The most common asymmetry is a lateral shift to one side.

The standing anterior view of the head-neck region (Figure 8-4) is helpful in confirming a torticollis, but the assessment for craniofacial asymmetries is more relevant to the temporomandibular examination. In children with congenital torticollis, the face is often shorter on the side of the cervical concavity. However, this usually improves, as head posture is corrected in the developing child.

In patients with moderate to severe FHP, there is often an associated retrognathia of the mandible (ie, horizontal deficiency of the lower jaw). The lateral view demonstrates a convexity of the lower third of the craniofacial region. This is seen in children who are mouth breathers and in patients with juvenile rheumatoid arthritis. The connection between this finding, dental malocclusion, and adults with temporomandibular disorders will be covered in a subsequent chapter.

A plumb-line or posture grid can also be used for greater accuracy in both the anterior and posterior assessment of standing posture.

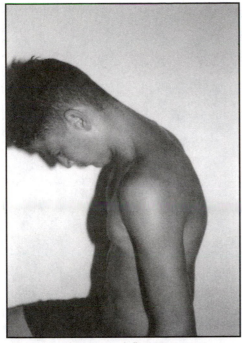

Figure 8-5a. Cervical flexion.

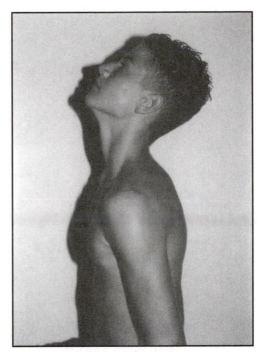

Figure 8-5b. Cervical extension.

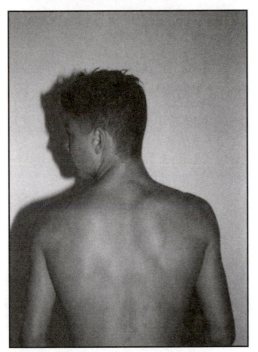

Figure 8-5c. Cervical rotation left.

Active Movements

The examination of active cervical movements can be performed with a variety of methods, including the CROM device, the universal goniometer, inclinometers, computerized motion diagnostics, visual estimation, etc. Though the CROM device is the preferred clinical goniometer for the cervical spine regarding reliability and validity,[3] therapists should learn the visual estimation method for two reasons. The first reason is that the CROM device is not available in all clinical situations. The second reason is that manual therapists need to develop the clinical skill of observing not only the quantity but also the quality of motion as discussed in Chapter 4. The skilled observer can detect things about human motion that a sophisticated goniometer or computer can never appreciate. It's true that outcomes are based upon numbers, but perhaps there are other numbers, in addition to degrees or centimeters, that are just as representative of improvement (eg, the Neck Disability Index, which looks at ten overall categories with all but two being directly related to functionality; the Northwick Park Neck Pain Questionnaire; the McGill Pain Questionnaire).

Returning to the visual examination of active cervical spine mobility, there are six movements that the patient is asked to perform (Figures 8-5a to 8-5f). They are: flexion, extension, rotation left and right, and side bending left and right. As with the remainder of the vertebral column, the therapist can refer to other texts for the normative values related to the quantity of each movement.

The salient points of the active cervical motion examination include the presence of impairment (minimal, moderate, severe), the reactivity of the tissues, areas of suspected hypo/hypermobility, neuromuscular coordination, and the willingness of the patient to perform the motion. This last item speaks to the patient's motivation and may, in some cases of severe apprehension, indicate the presence of tissue pathology and/or systemic disease. Under the special tests section of the cervical spine examination (S), the use of radiologic, neurologic, orthopaedic, and vascular proce-

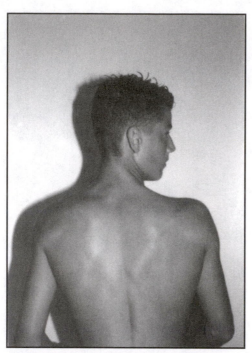

Figure 8-5d. Cervical rotation right.

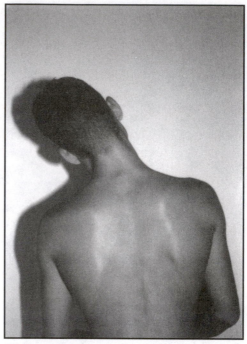

Figure 8-5e. Cervical side bending left.

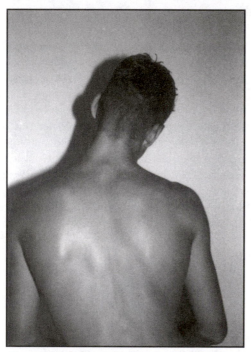

Figure 8-5f. Cervical side bending right.

dures will be discussed relative to the diagnosis of non-mechanical and systemic disease.

Repeated Movements Exam for Cervical Derangement (Phases 1 to 4)

During the interview process of the examination, indications of an intervertebral disc derangement become apparent. As discussed in Chapter 2, the hallmarks of a McKenzie derangement include the following:

1. Symptoms during movement as compared to a dysfunction that is at end-range.

2. Symptoms that may be constant and severe as compared to intermittent and mild to moderate.

3. Symptoms that start proximal, but with time become more distal (ie, below the elbow).

4. Symptoms that have neurologic features (ie, burning, tingling, shooting, sharp, piercing, etc).

5. The presence of an acute deformity (ie, torticollis or wryneck).

When the McKenzie cervical derangement syndrome is suspected, the therapist can then proceed to placing the patient in one of seven categories. An overview of these derangements is as follows:

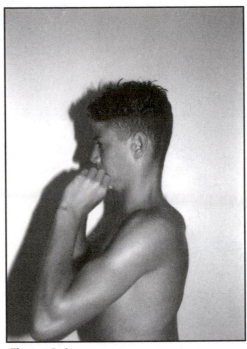

Figure 8-6a.

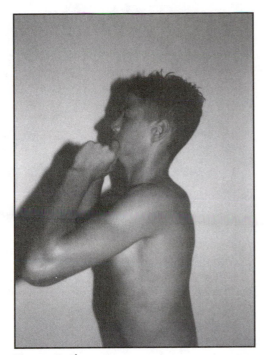

Figure 8-6b.

➠ Derangement one: Central or symmetrical pain across C5 to C7; rarely scapular or shoulder pain, no deformity.

➠ Derangement two: Central or symmetrical pain across C5 to C7 with or without scapular and/or shoulder pain. Deformity of flattened or flexed cervical spine.

➠ Derangement three: Unilateral or asymmetrical pain across C3 to C7 with or without scapular and/or shoulder pain. No deformity is present.

➠ Derangement four: Unilateral or asymmetrical pain across C5 to C7 with or without scapular and/or shoulder pain. With deformity of acute wryneck or torticollis.

➠ Derangement five: Unilateral or asymmetrical pain across C5 to C7 with or without scapular and/or shoulder pain. Arm pain extends below the elbow. No deformity.

➠ Derangement six: Unilateral or asymmetrical pain across C5 to C7 with or without scapular and/or shoulder pain. Arm pain extends below the elbow. Deformity of flattened or flexed cervical spine, acute wry neck, or torticollis.

➠ Derangement seven: Symmetrical or asymmetrical pain about C4 to C6 with pain occasionally referred to the anterior/anterolateral neck and throat. Obstruction of cervical flexion present.

According to Kramer,[4] 41% of cervical spine derangements are at C5,6 while 33% are at C6,7. The incidence of nerve root involvement is greatest at C6, followed by C7, C8, and C5 in decreasing order.

The purpose of the repeated movements examination is to determine the responsiveness of the derangement to mechanical therapy. Theoretically, a contained disc displacement, be it annular or nuclear, should respond to the correct mechanical intervention with the centralization phenomenon (ie, symptoms become more proximal and therefore less distal) with the eventual resolution of all signs and symptoms. On the contrary, a noncontained disc herniation, as occurs in disc rupture, would not be expected to respond favorably to mechanical therapy. As discussed under contraindications (see Chapter 3), patients with neurologic signs should not be treated, but referred to the physician for further consultation.

In the lower cervical spine, patients with derangements one through six are subjected to a series of mechanical phases, developed by the author, that begin with the simplest of procedures and progress to the more complex as needed. To achieve head-neck retraction, the index fingers and thumbs guide the motion; to prevent mandibular retrusion, the teeth are "lightly" clenched. Because derangement seven is rare, it will not be addressed in this introductory textbook.

Phase 1

a. Self-exam head-neck retraction. Upper cervical flexion/lower cervical extension (Figure 8-6a).

b. Self-exam head-neck retraction followed by head-neck extension (Figure 8-6b).

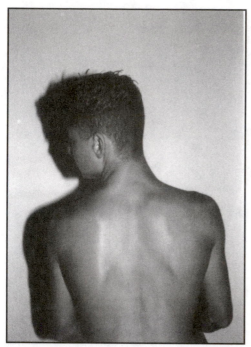

Figure 8-7a.

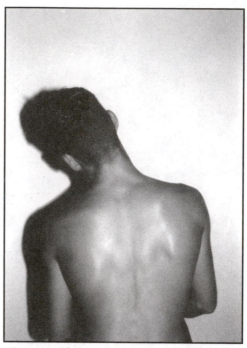

Figure 8-7b.

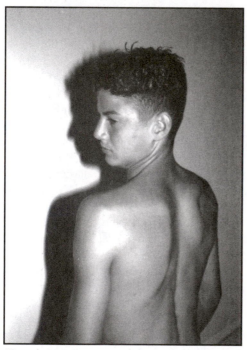

Figure 8-7c.

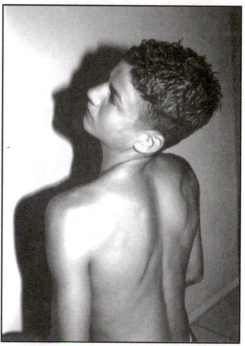

Figure 8-7d.

Phase 2

  a. Self-exam head-neck rotation (Figure 8-7a).

  b. Self-exam head-neck side bending (Figure 8-7b).

  c. Self-exam combined head-neck retraction, rotation, and side bending (Figure 8-7c).

  d. Self-exam combined head-neck retraction, extension, rotation, and side bending (Figure 8-7d).

Phase 3

  a. Self-exam head-neck retraction in supine (Figure 8-8a).

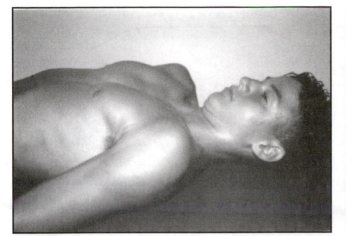

Figure 8-8a.

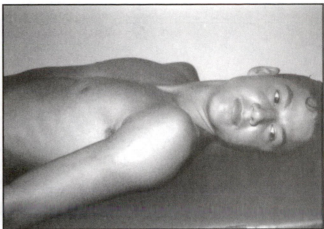

Figure 8-8b.

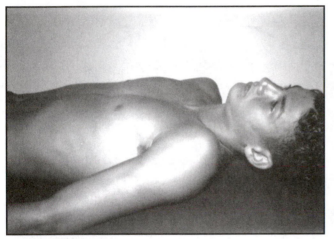

Figure 8-8c.

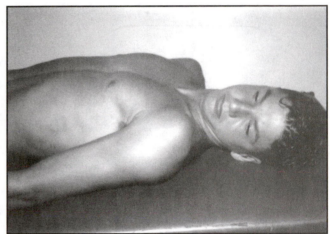

Figure 8-8d.

b. Self-exam head-neck rotation in supine (Figure 8-8b).

c. Self-exam head-neck side bending in supine (Figure 8-8c).

d. Self-exam combined head-neck retraction, rotation, and side bending (Figure 8-8d).

Phase 4

a. Therapist-assisted traction/retraction in sitting (Figure 8-9a).

b. Therapist-assisted traction/retraction in supine (Figure 8-9b).

c. Therapist-assisted traction/retraction/extension in supine (Figure 8-9c).

d. Therapist-assisted traction/retraction/extension/rotation in supine (Figure 8-9d).

Guidelines to follow when performing the repeated movements exam include the following:

1. Sagittal plane movements (retraction, extension) are attempted prior to lateral compartment movements (rotation, side bending).

2. Self-treatment is always attempted prior to therapist-assisted technique.

3. Sitting intervention is more functional than recumbent and should be attempted first.

4. After each set of 10 repetitions, the patient's symptoms are reassessed relative to the location and the intensity of the distal-most symptom. A 0 to 10 scale for rating intensity of the distal-most symptom is suggested. Any proximal migration of the distal-most symptom toward the cervical area (centralization) is considered a successful outcome and that motion(s) should be continued.

5. Progression to the next phase is suggested when the patient reaches a plateau.

6. If at any time the distal-most symptom is referred more distally (peripheralization), treatment should stop and the patient's intervention taken back to the previous phase if possible.

The repeated movements exam is used to accomplish the first goal of managing a derangement, which is to reduce it. The remaining three goals will be addressed in Chapter 11.

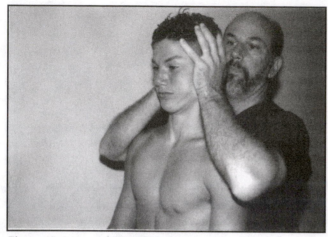

Figure 8-9a.

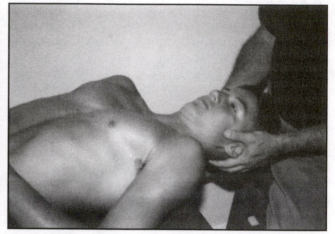

Figure 8-9b.

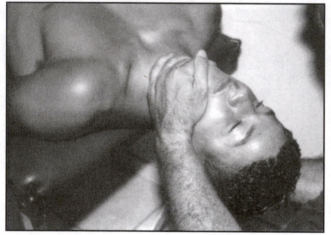

Figure 8-9c.

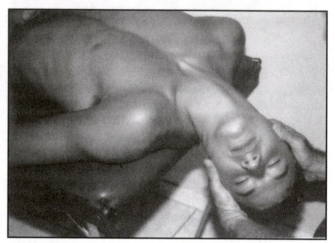

Figure 8-9d.

Apophyseal Joint
Opening/Closing (C2 to C7)

The following arthrokinematic examination of the apophyseal joints of the lower cervical spine was developed by Rocabado and is one of the most useful examination procedures available for the cervical spine. As mentioned in the preface, the arthrokinematic examination of the upper cervical spine is more suitable for advanced coursework and will not be covered at this time.

In Chapter 1, apophyseal joint kinematics, including facet opening and closing, were reviewed. The unilateral evaluation of cervical apophyseal joint motion is unlike any of the other spinal mobility tests in that the lower cervical region is the only area where the apophyseal or facet joints of the spine can be directly palpated. There are some guidelines that will hopefully elucidate the key aspects of this useful examination tool. The technique will be described for the patient's right side. The therapist stands on the right

side of the sitting patient; the therapist's left hand lightly palpates the C2,3 facets with the thumb and the distal phalanx of the middle finger over the right and left facets, respectively (the C2,3 facets are convex structures at the level of the spinous process of C2, between the sternocleidomastoid muscle, anteriorly, and the posterior cervical muscles, posteriorly). The therapist controls head-neck motion with the right hand over the cranial vertex. The key to the effectiveness of this procedure is proper localization to the appropriate joint level. For the assessment of C2,3 motion on the right, the head-neck region is rotated to the right until motion "arrives" at the left thumb. At this point, the therapist "rocks" the head-neck into combined extension/right side bending for the evaluation of facet "closing" (Figure 8-10a), then proceeds to "rock" the head-neck into combined flexion/left side bending for the evaluation of opening (Figure 8-10b). The patient's ears provide a useful landmark for establishing the direction of the forward and backward rocking motion (ie, the closing motion is in line with the right ear, while the opening motion is in

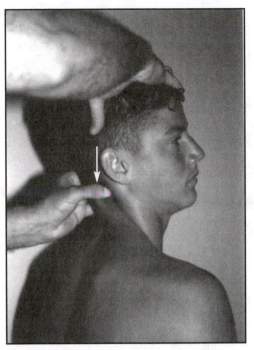

Figure 8-10a.

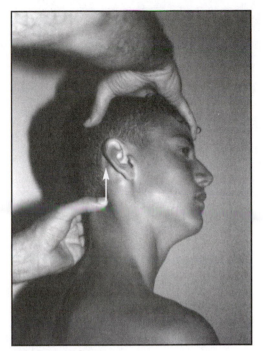

Figure 8-10b.

line with the left). This diagonal motion, induced with the right hand, is combined with translation of C3, with the left hand, in the opposite direction to achieve a "roll-glide" motion of the segment. Facet closing of C2,3 on the right is associated with translation of C3 to the left; opening with translation of C3 to the right. The information attained from this technique, as with other joint mobility tests, consists of the quantity and quality of motion and the end-feel.

To assess the remainder of the lower cervical spine, the head-neck is rotated down to each level and the process is repeated. To assess the left side, the patient's head-neck are rotated to the left and all contacts are reversed.

In the lower cervical spine, FRS and ERS impairments are common. There are no type 1 impairments from C2 to C7 because there is only type 2 mechanics. Applying the Rocabado sitting technique to our understanding of type 2 impairments, it can be said that a closing restriction represents an FRS impairment, whereas an opening restriction represents an ERS impairment. For example, the C4,5 segment is considered an FRS left when the right apophyseal joint is limited in closing on the right. Limitation in arthrokinematic closing on the right is associated with limitation in osteokinematic extension, rotation, and side bending to the right. If C4 cannot freely extend, rotate, and side bend to the right, then it must be FRS left (the cause of cervical spine closing restriction is controversial with such possibilities as apophyseal joint irregularity, disc derangement, and meniscoid entrapment). Conversely, limited opening of the right C2,3 facet results in impairment of combined flexion, rotation and side bending left of C2 on C3. Consequently, its position is opposite its restriction and is considered ERS right.

Ellis taught the FOES acronym for remembering the side of involvement in type 2 lesions. FOES stands for flexion opposite extension same. Consequently, the involved joint is on the opposite side with an FRS impairment, and the involved joint is on the same side with an ERS impairment.

The above sections on active cervical movements, repeated movements, and apophyseal joint kinematics are under the range of motion (R) category of the CHARTS examination. We will now proceed to tissue texture abnormality (T).

Soft Tissue Palpation

A review of cervical spine landmarks will prove helpful prior to the examination of relevant soft tissue structures in the head and neck region.

1. External occipital protuberance. Bony prominence on the occiput at the level of the superior nuchal line.

2. Inferior nuchal line. The inferior aspect of the occipital ridge.

3. Mastoid process. Bony temporal bone prominence behind the ear.

4. External jugular tubercle. Bony prominence on either side of the occiput just below the inferior nuchal line.

5. Spinous process of C2. The first palpable spinous process in the cervical spine (the posterior arch of atlas is not easily palpable).

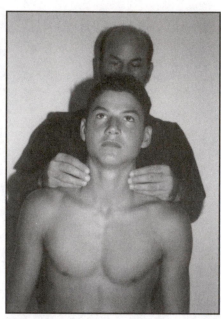

Figure 8-11.

6. Spinous process of C6. The next easily palpable spinous process in the cervical spine (the spinous processes of C3, C4, and C5 are small); upon extension of the head-neck, the spinous process of C6 translates forward.

7. Spinous process of C7 (vertebra prominens). The largest of the cervical spinous processes, which does not translate forward upon head-neck extension.

8. Transverse process of C1 (atlas). Midway between the angle of the mandible and the mastoid process.

9. Hyoid bone. Superior to the thyroid cartilage ("Adam's apple") in the anterior neck region.

The soft tissue examination of the cervical region inspects myofascial, articular, and neural structures for tissue texture abnormality. The presence of tenderness, tightness, and tone is recorded.

Anterior cervical palpation (Figure 8-11) includes the following structures:

1. Hyoid bone. Assess motion side to side.

2. Supra/infrahyoid muscles.

3. Sternocleidomastoid muscles from the mastoid process to both the sternal and clavicular attachments.

4. Scaleni muscles (anterior, middle, posterior). Palpated at the lateral edge of the midbelly of the sternocleidomastoid muscle. Contralateral side bending of the head-neck tightens the ipsilateral scaleni, making them easier to palpate.

5. Inferior clavicular region. Assessing attachment of the pectoralis major and fascia, clavipectoral fascia, superficial layer of the cervical fascia, subclavius muscle, and the coracoclavicular ligament (conoid and trapezoid ligaments).

6. Pectoralis minor tendon. The coracoid process is palpated in the deltopectoral groove and the pectoralis minor tendon is accessed inferior to the coracoid. A deep inhalation will tauten the tendon, making it easier to palpate.

Posterior cervical palpation includes the following structures:

1. Upper trapezius muscle. The therapist inspects for taut bands and myofascial trigger points.

2. Levator scapulae muscle. Palpated from the vertebral border of the scapula between the superior angle and root of the scapular spine, to the upper four vertebrae of the cervical spine.

3. Posterior cervical muscles (splenius capitis/cervicis, semispinalis capitis/cervicis, longissimus capitis/cervicis, multifidi, and rotators). No attempt is made to distinguish one individual muscle from another. Palpation proceeds from caudal to cranial.

4. Suboccipital muscles (rectus capitis posterior major/minor, inferior/superior oblique). Slight passive extension of the occiput relaxes the superficial muscles, allowing access into the deeper suboccipital region. No attempt is made at this point to identify the individual muscles.

5. Greater occipital nerve. There are four potential sites of impingement:

   a. In the upper trapezius

   b. In the semispinalis capitis

   c. Under the inferior oblique

   d. Between the occiput and posterior arch of C1 when the occipitoatlantal space is less than 4 mm[1]

The optimal site for testing irritability of the greater occipital nerve is where it becomes subcutaneous, approximately 2 to 3 cm inferior and lateral to the greater occipital protuberance. The forehead is stabilized with one hand; with the thumb or middle finger of the other hand, the nerve is compressed for approximately 10 seconds (Figure 8-12). Both sides are tested for irritability. A positive test consists of nerve-type discomfort (eg, burning, paresthesia, sharp pain) in the distribution of the nerve or over the ipsilateral eye where it has an anastomosis with the supraorbital branch of the ophthalmic division of the trigeminal nerve. A positive response is suggestive of a greater occipital neuralgia, which can be mistakenly diagnosed as migraine.

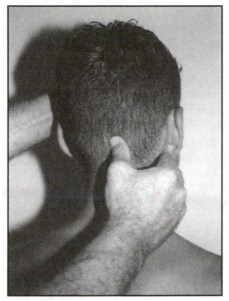

Figure 8-12.

Special Tests

For the sake of clarity, this section will be organized as follows:

1. Neurologic
   a. Myotomes (C1 to T1)
   b. Dermatomes (C2 to T2)
   c. Deep tendon reflexes (biceps, triceps, brachioradialis)
   d. Neurodynamic testing (upper limb neurodynamic tests 1, 2A, 2B, and 3)
   e. Upper motor neuron lesion (Babinski's sign)
   f. Valsalva's test (reveals space-occupying lesions in the cervical canal)
   g. Myelopathy hand
2. Orthopaedic
   a. Spurling's test (maximal cervical compression)
   b. Distraction test (relieves nerve root compression)
   c. Cervical rotation lateral flexion (CRLF) test for a superiorly subluxed first rib
   d. Functional assessment (ie, the Neck Disability Index)
   e. Fitz-Ritson test for cervicogenic dizziness (see Figures 12-3a and 12-3b)
   f. Nine-point Brighton scale for generalized hypermobility

3. Vascular
   a. Vertebrobasilar insufficiency (5 Ds method)
   b. Roos test for thoracic inlet (outlet) syndrome
4. Physician-based
   a. Radiologic (cervical x-ray series with mobility films, magnetic resonance imaging [MRI], computerized tomography [CAT] scan, myelogram, etc)
   b. Electrodiagnosis (electromyography [EMG], conduction velocity, etc)
   c. Lab work (complete blood cell count [CBC], erythrocyte sedimentation rate [ESR], rheumatoid factors, HLA-B27 antigen, Lyme test, Epstein-Barr virus, antinuclear antibodies, etc)
   d. Tissue biopsy
   e. Sleep studies (sleep apnea, fibromyalgia/chronic fatigue, etc)
   f. Psychiatric/psychological evaluation

The reader is referred to other textbooks listed in the bibliography (ie, Konin et al, Magee, and Gross et al) for a complete review of these tests and their clinical significance. The author would, however, like to comment on two of the above items. The subject of vertebral artery testing is a controversial one. It has never been the author's practice to teach techniques in an introductory level course that provoke transient ischemia to the brainstem and other structures of the posterior cranial fossa. When analyzing the risk-to-benefit ratio, there is not enough benefit to justify the risk. However, in advanced courses the risk is justified by the benefit. Consequently, at the basic level the 5 Ds approach of Coman[5] will suffice. Any patient who presents with undiagnosed dizziness, diplopia, drop attacks, dysarthria, or dysphagia should be seen by a neurologist to rule out vertebrobasilar insufficiency (VBI). Other symptoms of VBI may include nausea, blurred vision, lightheadedness, and perioral dysesthesia.[6] The relationship between VBI and the cervical spine is such that blood flow in the vertebral artery is reduced physiologically at the level of C1 when the head-neck region is rotated or rotated and extended to the contralateral side. This response is time-dependent; therefore, patients should not be placed in these positions for extended periods of time. In those patients diagnosed with VBI or in the elderly, the extremes of these positions should be avoided entirely. In patients with diagnosed benign paroxysmal positional vertigo (BPPV), therapy may include working through these positions that provoke dizziness,[7] but this should not be attempted without medical clearance.

Regarding the potential risks of cervical manipulation (eg, vertebral artery injury, tissue disruption), the tech-

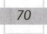

niques presented in this book do not involve high velocity thrust nor the excessive use of force; if the contraindications to manual therapy (discussed in Chapter 3) are respected, the patient is at no time placed at risk for serious injury.

The second item that warrants discussion, relative to special tests, is the need to identify clinical instability when it exists. As a general rule, vertebral horizontal translation of greater than 3.5 mm on a flexion or extension x-ray and/or angular vertebral rotation of more than 11 degrees indicates the presence of lower cervical segmental instability.[8,9] In the upper cervical spine, patients with rheumatoid arthritis, ankylosing spondylitis, Down's syndrome, and a history of macrotrauma must have the atlantodental interval (ADI) assessed with lateral radiographs, including a flexion view, for signs of hypermobility/instability. In a typical adult, the ADI should be no greater than 3 mm. Patients are typically placed in hard collars with an ADI of more than 4 mm and considered a candidate for spinal fusion when greater than 7 mm.

Adverse Effects of Forward Head Posture

In ideal human anatomy, the head is anteriorly positioned with respect to the vertebral column. The term *forward head* implies excessive displacement of the head relative to the spine whereby the presence of abnormal muscle tensions may develop. Rocabado[8] uses the term *tripodism* to describe the normal balance that exists in the lower cervical spine (ie, C2 to C7) when vertebral function takes place at the posterior third of the intervertebral disc and the two apophyseal joints are parallel. In this balanced state, each member of the "tripod" (ie, the intervertebral disc anteriorly and the two facet joints posteriorly) bears equal weight. With forward head posture (FHP), tripodism is lost as the upper cervical spine at the occipitoatlantal junction extends (ie, "backward head") and the lower cervical spine and cervicothoracic junction flex (ie, "forward neck"). Consequently, the lower cervical tripod shifts forward onto its anterior aspect and away from the apophyseal joints. The adverse effects of this shift include suboccipital compression; lower cervical hypermobility, especially from C3 to C6 due to slackening of the nuchal ligament; off-center loading on the nucleus pulposus; elevation of the first two ribs from increased scaleni tension; and posterior/superior

displacement of the mandible, which will be addressed in a subsequent chapter on the temporomandibular joint. With these pathophysiologic changes in alignment and function comes the possibility of developing cervicogenic headache, midcervical instability (leading to osteoarthrosis and spinal stenosis), cervical disc derangement, thoracic inlet (outlet) syndrome, and temporomandibular disorder.

In addition to the loss of physiologic tripodism, forward displacement of the head increases the torque on the cervical spine. For example, given that the average head weighs 10 pounds, the torque on the cervical spine will increase by a factor of 10 for every inch of forward displacement (ie, torque = force x distance). Consequently, a forward head of 3 inches results in the equivalent of 30 in. lbs. of torque, whereas a 5-in. anterior displacement of the head results in 50 in. lbs. of torque on the neck in the direction of flexion. This nonphysiologic posture, in turn, places excessive demands on the cervical erector spinae muscles, which must produce an equivalent counter-torque for postural support.[10]

Related to the global effects of FHP on the body, Alexander believed that the tensing of muscles in the neck (suboccipital/cervical extensors) results in the tensing of muscles of the whole body.[11] A simple experiment shows the veracity of this concept. In the forward head position, the extensors of the head-neck and spine can be felt to contract as far down as the lumbosacral junction. This appears to be a stabilizing response to gravity as the head-neck region is displaced forward. In addition, the larynx is pulled up and forward, the scapulae protracts, the anterior chest wall depresses, and the shoulders and ribs lose mobility. More indirect effects of FHP include hip internal rotation and rearfoot pronation of both feet.

Clinically, patients with FHP are at greater risk of developing swallowing impairment, impingement of the glenohumeral joints, reduced costal cage expansion during inhalation, and lower extremity problems related to hyperpronation (eg, ankle sprains, shin splints, patellofemoral pain).

Obviously, there is a large segment of the population that never experiences the untoward consequences of FHP as outlined above. However, as their adaptive potential is compromised as a result of aging, disease, emotional stress, cumulative microtrauma, and frank injury, the likelihood of developing these ailments becomes greater. Much of what is done to improve health and ameliorate suffering in this book is based upon the balance of head, neck, and spinal alignment and the reduction, if not the elimination, of FHP!

Connective Tissue Techniques and Stretching Procedures for the Cervical Spine

Lateral Neck Fascial Technique

This direct fascial technique (Figure 9-1) is useful for treating the levator scapulae, upper trapezius, and posterior cervical muscles. The patient's occiput is placed on a head block or towel roll to create space under the cervical concavity. The examiner stabilizes the patient's head-neck region by placing one hand on the patient's forehead, while the other hand "rakes" through the soft tissues in a cross-fiber direction. A small amount of Deep Prep II (Smith & Nephew, Germantown, Wisc) or similar soft tissue massage cream is useful.

The therapist begins in the upper thoracic region and progresses cephalward into the upper neck area. An oscillatory motion can be added for additional soft tissue relaxation.

Deep Neck Fascial Technique

This direct fascial technique (Figure 9-2) is directed toward the deeper spinal muscles in the medial groove of longissimus. With the patient's occiput resting on the therapist's anterior forearms, the flexed PIP joints of both hands once again "rake" through the soft tissues from the upper thoracic region to the craniovertebral region. Upon encountering increased tone or tightness, the therapist maintains a superiorly directed force with the addition of oscillatory motion until the tension and/or tightness has abated. At the end of the caudal to cranial "sweep," the therapist imparts a gentle traction force on the occiput to stretch the posterior occipitoatlantal space. Several cycles can be applied as tolerated. This technique is excellent preparation for inhibitive occipital distraction, which is to follow.

Inhibitive Occipital Distraction

This procedure (Figure 9-3) is a combination of direct fascial technique and manual traction. The first phase involves the use of digital compression for the purpose of inhibiting tone in the occipital extensors. The therapist supports the patient's occiput in his or her palms with the second through fifth digits making contact with the skull over the inferior nuchal line. The patient is asked to relax, breathe "in through the nose and out the mouth," and imagine a quiet and tranquil scene that will enhance overall relaxation. As the subcranial soft tissues soften, the therapist is ready to progress the patient to the second phase. Now that the tissues have "let go" of their contraction, the occiput is distracted away from C1 by pulling it along the table in a cephalward direction toward the therapist. In addition to a longitudinal elongation of the subcranial muscles, the therapist is encouraged to manually stretch these soft tissues in a lateral direction as well. This separation of the occiput from the atlas creates more space at the occipitoatlantal junction, posteriorly, and essentially decompresses the region, including the greater occipital nerve. This sequence of neuromuscular inhibition followed by occipital distraction is repeated several times until the tissue slack has been removed.

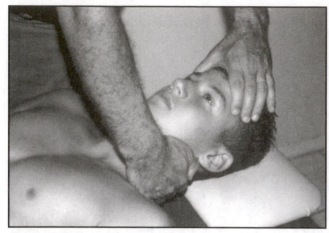

Figure 9-1.

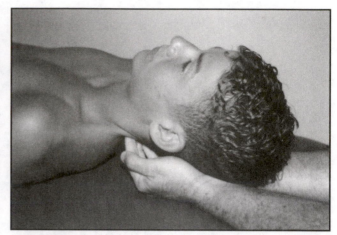

Figure 9-2.

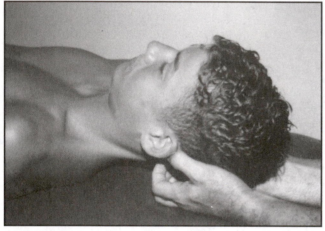

Figure 9-3.

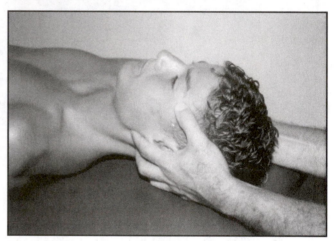

Figure 9-4.

Osteopathic practitioners describe a related technique known as condylar decompression.[12] In addition to the inhibitive distraction described above, they incorporate a lateral release of the area. This "lateral release" is achieved as the manual therapist increases bilateral forearm, wrist, and hand supination and brings both elbows together. The digital pressure is maintained until a release of tension is felt, especially the sensation of softening on each side of the occipital bone.

At this point, the patient is progressed to the third phase of the technique in which the occiput is lifted off the therapist's palms and supported solely on the distal finger pads of all the extended digits save the thumbs. This increase in pressure achieves further inhibition and allows additional separation of the occiput away from the atlas for maximal patient benefit. Progression to the third phase may not be possible in those individuals who find the increase in pressure uncomfortable (ie, pain, headache, and dizziness may result). Compression of the vertebral artery is avoided by maintaining pressure over the inferior nuchal line rather than between the occiput and atlas.

The author has modified the Paris technique of "Inhibitive Distraction" to arrive at its present form.[13]

Manual Traction/Functional Technique

The advantages of manual over mechanical traction include localization, feedback, specificity, and patient comfort. Some of the physiologic effects of traction include decompression of articular, neurologic, and vascular structures; soft tissue stretching; and mechanoreceptor stimulation for the relief of pain and reduction of muscle tone. It has been the author's experience that 5 minutes of effective manual traction is far superior to 20 minutes of mechanical traction.

To enhance the effectiveness of manual traction (Figure 9-4), the author has combined it with an osteopathic functional technique known as balance and hold. The purpose of this "indirect" maneuver[14] is to reduce neuromuscular tone to a minimum prior to the application of traction.

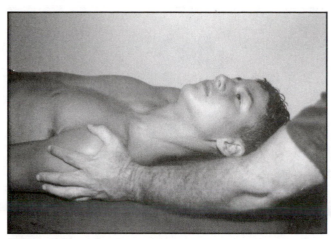

Figure 9-5.

This "preparation" phase will enhance the efficacy of traction in that the muscular resistance to traction is minimized. This is a major problem with mechanical traction, as a "tug of war" struggle between muscle tone and traction leaves the patient caught in the middle.

The therapist's fingers monitor head-neck muscle tone with the fifth fingers on the suboccipitals, the fourth fingers on the posterior cervicals, the third fingers on the scaleni, the second fingers on the sternocleidomastoids, and the thumbs on the temporalis muscles. At this point the therapist seeks "ease" in head-neck side bending, rotation, and flexion-extension. When "ease" is found in one plane (eg, side-bending right or left), the other motions are "stacked" one on the other in a final position of maximal tissue ease. This "preferred tissue pattern" represents the neuromuscular rest position of the head-neck region and is the optimal starting position for manual traction. For one patient, this position may consist of 5 degrees side bending right, 10 degrees rotation left, and 5 degrees extension. For another, this position may be 3 degrees side bending right, 6 degrees rotation right, and 5 degrees extension. There are as many neuromuscular rest positions as there are patients to assess and treat. It is this "tuning in" process that makes functional technique so interesting and effective.

The actual traction is performed along the adjusted vertical axis of the head-neck region in a cephalward direction. The therapist has a choice of grade 1 (ie, support of the head and neck), grade 2 (ie, to the end of the tissue slack), and grade 3 (ie, beyond the slack to patient tolerance). Between 5 to 10 repetitions of the appropriate grade should be applied in a "ramping" manner in both directions. The actual traction should be held for approximately 10 seconds.

At this point in the process, the "balance and hold" technique is repeated. As nociception and muscle splinting are reduced, the "adjusted vertical axis" and the true vertical axis of the head-neck approach each other. The therapist must, however, apply manual traction in "functional

neutral" and not force the head-neck region into "anatomic neutral." The therapist must also be careful not to squeeze the head too tight, especially during the more rigorous grade 3 traction.

The next five sections address specific stretches of the main muscle groups of the head-neck region. Each stretch will incorporate the postisometric relaxation concept (osteopathic muscle energy) for enhanced treatment efficacy. When performing these procedures, therapists need to be careful not to inflame a healed cervical disc derangement or create one through the use of excessive force. If at any time patients report a peripheralization of their symptoms, the stretch should be immediately stopped. All stretching techniques will be performed in the supine position.

Upper Trapezius Stretch

The author recommends the use of contralateral side bending to stretch the fibers of the upper trapezius muscle. A stretch (Figure 9-5) will be described for the left side. The patient's left shoulder is depressed until the slack is removed, at which time the head-neck region is passively right side bent to the restrictive barrier with the therapist's right hand. The patient is then given the command, "Don't let me move your left shoulder down." Following a submaximal, isometric contraction of the left upper trapezius of 6 seconds duration, the left shoulder is depressed further (ie, the slack is taken up). It is important to wait a few seconds before moving into the new range as this allows for maximal postfacilitation inhibition of the muscle. The contraction-relaxation cycle is repeated three times. To stretch the right upper trapezius muscle, all contacts and instructions are reversed accordingly. To avoid "technique-related" injury, the patient is never stretched to the point of pain; peripheral symptoms should not be permitted, especially on the stretched side; and the head-neck region is always returned slowly to the midline.

Scaleni Stretch

Kinesiologically, the anterior, middle, and posterior scalene muscles have been treated, for the most part, as one combined system.[15] However, Evjenth[16] functionally separates the anterior and middle from the posterior scalene muscle. He ascribes the movements of flexion, ipsilateral side bending, and contralateral rotation to the anterior and middle scalenes and extension, ipsilateral side bending, and ipsilateral rotation to the posterior scalene. Consequently, two different stretches will be performed—one for the anterior and middle and one for the posterior scalene.

The anterior and middle scalenes, together, affect all levels of the lower cervical spine (ie, C2 to C7). The opti-

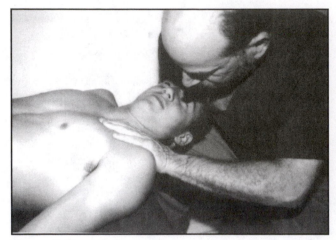

Figure 9-6a.

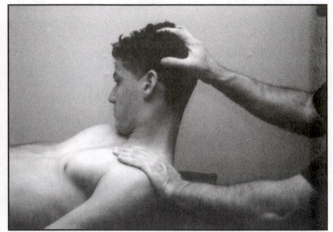

Figure 9-6b.

mal stretch of these two muscles is achieved with the head-neck region off the end of the table. To stretch the left side, the motions of head-neck retraction, right side bending, and left rotation are combined. The left first rib is held in depression by the patient grasping the left side of the table and the therapist stabilizing the first rib with his or her left hand. The patient is asked to resist passive side bending to the right; following the postisometric relaxation, the head-neck is repositioned in further right side bending. The greater the head-neck retraction off the end of the table, the more effective is the stretch. For additional effectiveness, the stretch should be coordinated with the exhalation phase of breathing (Figure 9-6a).

The posterior scalene affects the lower three levels of the cervical spine (C5, C6, and C7). To stretch the left side, the head-neck is flexed, right side bent, and right rotated as the patient's left hand grasps the table and the first two ribs are stabilized with the therapist's left hand. The therapist's command to the patient is, "Don't let me move you" as the therapist attempts to move further into this combined position. As the patient's extensors, left side benders, and left rotators relax, the head-neck is taken further into the range of motion. This stretch can also be coordinated with exhalation for enhanced effectiveness (Figure 9-6b).

Regarding the integration of different treatment approaches, hypertonicity and/or tightness of the anterior and middle scalenes are associated with both posterolateral cervical disc derangements and FRS impairment. Conversely, posterior scalene hypertonicity and/or tightness can be found with ERS impairments in the neck, specifically at C5,6 and C6,7 and occasionally at C7,T1. With ERS impairments, the side of the restricted facet joint correlates well with ipsilateral posterior scalene dysfunction. However, the relationship between FRS impairment, disc derangement, and anterior/middle scalene dysfunction is not as straight forward. It appears that anterior scalene tightness on the right results in an FRS left impairment at C2 through C5 and not FRS right as might be expected. The explanation relates to the anterior scalene's limiting affect on translation of the inferior vertebrae to the opposite side. The middle scalene has the same influence including the C6,7 motion segment. Regarding the influence of the scalenes on the first and second ribs, hypertonicity of the anterior scalene is thought to cause first rib superior subluxation, whereas posterior scalene hypertonicity is thought to contribute to a superiorly laterally flexed second rib.

Sternocleidomastoid Stretch

The unilateral sternocleidomastoid (SCM) stretch is similar to the anterior/middle scalene stretch. The difference is the occipital flexion component, which was unnecessary for the scaleni because they have no occipital attachment. To stretch the right SCM, the therapist places his or her right hand on the patient's forehead, while the left hand grasps the occiput. To stabilize the distal attachments, the patient's right hand holds the side of the table. The first phase of the stretch involves combined head-neck retraction, left side bending, and right rotation. The second phase incorporates occipital flexion, which is accomplished by a simultaneous "push" of the right hand and "pull" of the left hand (Figure 9-7). Care must be taken not to flex the lower cervical spine, as this will undermine the stretch.

The isometric component is directed toward occipital extension. This is accomplished by having the patient look up and back with his or her eyes. Following the 6 second contraction, the occiput is passively flexed. This cycle is repeated three times. If the technique is effective, the patient should feel a stretch at the right mastoid process. Because techniques involving a chin tuck may encroach upon the pharyngeal airway, patients need to indicate any respiratory distress immediately.

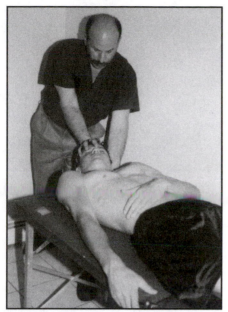

Figure 9-7.

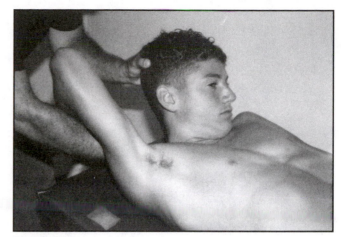

Figure 9-8.

Levator Scapulae Stretch

Tightness of the levator scapulae muscle adversely affects the scapulae, cervical spine, and shoulder complex. It, like the posterior scalene, can cause ERS dysfunction in the cervical spine, albeit at higher levels (ie, C2, C3, and C4) and can cause fixation of the atlas, resulting in headache and dizziness. In the shoulder complex, tightness of the levator scapulae will contribute to downward rotation of the scapula. If upward rotation of the scapula becomes impaired, subacromial impingement may occur due to poor clearance of these tissues under the coracoacromial arch. Consequently, normal length of the levator is "key" to normal upper quarter physiology.[17]

There are different options for stretching this muscle, but the author's preferred method is to incorporate scapular upward rotation and depression from below and combined head-neck flexion and contralateral rotation/side bending from above. Because pushing is preferable to pulling, this technique (Figure 9-8) involves guiding the head from below such that the head-neck region is pushed toward the contralateral side (nose to opposite hip). This follows the initial set-up in which the upper limb on the stretched side is elevated with the hand grasping the top of the table. To ensure scapular upward rotation and depression, the therapist holds the superior angle down with the radial aspect of the first MCP contact (lateral "knife-edge"). If possible, the therapist should attempt to add posterior scapular tilt to depression/upward rotation with the first MCP contact (anterior and posterior tilting of the scapula were discussed in Chapters 4 and 5). The head-neck region is then flexed

to the contralateral side to the motion barrier. The patient is then asked to resist further motion for a count of 6 seconds followed by movement of the head-neck region to the new barrier while the scapula is prevented from elevating and downwardly rotating. Of all the neck stretches, the levator stretch has the most potential to cause disc injury secondary to lower cervical flexion with contralateral rotation. Consequently, the patient must be monitored continuously for radicular symptoms. As usual, the cervical spine must be returned to neutral slowly to avoid facet joint compression.

Occipital Extensor Stretch

The restoration of Alexander's primary control (ie, optimal and tension-free alignment of the head, neck, and upper back) is dependent on restoring normal length to the occipital extensors. Prior to restoring length to these muscles, the requisite myofascial extensibility, covered previously, should be attained.

The therapist uses a force-couple contact (as explained with the SCM stretch) with one hand under the occiput and the other hand placed on the forehead with the fingers directed caudally. The motion is that of occipital flexion, with the lower cervical spine in a neutral position on the table. The isometric contraction of the occipital extensors is achieved with the patient's eyes looking up and back against therapist resistance for 6 seconds.

The technique (Figure 9-9) is complete after three hold-relax-stretch cycles. As with the SCM stretch, the patient's pharyngeal airway must not be unduly compressed. A useful option to the bilateral stretch is to bias the force to the more restricted side. Some therapists use this unilateral technique as a form of occipitoatlantal flexion mobilization. When used as either a bilateral or unilateral flexion mobilization, both hands participate simultaneously.

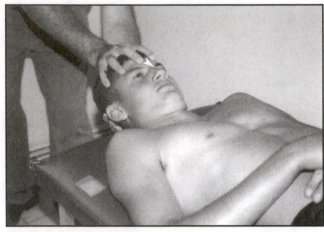

Figure 9-9.

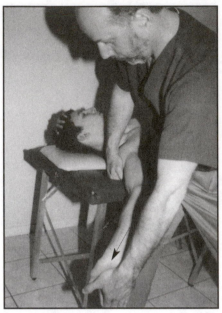

Figure 9-10a.

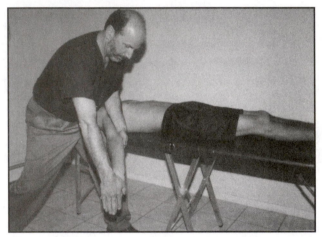

Figure 9-10b.

Neural Mobilization (Median, Radial, and Ulnar Nerves)

The upper limb neurodynamic tests (ULNT) 1, 2A, 2B, and 3 were mentioned under special tests but were not described or illustrated. Consequently, this section will provide information related to both the examination and intervention of adverse neural tension in the brachial plexus. Consistent with the philosophy of this textbook, this presentation will be streamlined to provide only the essentials on the topic.

Neurodynamic testing/intervention of the upper limb is recommended for patients presenting with nonirritable conditions of the head, neck, thoracic spine, and upper extremities.[18,19] It consists of various positions designed to put stress on neural structures, but in so doing other extra-neural soft tissue structures are stressed as well. Contraindications include irritable conditions, inflammation, spinal cord signs, malignancy, nerve root compression, peripheral neuropathy, and complex regional pain syndrome (ie, reflex sympathetic dystrophy).

Median Nerve

Two positions for the right median nerve will be described and illustrated, one in which shoulder elevation is blocked (ie, ULNT 1) and the other (ULNT 2A) in which shoulder girdle depression is utilized. In the ULNT 1 (Figure 9-10a), the supine patient's right upper limb is positioned sequentially as follows: shoulder abduction of 110 degrees with restraint on shoulder girdle elevation, elbow extension, shoulder external rotation/forearm supination, wrist extension, and finger/thumb extension. Contralateral cervical side bending can be added if additional tension is needed.

The production of symptoms alone is not noteworthy (eg, deep ache, tingling, stretch), but rather the reproduction of the patient's symptoms. The earlier in the sequence the symptoms occur, the greater the likelihood of neural impairment. The intervention has been described as a "flossing" motion in which the affected nerve(s) are stretched in a gentle "on/off" manner without sustained stretching for approximately 1 minute.

The ULNT 2A again stresses the median nerve, but this time shoulder girdle depression is included (Figure 9-10b). The supine patient is positioned diagonally such that the right shoulder is at the edge of the table with the feet pointed to the left. The movement sequence of the right upper limb is as follows: left shoulder girdle depression in slight abduction, elbow extension, forearm supination, wrist extension, and finger/thumb extension. Contralateral cervical side bending can be added as above, if necessary. In the presence of neural impairment, the "flossing" maneuver is again utilized for approximately 1 minute.

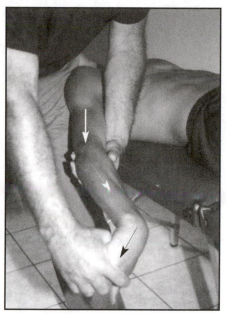

Figure 9-11.

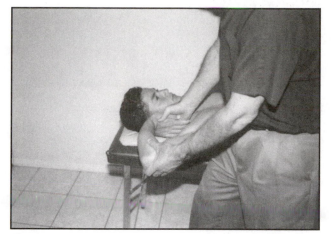

Figure 9-12.

Radial Nerve

To perform a test/intervention of the right radial nerve a supine patient is positioned as above for the ULNT 2A. The therapist incorporates the following movements in sequential order: shoulder girdle depression, elbow extension, shoulder internal rotation/forearm pronation, wrist flexion, ulnar deviation, and thumb flexion. As above, it is the reproduction of the patient's symptoms that is significant. "Flossing" of the radial nerve is the recommended intervention if impairment is noted. This maneuver is referred to as the ULNT 2B (Figure 9-11).

Ulnar Nerve

This maneuver is known as the ULNT 3. The patient is positioned in supine without being placed diagonally. For the right upper limb, the movement sequence is as follows:

wrist extension, forearm pronation, elbow flexion, shoulder external rotation/abduction, and shoulder girdle depression. As above, a neural "on/off" gliding motion is performed as necessary for approximately 1 minute (Figure 9-12).

As mentioned previously, contralateral head-neck side bending can be used to enhance all the above gliding movements for both examination and intervention purposes. Regarding neural mobilization, the therapist is advised to perform the "floss" within the symptom-free range of the nerve and to gauge the number of sets and repetitions to the nerve's reactivity. Overstretching a muscle may cause temporary discomfort, but overstretching a nerve is not a good idea!

The therapist must also keep in mind that peripheral nerves traverse tunnels, spaces, myofascial tissues, etc. Consequently, connective tissue techniques are usually necessary in conjunction with neural mobilization in order to achieve the desired restoration of normal mobility in the nervous system.

Cervical Spine Manipulation

As previously mentioned, manipulation of the cervical spine will not include the occipitoatlantal and atlantoaxial joints. The examination and treatment of the upper cervical spine is usually taught to students and therapists who have completed coursework in basic spinal manual therapy. The reasons for this are many and include the complexity of craniovertebral kinematics, the influence of craniovertebral motion on vertebrobasilar circulation, the risk of treating undiagnosed upper cervical instability, and the relationship between the high cervical segments and the upper cervical spinal cord. However, the author is confident that the interventions covered in this textbook will enable the treating therapist to successfully manage the majority of cases seen without incurring the risk of the advanced upper cervical procedures.

Apophyseal Joint Closing Restriction (Flexed, Rotated, and Side Bent Impairment)

The restriction of apophyseal joint closing from C2 through C7 is managed similarly to the examination technique described in Chapter 8. However, the intervention, unlike the examination, involves the use of postisometric relaxation (ie, muscle energy technique) as well as graded mobilization against the restrictive motion barrier. The

manual traction/functional technique, described in the previous chapter, is an effective means of preparing the facet joints for FRS correction (it must be kept in mind that the "closing" of a spinal facet joint must be performed carefully because of the associated compression and with minimal force lest symptoms become exacerbated).

For the successful management of a C2,3 FRS left, the therapist localizes the combined motions of extension, rotation, and side bending to the right to the "feather edge" of the restrictive barrier (Figures 10-1a and 10-1b). The command given to the patient is, "Don't let me move you," as the therapist attempts to move the head-neck down and to the right (ie, the patient attempts to move the left ear to the left axilla but is prevented from doing so). This 6-second isometric contraction is followed by a relocalization against the closing barrier of C2,3 and repeated for a total of three cycles. Following the "muscle energy technique," graded mobilization for 30 to 60 seconds is performed. It is important to move the joint surfaces over the previously underutilized portion of the range of motion. The preferred mobilization involves a "roll-glide" in which C2 is rolled over C3 in a diagonal plane to the right, as C3 is translated under C2 diagonally to the left. In addition, it is always helpful to follow passive manipulations with an active movement in the same direction for the purpose of integrating the additional range into the sensorimotor learning process. This, however, must be done slowly and under therapist supervision.

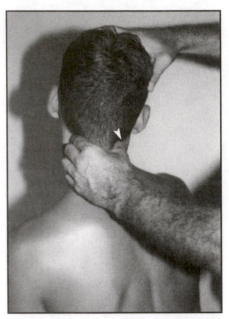

Figure 10-1a.

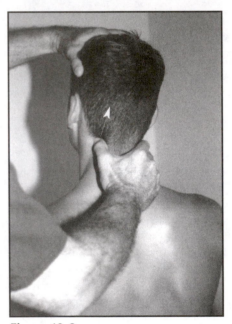

Figure 10-2a.

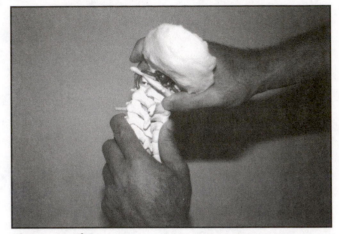

Figure 10-1b.

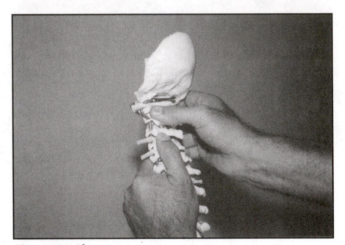

Figure 10-2b.

Apophyseal Joint Opening Restriction (Extended, Rotated, and Side Bent Impairment)

The treatment of an ERS left impairment at C2,3 is similar to the examination procedure for an apophyseal joint opening restriction. Once the head-neck region is localized to the "feather edge" of the restrictive barrier in C2,3 opening on the left, the therapist proceeds with the muscle ener-gy component followed by the graded mobilization (Figures 10-2a and 10-2b).

Students often question the head-neck position in this technique. Though it is true that the combined motions of C2 flexion, rotation, and side bending to the right are used to achieve apophyseal joint opening at C2,3 on the left, it is also true that rotation of the head to the left in no way interferes with the mechanics of this technique. This is because upper cervical kinematics are out of phase with those of the lower cervical spine, and even though the head is rotated left, the mechanics at C2,3 will necessitate that right side bending be associated with right rotation (type 2 mechanics). Although it is possible to perform this technique with the head rotated to the right, the principles of localization, balance, and control are optimal when performed as illustrated with the head rotated to the left.

The "roll-glide" mobilization involves a roll of the head-neck to the right (ie, right ear to right axilla) as C3 is translated to the left in the opposite direction. The passive manipulation is followed by an active movement in the same direction for the purpose of sensorimotor training.

This Rocabado sitting technique is used as an intervention for all FRS and ERS impairments from C2 through C7. Though the supine muscle energy techniques can be equally effective, with the advantage of reduced muscle activity, the sitting approach has the advantage of ease of application (ie, no table required) and optimal three-dimensional control of the cervical structures. In addition, people tend to spend more time sitting than recumbent; therefore, sitting interventions are more functionally oriented.

11

Therapeutic and Home Exercises for the Cervical Spine

Chin Tuck

There are two variations of the chin tuck that are taught to patients: the basic chin tuck and the "corkscrew" chin tuck. The basic chin tuck is a simple way of achieving occipital flexion and elongation of the occipital extensors. The patient should be positioned in standing with his or her back to the wall. The patient is asked to imagine a "rope" attached to the back of the head, approximately half-way between the top of the head and the most inferior aspect of the occiput (anatomically, this corresponds to the junction of the sagittal and lambdoid sutures known as lambda). This rope, when tightened, pulls the occiput out of "downward pull" in a "forward and up" direction and simultaneously causes the chin to move back and slightly down toward the hyoid bone, which is just above the Adam's apple in the throat. According to Alexander,[11] this restoration of "primary control" has the effect of lengthening and widening the torso (Figure 11-1).

The patient's head-neck region is in contact with the wall at all times. The stretch is held for 30 seconds at the point where the tissues at the back of the skull begin to feel the stretch (as with the other self-stretches, the patient is begun with a 5 to 10 second stretch and progressed up to 30 seconds as tolerated). The basic chin tuck is performed three times and repeated every 2 hours. As with all self-stretches, the patient must not elicit pain at any time. The most common error seen among patients is that they flex not at the occipitoatlantal junction but in the midcervical region. This movement is not only ineffective in restoring

normal head, neck, and spinal alignment, but contributes to the problem of midcervical hypermobility. To avoid this, the patient is given a visual aide to assist with occipitoatlantal flexion. The patient is asked to place an imaginary "axis" through the ears as he or she rotates around it. This, in conjunction with keeping the eyes level and not looking down toward the floor, ensures that the motion occurs in the upper and not lower cervical area.

The advanced variation, known as the "corkscrew" chin tuck, is so named because of how it resembles the workings of a corkscrew (Figures 11-2a and 11-2b). As illustrated, the "head," "neck," and "spine" of the corkscrew are driven cephalward into length by depression of its "shoulder complex" as per Newton's Third Law (ie, "To every action there is always an equal and opposing reaction."). In the human structure, this "ratcheting up" of the head, neck, spine, and sternum is believed to be a function of the ribs. As the shoulder girdle is depressed/retracted, the rib angles are depressed. However, the costovertebral, costotransverse, and costosternal joints move in a cephalward direction, providing a "lift" to the spine and sternum in the opposite direction. The converse is also true: shoulder girdle elevation/protraction allows these same structures to descend, causing the torso to functionally "shorten." The clavicles at the sternoclavicular joints most likely contribute to this corkscrew mechanism as well (ie, with shoulder girdle depression/re-traction, the sternal end of the clavicles provides a "lift" to the trunk, whereas with elevation/protraction of the shoulder girdle they allow a "collapsing" down of the trunk).

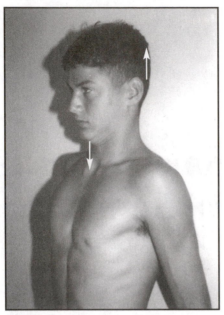

Figure 11-1.

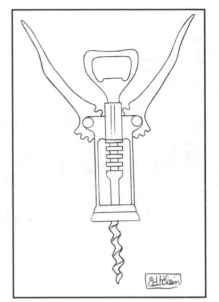

Figure 11-2a. Spinal "cork-screw" principle. The spine is shortened. (Illustration by Ed Klein)

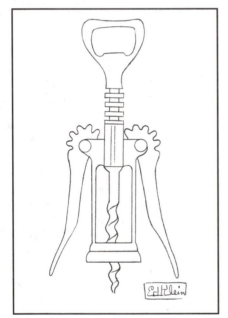

Figure 11-2b. Spinal "corkscrew" principle. The spine is lengthened. (Illustration by Ed Klein)

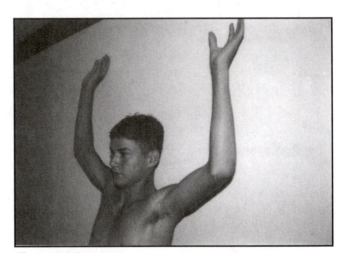

Figure 11-3a.

As the spine functionally "lengthens" in response to shoulder girdle depression/retraction, the occiput naturally flexes on the cervical spine. This is because the lower cervical spine extends with spinal lengthening, causing the upper cervical spine to flex (the upper and lower cervical spine are out of phase such that upper cervical flexion causes lower cervical extension and vice versa). Consequently, there is a correlation between depression/retraction of the shoulder girdle and flexion of the craniovertebral region.

The corkscrew chin tuck exercise is similar to the basic chin tuck except for the shoulder girdle component (Figures 11-3a and 11-3b). As the patient performs a "framing the doorway" motion of the upper extremities, he or she again imagines a rope pulling the back of the head forward and up as the chin approaches the hyoid bone just superior to the thyroid cartilage. It is believed that the descending shoulders and scapulae enhance the chin tuck as hypothesized in the spinal "corkscrew" principle described above. This exercise can be performed as a stretch or as a strengthening maneuver. When performed for strengthening purposes, it is done 10 times, with a hold of 5 to 10 seconds, three times per day.

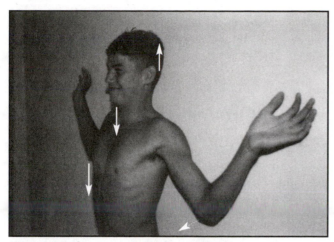

Figure 11-3b.

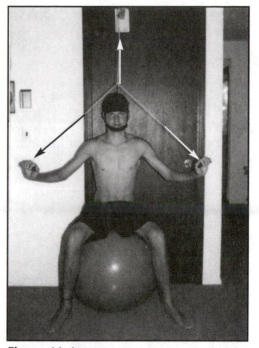

Figure 11-4a.

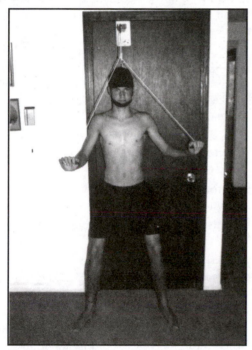

Figure 11-4b.

Based upon the spinal "corkscrew" principle, an exercise device (Patent Pending US and Canada) has been developed by the author. As illustrated (Figures 11-4a and 11-4b), it is designed to lengthen the spine and therefore improve postural alignment by directing the occiput up and forward on the neck as the shoulder girdle is simultaneously directed down and back. In addition to its obvious mechanical effects, this newly developed system helps to break poor postural habits while establishing new ones.

Management of Cervical Derangement (Phases 1 to 4)

The self-treatment model for a lower cervical derangement is based upon the patient's response to the repeated movements exam previously covered in Chapter 8. Because the photographs of the various phases (1 to 4) are the same for both examination and treatment, those taken previously will not be repeated here. The reader is, therefore, encouraged to cross-reference the appropriate treatment phase with the corresponding photograph in Chapter 8.

The management of a disc derangement is more of an art than a science. The author trusts that the following suggestions will serve as guidelines for the treating therapist:

1. The patient must be responsive to this intervention (ie, the patient must demonstrate the McKenzie centralization phenomenon during the repeated movements exam).

2. The phase selected for the home program is ideally phase 1. The intervention phase is escalated to the higher phases only when more force is required.

3. The patient must demonstrate proficiency with self-treatment in the clinic before he or she can be trusted to perform it at home.

4. The patient must stop the exercises if the symptoms peripheralize; however, a mild increase in intensity is permitted as long as it is in a centralized direction.

5. Head-neck extension in supine is permissible only under therapist supervision and not at home. This is because of the adverse effect of cervical backward bending on vertebral artery blood flow as well as possible spinal canal narrowing in those with spinal stenosis. In the clinic, signs of distress can be monitored, but at home, over the end of the bed, serious complications without assistance may ensue. Sitting extension at home is permitted (phase 2) because the patient can easily alter head and neck position without difficulty, if necessary.

6. Therapist-assisted technique (phase 4) is used as a last resort. Self-treatment is always the preferred approach with McKenzie.

7. The patient must be committed to performing the home program every 2 hours. The number of repetitions depends on the response to treatment. At least three sets of 10 repetitions are recommended; however, additional repetitions are allowed, providing the symptoms are improving.

8. In addition to the repeated movements component of derangement reduction, the patient needs to concentrate on maintaining the reduction in order to allow healing to occur. In this regard, instruction in proper posture (eg, avoid forward head positions) and the use of a cervical support pillow are mandatory. It is imperative that the cervical lordosis be preserved day and night lest the deranged tissue be reinjured. There are many such pillows on the market. There are three, in particular, that the author currently recommends. The Tempur-Pedic Swedish neck pillow (Tempur-Pedic Inc, Lexington, Ky), the Mediflow water-base pillow (Mediflow Inc, Markham, Ontario, Canada), and the McKenzie roll (OPTP, Minneapolis, Minn).

Once the derangement is reduced and stabilized, the final goals are to recover lost function and prevent recurrence. The recovery of function will be addressed in subsequent home exercises. The prevention of recurrence is multifactorial, including postural correction, normalizing strength of the weak phasic muscles, addressing ergonomic factors at home and in the workplace, stress management, etc.

Regarding the management of derangements that do not respond to mechanical therapy, the next step would be pain management for those patients who are not surgical candidates. For those patients who are surgical candidates, referral to a spinal surgeon is the next step. The indications for surgery include intractable pain and suffering; frank neurologic signs (ie, sensory loss, reflex changes, muscle weakness, atrophy, Babinski's sign, etc); diagnostic confirmation of pathology with MRI, MRA, CAT scan, discography, myelography, etc; and failed conservative therapy. This final item does not mean the use of pain-relieving modalities alone, but in conjunction with manual therapy and therapeutic exercise. The decision regarding spinal surgery is often a difficult one and requires the combined input of a team of professionals working together for the good of the patient.

Active Cervical Range of Motion

The use of cardinal plane active range of motion exercises is especially useful for those patients who cannot tolerate the other home exercises described in this chapter. Patients who are elderly and/or those with pathology of the spine, such as rheumatoid arthritis, ankylosing spondylitis, severe osteoporosis, etc, can experience the benefit of movement therapy without the risk of tissue disruption or injury (providing that their condition is not so severe as to preclude the use of active motion). The patient's instructions include the following:

1. Assume an upright head-neck position in either sitting or standing.

2. Turn slowly to the right until a slight stretch is experienced; return to the midline position and repeat three times.

3. Turn slowly to the left until a slight stretch is experienced; return to the midline position and repeat three times.

4. Tilt the head-neck region to the right (ie, ear to shoulder) and repeat three times.

5. Tilt the head-neck region to the left and repeat three times.

6. Bend the head-neck forward beginning with a **chin tuck** and repeat three times.

7. Perform a chin tuck followed by backward bending of the head-neck region; repeat three times. If at any time the patient becomes dizzy or apprehensive when tilting his or her head backward, he or she is to stop immediately. These symptoms may be the early warning signs of cerebral anoxia.

These exercises are to be performed at least three times per day, but this can be modified by the therapist as indicated.

The photographs of the active cervical movement exam in Chapter 8 (see Figures 8-5a to 8-5f) will serve to illustrate the movements performed in the above home program as well.

Upper Trapezius Self-Stretch

To stretch the left side (Figure 11-5), the sitting patient is instructed to grasp the bottom of the chair with the left hand. With the right hand, the patient pulls the head-neck

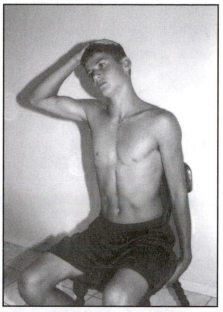

Figure 11-5.

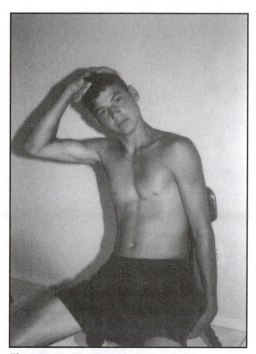

Figure 11-6a.

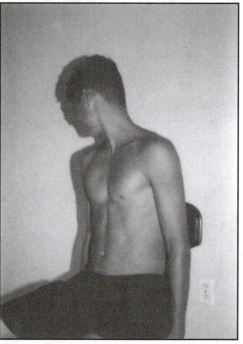

Figure 11-6b.

region toward the right shoulder (the motion involves straight side bending to the side opposite the stretch). The patient is instructed to stop at the first indication of a stretch, hold for 30 seconds, return slowly to the start position, and repeat three times every 2 hours. At no time should peripheral symptoms in the left upper limb be experienced. Experiencing these symptoms would suggest either

an active derangement and/or adverse neural tension that should be avoided in this simple muscle stretch.

For the more coordinated and intelligent patient, a self-muscle energy component can be added to the stretch for enhanced efficacy (eg, a 6-second isometric contraction of the left upper trapezius followed by the stretch).

Scaleni Self-Stretch

As with the distinction in function made between the anterior and middle with the posterior scalene in Chapter 9, so too the self-stretch for the scalene muscles must separate the anterior and middle components from the posterior one. The self-stretch for the left anterior and middle scalenes is similar to the upper trapezius stretch described above; however, the patient's head-neck region is positioned in retraction (upper cervical flexion and lower cervical extension), side bending right, and slight rotation left (Figure 11-6a).

The left posterior scalene self-stretch involves head-neck flexion, side bending, and rotation to the right (Figure 11-6b). The purpose of grasping the chair with the left hand is to maintain first and second rib depression during the stretch. Both stretches are held for 30 seconds and repeated three times every 2 hours. Again, the patient must be careful not to overstretch and should stop immediately if symptoms peripheralize.

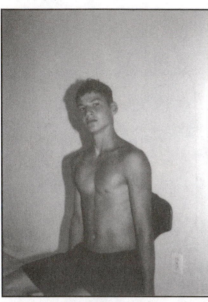

Figure 11-7a.

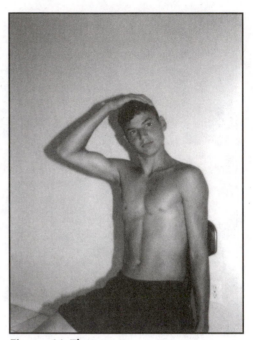

Figure 11-7b.

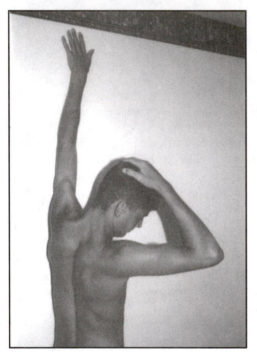

Figure 11-8a.

Sternocleidomastoid Self-Stretch

To stretch the left sternocleidomastoid (SCM), the patient's left hand grasps the bottom of the chair. The initial phase is to tilt the head-neck region to the right shoulder in a position of retraction and slight left rotation (Figure 11-7a). The next phase is what separates the SCM from the anterior/middle scalene stretch. The patient, who is already in a slight chin tuck, accentuates it further, while simultaneously pulling the head into further right side bending/left rotation with the right hand, until a stretch can be felt at the left mastoid process (Figure 11-7b). As with previous stretches, the patient must proceed to the point of the initial stretch and go no further. The stretch is repeated three times, holding each stretch for 30 seconds, every 2 hours (this number of sessions through the day may not be feasible for some patients, but it emphasizes the need to do them often).

Levator Scapulae Self-Stretch

The last of the self-stretches concludes with the levator stretch. To stretch the left side, the standing patient places the left arm against the wall in full abduction. This places the left scapula in upward rotation. With the right hand, the patient pulls the head-neck into combined flexion, rotation, and side bending to the right (Figure 11-8a). If there is a coexisting shoulder condition that precludes full abduction, the levator self-stretch can be modified to include scapular depression instead. This is achieved by having the sitting patient grasp the bottom of the chair as with the other stretches (Figure 11-8b).

Because the posterior scalene and levator scapulae stretches incorporate lower cervical flexion, the therapist and patient need to exercise caution. It is possible to exacerbate a latent derangement on the stretched side. Therefore, the patient must not overstretch, stop at the first indication of peripheral symptoms, return slowly to the start position, and perform a few prophylactic neck retractions to protect against disc disturbance.

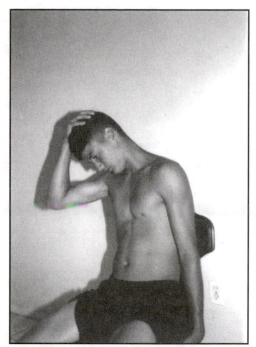

Figure 11-8b.

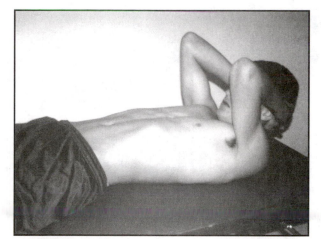

Figure 11-9a.

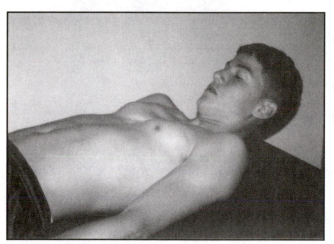

Figure 11-9b.

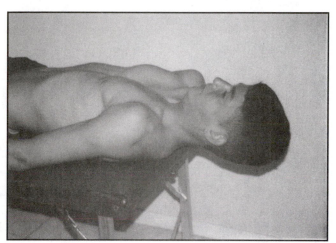

Figure 11-9c.

Cervical Strengthening Exercises

The phasic muscles that require strengthening in the cervical region are the upper cervical flexors and the lower cervical segmental extensors. It is only when these muscles are active and strong that the tendency towards FHP (ie, "backward head/forward neck") can be overcome.

To strengthen the occipital or upper cervical flexors (ie, rectus capitis anterior and longus capitis muscles), the supine patient is instructed to perform passive upper cervical spine flexion followed by lower cervical flexion with his or her fingers interlocked behind the occiput (Figure 11-9a). The patient then progresses from passive to active assisted to active flexion without the assist from his or her hands (Figure 11-9b). To improve the endurance of the upper cervical flexors, which is often poor in patients with chronic headache,[20] the patient is asked to maintain a chin-tuck position over the end of the table for 10 to 30 seconds (Figure 11-9c).

To strengthen the lower cervical segmental extensors (ie, semispinalis, multifidus, and rotatores), the prone patient's head-neck region is placed over the end of the table as the therapist localizes axial extension to the C4 through C7 levels, one segment at a time (Figure 11-9d). Once properly localized to the barrier of bilateral apophyseal joint extension, the therapist withdraws his or her forehead support and the patient performs an isometric contraction of the segmental extensor muscles. The patient can then be progressed to an isotonic mode by beginning from the flexed position of the head-neck and working segmentally upward (Figure 11-9e). Through bilateral facet palpation, the therapist ensures that the patient activates the desired segmental extensor muscles. Similar segmental extensor training can be performed in sitting as well (Figure 11-9f).

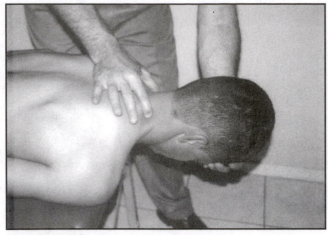

Figure 11-9d.

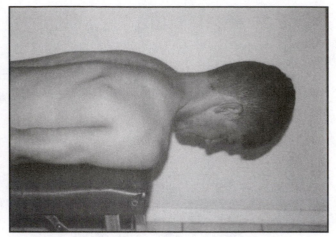

Figure 11-9e.

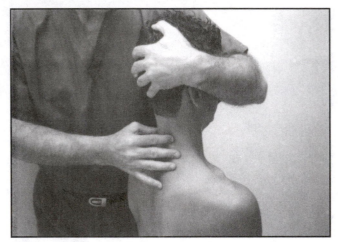

Figure 11-9f.

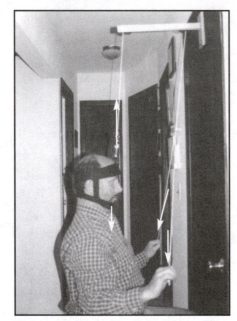

Figure 11-10.

For either the upper cervical flexors and/or the lower cervical segmental extensors, the patient, following competency in the clinic, can perform self-strengthening at home. He or she can do 10 repetitions, holding each repetition for 5 to 10 seconds, repeating three times per day.

In addition to the postural realignment function of the exercise device mentioned previously in this chapter, the same device is used to enhance the strength of the occipital flexor muscles, lower cervical segmental extensors, and the lower scapular stabilizers, simultaneously. As illustrated in Figure 11-10, the patient merely turns around to face the door. With the rope now pulling the occiput into extension rather than flexion, the patient performs a combination of isometric, isotonic, and eccentric exercises of the aforementioned muscle groups.

Another device, the Stabilizer (Chattanooga Group Inc, Chattanooga, Tenn), has an air-filled pressure sensor that monitors the slight flattening of the cervical lordosis associated with contraction of the longus colli muscle. It, too, is useful in retraining the upper cervical flexor/lower cervical segmental extensor muscles.[21]

The Role of the Cervical Spine
in Headache and Dizziness

Headache and dizziness are common features of cervical impairment, injury, or disease. Their cervical causes are of great interest to manual therapists. In this chapter, the role of the cervical spine in both headache and dizziness will be explored. The purpose of this overview is to underscore the significant contribution made by cervical structures in both of these common clinical conditions. Porterfield and DeRosa[22] state, "The neurosciences of the cervical spine have a degree of complexity found in no other region of the axial skeleton." We will certainly be exposed to some of this complexity in this chapter.

Headache

Although headache of cervical origin (ie, cervicogenic headache) is found in approximately 14% of chronic headache sufferers,[23] up to 70% of headache sufferers overall have impairment of the cervical spine.[24]

To better understand the role of the cervical spine in cervicogenic headache and its contribution to other forms of chronic headache, it is necessary to review our current understanding of the neuroanatomy of the upper cervical spinal cord.

The spinal nucleus of the trigeminal nerve (ie, fifth cranial nerve) consists of three parts: pars oralis, pars interpolaris, and pars caudalis (Figure 12-1). The pars caudalis is the most caudal of the three and merges imperceptibly with the dorsal horns of the upper three cervical spinal cord segments, consisting of the marginal zone, substantia gelatinosa, and the nucleus proprius. The spinal tract of the trigeminal nerve descends caudally through the medulla oblongata as far as the C4 level. Fibers from the spinal tract terminate in the gray matter of the pars caudalis and upper three cervical cord segments. Bogduk[25] refers to this continuous column of interconnecting gray matter of the pars caudalis and the upper cervical dorsal horns as the trigeminocervical nucleus. This nucleus is defined not by intrinsic features but by the afferent input it receives from the spinal tract of the fifth cranial nerve. Because it incorporates the neuroanatomic structures responsible for pain transmission and receives afferent input from trigeminal and upper cervical nerves, the trigeminocervical nucleus can be seen as the nociceptive nucleus for the entire head and upper neck. In addition, Mannheimer and Rosenthal[26] report that the entire trigeminocervical complex includes not only the fifth cranial nerve, but also receives input from the 7th, 9th, 10th, 11th, and 12th cranial nerves as well.

The clinical significance of these scientific discoveries is summarized by Jull[27] who states, "Through the convergence of cervical and trigeminal afferents on common neurons in the trigeminal nucleus, any structure innervated by any of the upper three cervical nerves may refer pain into the head and face." To support the concept of upper cervical pain referral into the head and face, Bogduk[25] cites several studies in this regard and then states the following, "These experiments clearly demonstrate the capacity of experimental painful stimuli in the upper neck to produce pain in the head. It is possible, therefore, that pathological painful lesions of any of the structures innervated by the upper cervical nerves are equally capable of producing such referred pain" (Figure 12-2).

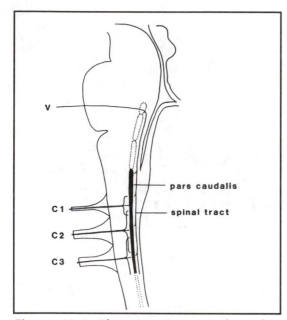

Figure 12-1. The trigeminocervical nucleus (reprinted with permission from Bogduk N. Cervical causes of headache and dizziness. In: *Grieve's Modern Manual Therapy*. 2nd ed. New York, NY: Churchill Livingstone; 1994).

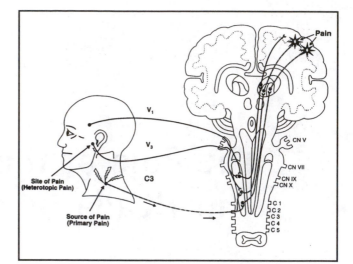

Figure 12-2. Head and temporomandibular joint/facial pain of cervical origin (reprinted with permission from Okeson J. *Orofacial Pain: Guidelines for Assessment, Diagnosis, and Management*. Chicago, Ill: Quintessence Publishing; 1996).

When considering the role of the cervical spine in headache, there are two possible connections. The first involves direct pain referral from upper cervical spine disease and/or somatic impairment referred to as cervicogenic headache. The second involves the indirect role of the upper cervical region in other forms of chronic headache, including tension-type, migraine with and without aura, post-traumatic headache, and analgesic rebound or abuse headache. The role of the cervical spine in temporomandibular disorders (TMD) will be addressed in a subsequent chapter.

Cervicogenic headache (CGH) is a headache arising from painful dysfunction and/or disease of the cervical spine, particularly the upper three segments. Although the International Headache Society (IHS) has not yet given CGH an official classification, there is growing support from around the world. The first attempt to establish diagnostic criteria for CGH was in 1990; as recently as 1998, the Cervicogenic Headache International Study Group has updated the criteria.[28]

Women are affected more than men. There is often a history of head and/or neck trauma. CGH is, in principle, a unilateral headache, but it may become bilateral over time. Signs and symptoms of CGH include precipitation of headache by neck movement, sustained awkward head positioning, and/or external pressure over the cervical or occipital region on the symptomatic side; restriction of range of motion in the neck; and ipsilateral neck, shoulder, or arm pain of a radicular or nonradicular nature. Headache

characteristics include moderate to severe, nonthrobbing, and nonlancinating pain, usually starting in the neck and eventually spreading to the oculofrontotemporal area on the symptomatic side. The frontotemporal pain may at times exceed the neck/occipital pain. In the initial phase, the headache is usually episodic; later it becomes chronic with a fluctuating quality. Occasionally, patients with CGH also report nausea, phonophobia/photophobia, dizziness, blurred vision, difficulty swallowing, and ipsilateral edema in the periocular area. However, these "attack-related phenomena" are not the major features of this headache. Diagnostic anesthetic blockade of the greater/lesser occipital nerves, C2 and C3 roots, third occipital nerve, facet joints, and lower cervical roots and branches on the symptomatic side should temporarily abolish the pain of CGH. Of the three spinal segments involved with CGH (ie, OA, AA, and C2,3), the C2,3 facet joints are thought to play the most significant role.[29]

Studies have shown a connection between cervicogenic headache, poor posture, weak cervical flexors, facet joint arthropathy, cervical spine trauma, and joint hypo/hypermobility.[30] Consequently, the role of manual therapy as an intervention for CGH is gaining momentum. In fact, the *Evidence Report: Behavioral and Physical Treatments for Tension-Type and Cervicogenic Headache* from the Duke University Evidence-Based Practice Center published in 2001 concluded the following: "Cervical spine manipulation was associated with significant improvements in headache outcomes in trials involving patients with neck pain and/or neck dysfunction and headache."[31] Schoensee et al,[29] investigating the effect of upper cervical mobilization on the frequency, duration, and intensity of cervical headaches, concluded that manual therapy was effective as an intervention for headaches of cervical origin.

There is much controversy regarding the role of the cervical spine in other forms of primary headache. There is, however, a growing body of knowledge suggesting that the musculoskeletal system does play a role in the pathogenesis and management of migraine.[32] Hack et al[33] identified a fibrous connection between the rectus capitis posterior minor muscle and the posterior atlanto-occipital membrane, which then attaches to the cranial dura mater. This finding may shed light on the connection between subcranial muscle tension and migraine. In the study by Marcus et al,[34] postural abnormalities were more prevalent in patients with migraine and tension-type headache then in the controls. In the Karpouzis et al study,[35] a history of head, neck, and back injury was the most commonly reported circumstance related to the onset of chronic headache in 1013 patients. In the Silberstein et al study,[36] patients with migraine responded favorably to pericranial injection of botulinum toxin type A with reduced migraine frequency, severity, acute medication usage, and associated vomiting. Whereas most neurology-based textbooks and articles view muscle contraction as a consequence of migraine, Silberstein et al raise the possibility that muscle contraction may play a role in migraine pathogenesis through some "as of yet unknown effect on the sensory system."

Moskowitz[37] proposed a mechanism whereby an upper cervical impairment can give rise to a throbbing vascular headache. This mechanism involves the activation of trigeminal sensory fibers in the brainstem, which in turn triggers an efferent pathway through the facial nerve to the greater superficial petrosal nerve. It is the greater superficial petrosal nerve that provides the autonomic connection by innervating autonomic pathways in the cranial vasculature. Some have used this and other similar physiologic mechanisms[38] to suggest a major role of the cervical spine in migraine. However, the literature does not support this concept. A more plausible argument, and the one to which the author subscribes, is that the cervical spine is one of many factors in migraine pathogenesis. Similar to the role of emotional stress, dietary triggers, sleep deprivation, hypoglycemia, hormonal factors in women, etc, the presence of upper cervical impairment contributes to the excitability of the trigeminocervical nucleus, the nociceptive nucleus, for the entire head and upper neck.

Whereas migraine was once thought to be a function of intracranial/extracranial vasodilatation (ie, Wolff's vascular theory), it is now believed that migraine is a complex disorder of central nervous system regulation of pain-producing intracranial structures (neurovascular theory). It is beyond the scope of this chapter to provide a detailed theoretical analysis of migraine pathophysiology. However, it is important for manual therapists to realize that migraine is enormously complex and that the presence of cervical impairment is not the "whole ball of wax." In addition to

abnormal afferent input from the upper cervical area (mainly through the first division of the trigeminal nerve), the trigeminocervical nucleus receives afferent input from the extensive trigeminovascular system, which is thought to be abnormal in patients suffering from migraines. There is strong evidence to suggest that serotonin (5-HT) plays a key role in this neurovascular abnormality. Plasma serotonin has been shown to fall at the onset of a migraine attack, and the fact that reserpine (a serotonin-depleting agent) precipitates migraine is further evidence that falling serotonin and migraine are related. In addition, the relief that migraine sufferers obtain from the 5-HT agonists (Imitrex [GlaxoSmithKline, Research Triangle Park, NC], Maxalt [GlaxoSmithKline, Research Triangle Park, NC], Amerge [Merck, Whitehouse Station, NJ], etc) is another indication of the serotonin-migraine connection.

The take-home message from this crash-course in brain neurochemistry is that migraine is multifactorial. The input from an impaired upper cervical region is one of many factors. Migraine, whether with or without aura, is primarily a disturbance within the trigeminal system, with the greatest pathology emanating from the trigeminovascular junctions at the base of the brain and in the dura mater. There is little to no benefit of manual therapy during an attack of migraine, but between episodes there is significant benefit. By correcting somatic impairment throughout the head, neck, TMJ, and upper back, there will be less nociceptive input into the trigeminocervical nucleus. This "defacilitation" will have the net effect of raising the central pain-threshold for the head and upper neck region and will hopefully have a beneficial effect on the frequency, duration, and severity of migraine.

There is an effective nonmedicinal strategy that can be employed to abort an extracranial vascular headache. According to Willis,[39] a tourniquet is applied around the head just above the ears. The best time to use this method is just prior to the headache, but it can be used during the migraine, providing that the scalp is not overly sensitive to pressure. The tightness of the tourniquet is to be moderate in nature and it can be left in place for several hours. The principle behind this method is based upon Laplace's law, where $T = Pr$. T represents the circumferential tension within the vessel wall, P represents the pressure gradient across the vessel, and r stands for the radius of the vessel. Because vasodilatation increases T during migraine, the arterial wall is stretched and becomes inflamed and painful. When T is decreased with the tourniquet by decreasing P and r, the stretch on the vessel wall is removed and the headache diminishes. This is a useful method in patients who cannot tolerate migraine medication.

Regarding the role of the cervical spine in other forms of chronic headache, there are implications for tension-type, post-traumatic, cluster, and analgesic abuse or drug rebound headache. Many researchers and clinicians believe that migraine and tension-type headaches are related. This connection is supported by the fact that platelet serotonin content is also low in patients with chronic tension-type headache. As with migraine, facilitation of the trigeminocervical nucleus is an integral component of tension-type headache (TTH). Consequently, the manipulative improvement of somatic impairment in the head, neck, TMJ, and scapulothoracic region should theoretically diminish the nociceptive afferent input into the trigeminocervical nucleus and improve symptoms.

Hanten et al[40] demonstrated the effectiveness of the craniosacral technique, CV-4, for the treatment of TTH. There was significant improvement in both headache intensity and affect scores as compared to the no-treatment control. However, Bove and Nilsson[41] failed to demonstrate the effectiveness of spinal manipulation in the treatment of episodic TTH (fewer than 15 episodes per month). The different outcomes between these two studies may be found in the fact that Hanten et al included both chronic and episodic TTH patients, whereas Bove and Nilsson restricted their sample to only episodic TTH. It is expected that the trigeminocervical nucleus would be more chronically facilitated with chronic versus episodic TTH and thus therapy aimed at reducing its excitability (ie, manual therapy and therapeutic exercise) should, theoretically, result in symptom reduction as shown in the Hanten et al study.

Regarding post-traumatic headache (PTH), the role of the cervical spine cannot be ignored. Though there is a strong correlation between mild head injury and PTH, there is also a large percentage of PTH patients who have a history of cervical spinal injury as well. The term post-traumatic migraine has been used to describe the onset of migraine following mild head injury. However, according to Packard,[42] "trauma probably never causes migraine." Instead he attributes the onset of migraine following head injury to a temporary worsening of pre-existing migraine related to a nonspecific stress reaction or to a "complicating neck sprain," which may aggravate pre-existing migraine as well. Because the symptoms of PTH include physical, psychological, and cognitive aspects, its management must involve a multidisciplinary approach. Jensen et al[43] demonstrated a superior effect of manual therapy over cold packs in the treatment of PTH. Using a combination of spinal mobilization, high velocity thrust, and muscle energy techniques, the manual therapy group demonstrated a more rapid decline in the pain index and overall use of analgesics compared with the cold pack group.

There are two remaining chronic headache types to discuss relative to the role of the cervical spine. The first is cluster headache and the second is analgesic abuse headache. Though the exact mechanism of cluster headache remains uncertain, Hildebrandt and Jansen[44] reported on two middle age males in whom chronic intermittent hemicrania associated with ciliary injections, lacrimation, and rhinorrhea (typical symptoms of cluster headache) were successfully treated with surgical decompression of the C2 and C3 nerve roots. In one case, a pannus-like layered network of veins with arterial supply was the culprit; in the other case, it was a network of veins. This study illustrates the point that there may be an upper cervical component in some cases of cluster headache. Whether somatic impairment can cause the symptom complex noted in the above two cases of vascular compression is unknown, but certainly the possibility exists.

The abuse of both over-the-counter and prescription analgesics for chronic headache management is a serious health problem. Srikiatkhachorn et al[45] demonstrated that chronic paracetamol administration in laboratory animals resulted in 5-HT depletion that, in turn, produced readaptation of the 5-HT 2a receptor. This change in the 5-HT 2a serotonin receptor may be an important mechanism related to the loss of analgesic efficacy, ultimately resulting in the daily complaints associated with analgesic abuse. Analgesic abuse headache is finally receiving the attention it deserves and may be prevented or reversed by avoiding the chronic use of analgesic medication.[46] This means that therapists must do a better job of providing nonmedicinal headache relief to their patients. The normalization of head, neck, TMJ, and spinal function will go a long way toward achieving this goal and consequently spare at least some, if not many, the nightmare of the chronic head, neck, and face pain, in addition to the many other adverse effects associated with analgesic abuse (eg, gastrointestinal, kidney, and liver damage).

The author, as with much of this textbook, has intentionally not included an extensive review of the basic science material on this topic. The reader is encouraged to scan the references and bibliography in order to broaden his or her knowledge of the subject.

Dizziness

Another common complaint originating in the cervical spine is dizziness. The term dizziness will be used, generically, in this chapter to include the following symptoms:

1. Vertigo: A sensation that the environment is spinning (external), or that the individual is spinning (internal).

2. Presyncopal lightheadedness: A feeling that one is about to pass out.

3. Disequilibrium: A sensation of imbalance or unsteadiness (more prominent in standing).

Dizziness can have central, peripheral, or systemic causes.[47] Peripheral causes include peripheral vestibulopathy, benign paroxysmal positional vertigo (BPPV), Meniere's disease, labyrinthitis, labyrinthine concussion, vestibulotoxic drugs, perilymph fistula, etc. Central causes include demyelinating disease, tumors, seizures, vertebrobasilar insufficiency (VBI), migraine-related vertigo, transient

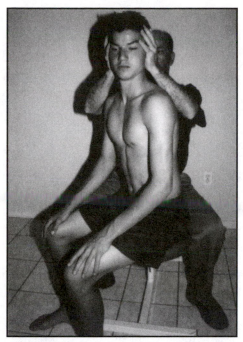

Figure 12-3a.

ischemic attack, and cervicogenic dizziness. Systemic causes of dizziness include endocrine disease (hypothyroidism, diabetes), pharmacologic side effects (anticonvulsants, antihypertensives, tranquilizers, analgesics, muscle relaxants, etc), and the many causes of presyncope (eg, hypoglycemia, panic, vasovagal episode, hypotension, cardiac arrhythmias, Valsalva's maneuver, etc).

Generally, true vertigo indicates a disorder of the inner ear, vestibular nerve, brainstem, or cerebellum, whereas vertebrobasilar insufficiency and cervicogenic dizziness are most often associated with disequilibrium.

The diagnosis of VBI is straight forward when the 5 Ds[5] are present (see special tests section of Chapter 8). However, when only dizziness is present (which is sometimes the case) diagnosis is difficult. The diagnosis of BPPV is straight forward. It is common in middle age, but in about 15% of cases there is a relationship to head trauma.[48] The patient typically develops severe vertigo when turning over or first lying in bed. The episodes last less than a minute and the patient can find another position in which he or she is asymptomatic. As soon as he or she moves, however, another attack is provoked. The Hallpike-Dix maneuver is used to test patients suspected of having BPPV.[49] The patient sits on an examining table and turns his or her head 40 degrees to one side. The examiner grasps the patient's head and briskly lowers him backward into a supine position with the head over the end of the bed 40 degrees below the horizontal. The patient's head is maintained in a rotated position with the eyes directed toward the floor. In the presence of BPPV, there will be an asymptomatic latent period of several seconds, followed by a sudden onset of

severe vertigo and rotatory nystagmus. When the patient looks toward the ceiling, the nystagmus becomes vertical. The symptoms and nystagmus last 30 to 50 seconds and then cease. When the patient sits up, there may be brief, milder vertigo and nystagmus in the opposite direction. With repeated testing, the reflex fatigues and the symptoms and nystagmus are less and finally cease. The maneuver should be performed to both sides.

Cervicogenic dizziness is a sensation of altered orientation in space and disequilibrium, originating from abnormal afferent activity from the neck. Cervicogenic dizziness does not result from vestibular dysfunction and, therefore, rarely results in true vertigo. Cervicogenic dizziness is often associated with flexion-extension injuries and has been reported in advanced cases of cervical arthritis, herniated cervical discs, and head trauma. In these patients, complaints of ataxia, unsteadiness of gait, and/or postural disequilibrium are the most common.[49]

The pathophysiology of cervicogenic dizziness appears to involve abnormal afferent input to the vestibular nuclei from damaged joint receptors in the upper cervical region. Aspinall[47] attributes cervicogenic dizziness to a disturbance of the tonic neck reflexes from a distortion of the normal afferent input to the vestibular nuclei from the neck. Herdman[49] suggests that inflammation or irritation of the cervical roots or facet joints would lead to a mismatch among vestibular, visual, and cervical inputs. This "multi-sensory mismatch" would then give rise to the symptoms of cervicogenic dizziness, especially during movements of the head-neck region. Isaacs and Bookhout[50] relate cervicogenic dizziness to abnormal muscle tone in cervical musculature or following mobilization of the cervical spine, when proprioceptive feedback does not match ocular and vestibular sensations. Wapner et al[51] discovered that the sensation of tilting or falling could be evoked by electrical stimulation of the cervical muscles. Gray[52] found that cervicogenic dizziness could be relieved by injecting local anesthetic into the posterior cervical muscles. Both studies support the claim that abnormal afferent input from the cervical region results in patient-perceived dizziness. Herdman[49] states that she doubts whether cervical lesions have a "profound effect" on the oculomotor and vestibular systems, but goes on to say, "There is evidence that treatment of cervical dysfunctions can lead to decreased symptoms of dizziness and improvements in postural stability." The author would add that for the patient whose dizziness improves, even a small amount, that is profound enough for him or her!

This discussion will conclude with a description of a clinical assessment tool for cervicogenic dizziness developed by Fitz-Ritson,[53] who in a study of 235 traumatized neck patients, found that 46.7% had cervicogenic dizziness. The patient is seated on a stool that rotates (Figures 12-3a and 12-3b). The therapist stands behind the patient and holds the patient's head steady. Fitz-Ritson suggests using slight cephalad traction to prestretch the cervical muscula-

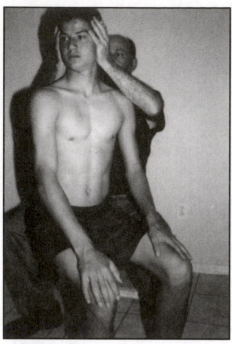

Figure 12-3b.

ture. With the patient's eyes closed, the body is rotated to either side with the feet. This motion essentially rotates the neck to either side while the semicircular canals are motionless. Any resulting dizziness must therefore be of cervical spine origin. Fitz-Ritson found that the patients who responded best to manipulative treatment were those who suffered upper cervical joint problems, along with muscle trauma in that region. This supports the theory that cervicogenic dizziness arises from abnormal afferent input from the receptors of the upper cervical spine.

When dealing with cervical spine impairment that is refractory to local methods of intervention, the therapist must be cognizant of the multiple inputs and influences that affect the somatic structures of the neck. They include vestibular,[49] visual,[54] limbic,[55] craniofacial,[56] respiratory,[57] and visceral.[12] In addition, migraine headache is known to evoke cervical muscle tightness of a reflexive nature.[46] Consequently, all potential causes of cervical spine impairment must be identified and managed if the patient's condition is to improve. In some cases, this may necessitate the expertise of a neurologist, ophthalmologist, optometrist, dentist, oral and maxillofacial surgeon, ear-nose-throat specialist, psychiatrist, psychologist, etc. In a related sense, it has been demonstrated that normal motor function of the cervical musculature may be contingent upon optimal craniofacial and occlusal relationships.[58]

References and Bibliography

References

1. Rocabado M. Diagnosis and treatment of abnormal craniocervical and craniomandibular mechanics. In: Solberg WK, Clark GT, eds. *Abnormal Jaw Mechanics: Diagnosis and Treatment*. Chicago, Ill: Quintessence Publishing; 1984.

2. Hickey ER, Rondeau MJ, Corrente JR, Abysalh J, Seymour CJ. Reliability of the cervical range of motion (CROM) device and plumb-line techniques in measuring resting head posture (RHP). *Journal of Manual & Manipulative Therapy*. 2000;8(1): 10-17.

3. Youdas JW, Carey JR, Garrett TR. Reliability of measurements of cervical spine range of motion-comparison of three methods. *Phys Ther*. 1991;71:98-104.

4. Kramer J. *Intervertebral Disc Diseases: Causes, Diagnosis, Treatment, and Prophylaxis*. 2nd ed. New York, NY: Thieme Medical Publishers; 1990.

5. Coman WB. Dizziness related to ENT conditions. In: Grieve GP, ed. *Modern Manual Therapy of the Vertebral Column*. Edinburgh: Churchill Livingstone; 1986.

6. Meadows J. *Orthopedic Differential Diagnosis in Physical Therapy*. New York, NY: McGraw-Hill; 1999.

7. Herdman SJ. Treatment of benign paroxysmal positional vertigo. *Phys Ther*. 1990;70(6):381-388.

8. Rocabado M. The importance of soft tissue mechanics in stability and instability of the cervical spine: a functional diagnosis for treatment planning. *J Craniomandibular Pract*. 1987;5(2): 130-138.

9. Weinstein JN, Rydevik BL, Sonntag VKH, eds. *Essentials of the Spine*. New York, NY: Raven Press; 1995.

10. Calliet R. *Soft Tissue Pain and Disability*. 3rd ed. Philadelphia, Pa: FA Davis; 1996.

11. Conable B, Conable W. *How to Learn the Alexander Technique*. Columbus, Ohio: Andover Road Press; 1992.

12. Greenman PE. *Principles of Manual Medicine*. 2nd ed. Philadelphia, Pa: Lippincott Williams & Wilkins; 1996.

13. Paris SV. *Course Notes, The Spine: Etiology and Treatment of Dysfunction Including Joint Manipulation*. Atlanta, Ga: Author; 1979.

14. Chaitow L. *Positional Release Techniques*. Edinburgh: Churchill Livingstone; 2002.

15. Kendall FP, McCreary FP, Provance PG. *Muscles: Testing and Function*. 4th ed. Baltimore, Md: Williams & Wilkins; 1993.

16. Evjenth O, Hamberg J. *Muscle Stretching in Manual Therapy: A Clinical Manual. Vol. II, The Spinal Column and Temporomandibular Joint*. Alfta, Sweden: Scand; 1984.

17. Kuzmich D. The levator scapulae: making the con-neck-tion. *Journal of Manual & Manipulative Therapy*. 1994;2(2):43-54.

18. Butler DS. *Mobilization of the Nervous System*. Melbourne: Churchill Livingstone; 1991.

19. Butler DS. *The Sensitive Nervous System*. Adelaide: Noigroup Publications; 2000.

20. Placzek JD, Pagett BT, Roubal PJ, et al. The influence of the cervical spine on chronic headache in women: a pilot study. *Journal of Manual & Manipulative Therapy*. 1999;7(1):33-39.

21. Jull G, Trott P, Potter H, et al. A randomized controlled trial of exercise and manipulative therapy for cervicogenic headache. *Spine*. 2002;27(17):1835-1843.

22. Porterfield JA, DeRosa C. *Mechanical Neck Pain: Perspectives in Functional Anatomy*. Philadelphia, Pa: WB Saunders; 1995.

23. Pfaffenrath V, Kaube H. Diagnostics of cervicogenic headache. *Funct Neurol*. 1990;5:159-164.

24. Pfaffenrath V, Dandekar R, Mayer G, Hermann G, Pollmann W. Cervicogenic headache: results of computer-based measurements of cervical spine mobility in 15 patients. *Cephalgia.* 1988;8:45-48.

25. Bogduk N. Cervical causes of headache and dizziness. In: Grieve GP, ed. *Modern Manual Therapy of the Vertebral Column.* 2nd ed. Edinburgh: Churchill Livingstone; 1994.

26. Mannheimer JS, Rosenthal RM. Acute and chronic postural abnormalities as related to craniofacial pain and temporomandibular disorders. *Dent Clin North Am.* 1991;35(1):185-208.

27. Jull GA. Headaches of cervical origin. In: Grant R, ed. *Physical Therapy of the Cervical and Thoracic Spine. Clinics in Physical Therapy.* London: Churchill Livingstone; 1988.

28. Sjaastad O, Fredriksen A, Pfaffenrath V. Cervicogenic headache: diagnostic criteria. *Headache.* 1998;38:442-446.

29. Schoensee SK, Jensen G, Nicholson G, Gossman M, Katholi C. The effect of mobilization on cervical headaches. *J Orthop Sports Phys Ther.* 1995;21(4):184-190.

30. Swerdlow B. *Whiplash and Related Headaches.* Boca Raton, Fla: CRC Press; 1999.

31. McCrory DC, Penzien DB, Hasselblad V, Gray RN. *Evidence Report: Behavioral and Physical Treatments for Tension-Type and Cervicogenic Headache.* Durham, NC: Duke University Evidence-Based Practice Center; 2001.

32. Saper JR. Chronic daily headache: a clinician's perspective. *Headache.* 2002;42(6):538-542.

33. Hack GD, Koritzer RT, Robinson WL, Hallgren RC, Greenman PE. Anatomic relation between the rectus capitis posterior minor muscle and the dura mater. *Spine.* 1995;20(23):2484-2486.

34. Marcus DA, Scharff L, Mercer S, Turk DC. Musculoskeletal abnormalities in chronic headache: a controlled comparison of headache diagnostic groups. *Headache.* 1999;39:21-27.

35. Karpouzis KM, Spierings E. Circumstances of onset of chronic headache in patients attending a specialty practice. *Headache.* 1999;39:317-320.

36. Silberstein S, Mathew N, Saper J, Jenkins S. Botulinum toxin type A as a migraine preventive treatment. *Headache.* 2000;40:445-450.

37. Moskowitz MA. The neurobiology of vascular head pain. *Ann Neurol.* 1984;16:156-168.

38. Olesen J. Clinical and pathophysiological observations in migraine and tension-type headache explained by integration of vascular, supraspinal, and myofascial inputs. *Pain.* 1991;46:125-132.

39. Willis GC. *Headache.* Lecture notes, Maizuru General Hospital, Kyoto Prefecture, Japan, 1990.

40. Hanten WP, Olson SL, Hodson JL, Imler VL, Knab VM, Magee JL. The effectiveness of CV-4 and resting position techniques on subjects with tension-type headaches. *Journal of Manual & Manipulative Therapy.* 1999;7(2);64-70.

41. Bove G, Nilsson N. Spinal manipulation in the treatment of episodic tension-type headache. *JAMA.* 1998;280(18):1576-1579.

42. Packard RC. Post-traumatic headache: more than just a headache. *Headache Quarterly.* 2001;12:99-100.

43. Jensen O, Nielsen F, Vosmar L. An open study comparing manual therapy with the use of cold packs in the treatment of post-traumatic headache. *Cephalgia.* 1990;10:241-250.

44. Hildebrandt J, Jansen J. Vascular compression of the C2 and C3 roots—yet another cause of chronic intermittent hemicrania? *Cephalgia.* 1984;4:167-170.

45. Srikiatkhachorn A, Tarasub N, Govitrapong P. Effect of chronic analgesic exposure on the central serotonin system: a possible mechanism of analgesic abuse headache. *Headache.* 2000;40:343-350.

46. Saper JR, Silberstein S, Gordon CD, Hamel RL. *Handbook of Headache Management: A Practical Guide to Diagnosis and Treatment of Head, Neck, and Facial Pain.* Baltimore, Md: Williams & Wilkins; 1993.

47. Aspinall W. Clinical testing for cervical mechanical disorders which produce ischemic vertigo. *J Orthop Sports Phys Ther.* 1989;11(5):176-182.

48. Willis GC. *Acoustic Nerve: Deafness, Tinnitus, and Vertigo. Neuroanatomy of the VIIIth Nerve and its Connections.* Lecture notes, Maizuru General Hospital, Kyoto Prefecture, Japan, 1990.

49. Herdman SJ. *Vestibular Rehabilitation.* 2nd ed. Philadelphia, Pa: FA Davis; 2000.

50. Isaacs ER, Bookhout MR. Screening for pathologic origins of head and face pain. In: Boissonnault WG, ed. *Examination in Physical Therapy Practice, Screening for Medical Disease.* 2nd ed. New York, NY: Churchill Livingstone; 1995.

51. Wapner S, Werner H, Chandler KA. Experiments on the sensory-tonic field theory of perception: effect of extraneous stimulation of the visual perception of verticality. *J Exp Psych.* 1951;42:351-357.

52. Gray LP. Extralabyrinthine vertigo due to cervical muscle lesions. *Journal of Laryngology.* 1956;70:352-361.

53. Fitz-Ritson D. Assessment of cervicogenic vertigo. *J Manipulative Physiol Ther.* 1991;14(3):193-198.

54. Vernon H. *Upper Cervical Syndrome: Chiropractic Diagnosis and Treatment.* Baltimore, Md: Williams & Wilkins; 1988.

55. Janda V. Muscles and cervicogenic pain syndromes. In: Grant R, ed. *Physical Therapy of the Cervical and Thoracic Spine.* New York, NY: Churchill Livingstone; 1988.

56. Urbanowicz M. Alteration of vertical dimension and its effect on head and neck posture. *J Craniomandibular Pract.* 1991;9(2):174-179.

57. Makofsky HW. Snoring and obstructive sleep apnea: does head posture play a role? *J Craniomandibular Pract.* 1997;15(1):68-73.

58. Chakfa AM, Mehta NR, Forgione AG, Al-Badawi EA, Lobo Lobo S, Zawawi KH. The effect of stepwise increases in vertical dimension of occlusion on isometric strength of cervical flexors and deltoid muscles in nonsymptomatic females. *Cranio.* 2002;20(4):264-273.

Bibliography

Aprill C, Dwyer A, Bogduk N. Cervical zygapophyseal joint pain patterns II: a clinical evaluation. *Spine.* 1990;15(6):458-461.

Beighton PH, Grahame R, Bird H. *Hypermobility of Joints.* 3rd ed. London: Springer-Verlag; 1999.

Bland JH. *Disorders of the Cervical Spine: Diagnosis and Medical Management.* Philadelphia, Pa: WB Saunders; 1987.

Cady R, Schreiber C, Farmer K, Sheftell F. Primary headaches: a convergence hypothesis. *Headache*. 2002;42:204-216.

Campbell DG, Parsons CM. Referred head pain and its concomitants. *J Nerv Ment Dis*. 1944;99:544-551.

Caputi CA, Firetto V. Therapeutic blockade of greater occipital and supraorbital nerves in migraine patients. *Headache*. 1997;37:174-179.

Coppieters MW, Stappaerts KH, Everaert DG, Staes FF. Addition of test components during neurodynamic testing: effect on range of motion and sensory responses. *J Orthop Sports Phys Ther*. 2001;31(5):226-237.

Darnell MW. A proposed chronology of events for forward head posture. *J Craniomandibular Pract*. 1983;1(4):50-54.

DiFabio RP. Manipulation of the cervical spine: risks and benefits. *Phys Ther*. 1999;79(1):50-65.

Dowling DJ. Progressive inhibition of neuromuscular structures (PINS) technique. *J Am Osteopath Assoc*. 2000;100(5):285-298.

Dreyfuss P, Michaelsen M, Fletcher D. Atlanto-occipital and lateral atlantoaxial joint pain patterns. *Spine*. 1994;19(10):1125-1131.

Dwyer A, Aprill C, Bogduk N. Cervical zygapophyseal joint pain patterns I: a study in normal volunteers. *Spine*. 1990;15(6):453-457.

Edeling J. Cervicogenic, tension-type headache with migraine: a case study. *Journal of Manual & Manipulative Therapy*. 1997;5(1):33-38.

Erhard RE, Hagan BF. Evaluation of acute torticollis in an adult with a history of childhood torticollis. *Journal of Manual & Manipulative Therapy*. 1997;5(3):107-113.

Feinstein B, Langton JBK, Jameson RM, Schiller F. Experiments on referred pain from somatic tissues. *J Bone Joint Surg*. 1954;36A:981-997.

Gross J, Fetto J, Rosen E. *Musculoskeletal Examination*. 2nd ed. Cambridge, Mass: Blackwell Science; 2002.

Hanten WP, Olson SL, Ludwig GM. Reliability of manual mobility testing of the upper cervical spine in subjects with cervicogenic headache. *Journal of Manual & Manipulative Therapy*. 2002;10(2):76-82.

Hamilton J, Dagg K, Sturrock, R, Anderson J, Banham S. Sleep apnea caused by rheumatoid arthritis. *Rheumatology*. 1999;38:679.

Horn C, Smith KL. Cervicogenic headache part II: clinical examination, findings, and approaches to management. *Journal of Manual & Manipulative Therapy*. 1997;5(4):171-175.

Isaacs ER, Bookhout MR. *Bourdillon's Spinal Manipulation*. 6th ed. Boston, Mass: Butterworth-Heinemann; 2002.

Jonsson H, Cesarini K, Sahlstedt B, Rauschnig W. Findings and outcome in whiplash-type neck distortions. *Spine*. 1994;19(24):2733-2743.

Konin JG, Wiksten DL, Isear JA, Brader H. *Special Tests for Orthopedic Examination*. 2nd ed. Thorofare, NJ: SLACK Incorporated; 2002.

Lord S, Barnsley L, Wallace B, Bogduk N. Third occipital nerve headache: a prevalence study. *J Neurol Neurosurg Psychiatry*. 1994;57:1187-1190.

Magee DJ. *Orthopedic Physical Assessment*. 4th ed. Philadelphia, Pa: Saunders; 2002.

Makofsky HW. Update on headache classification and the implications for orthopaedic physical therapists. *Journal of Manual & Manipulative Therapy*. 1994;2(1):7-10.

McKenzie RA. *The Cervical and Thoracic Spine: Mechanical Diagnosis and Therapy*. New Zealand: Spinal Publications; 1990.

Meloche JP, Bergeron Y, Bellavance A, Moland M, Huot J, Belzile G. Painful intervertebral dysfunction: Robert Maigne's original contribution to headache of cervical origin. The Quebec Headache Study Group. *Headache*. 1993;33:328-334.

Mercer S. The menisci of the cervical synovial joints. In: Boyling JD, Palastanga N, eds. *Grieve's Modern Manual Therapy*. 2nd ed. Edinburgh: Churchill Livingstone; 1994.

Mitchell FL, Mitchell PKG. *The Muscle Energy Manual, Vol. 1, Concepts and Mechanisms, the Musculoskeletal Screen, Cervical Region Evaluation and Treatment*. East Lansing, Mich: MET Press; 1995.

Moeti P, Marchetti G. Clinical outcome from mechanical intermittent cervical traction for the treatment of cervical radiculopathy: a case series. *J Orthop Sports Phys Ther*. 2001;31(4):207-213.

Nicholson GG. Cervical headache. *J Orthop Sports Phys Ther*. 2001;31(4):184-193.

Norris JW, Beletsky V, Nadareishvili ZG. Sudden neck movement and cervical artery dissection. *CMAJ*. 2000;163(1):38-40.

Ono K, Ebara S, Fuji T, Yonenobu K, Fujiwara K, Yamashita K. Myelopathy hand. New clinical signs of cervical cord damage. *J Bone Joint Surg*. 1987;69B(2):215-219.

Oostendorp R, VanEupen A, VanErp J, Elvers H. Dizziness following whiplash injury: a neuro-otological study in manual therapy practice and therapeutic implication. *Journal of Manual & Manipulative Therapy*. 1999;7(3):123-130.

Pearce JMS. The importance of cervicogenic headache in the over-fifties. *Headache Quarterly*. 1995;6(4):293-296.

Rocabado M. Biomechanical relationship of the cranial, cervical, and hyoid regions. *J Craniomandibular Pract*. 1983;1(3):61-66.

Smith KL, Horn C. Cervicogenic headache part I: an anatomic and clinical overview. *Journal of Manual & Manipulative Therapy*. 1997;5(4):158-170.

Van Suijlekom JA, De Vet HCW, Van de Berg SGM, Weber WEJ. Interobserver reliability of diagnostic criteria for cervicogenic headache. *Cephalgia*. 1999;19:817-823.

Vernon H, Mior S. The neck disability index: a study of reliability and validity. *J Manipulative Physiol Ther*. 1991;14:411.

Vincent MB, Luna RA. Cervicogenic headache: a comparison with migraine and tension type headache. *Cephalgia*. 1999;19(Suppl 25):11-16.

Viti JA, Paris SV. The use of upper thoracic manipulation in a patient with headache. *Journal of Manual & Manipulative Therapy*. 2000;8(1):25-28.

Watson D, Trott P. Cervical headache: an investigation of natural head posture and upper cervical flexor muscle performance. *Cephalgia*. 1993;13:272-284.

Wrisley DM, Sparto PJ, Whitney SL, Furman JM. Cervicogenic dizziness: a review of diagnosis and treatment. *J Orthop Sports Phys Ther*. 2000;30(12):755-766.

Zwart JA. Neck mobility in different headache disorders. *Headache*. 1997;37:6-11.

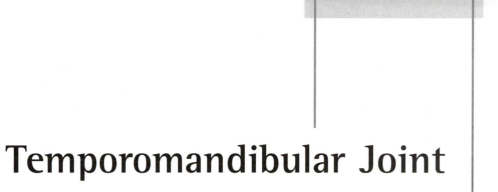

Temporomandibular Joint

Examination and Evaluation of the Temporomandibular Joint

Posture

The analysis of craniomandibular alignment or posture is a complex science that requires expertise in general dentistry, orthodontics, oral and maxillofacial surgery, as well as in physical medicine. For those therapists with advanced training in the temporomandibular joint (TMJ), including an understanding of cranial osteopathy, the analysis of craniofacial structure is an essential component of the examination. However, there is more emphasis placed on the analysis of mandibular range of motion, soft tissue palpation, and the influence of the cervical spine at the introductory level then on structural alignment, including the assessment of dental occlusion. However, a basic examination of the TMJ/facial region should note deviations from the normal orthognathic position, including horizontal deficiency of the lower jaw (ie, retrognathia) resulting in a lower facial convexity, horizontal excess of the mandible (ie, prognathia) resulting in a lower facial concavity, and coronal plane asymmetry of the craniofacial region in which one side of the face is convex and the other concave (ie, facial "scoliosis").

As mentioned, the examination of dental occlusion is beyond the scope of this introductory textbook. However, certain dental concepts are useful in terms of understanding the role of head-neck posture in both craniomandibular kinesiology and pathokinesiology. The term *maximum intercuspation* (MIP) refers to the position of the upper and lower teeth in the fully clenched state of the upper and lower jaws. It is a function of tooth anatomy and geometry and is unaffected by transient changes in head-neck position. The term *vertical dimension of occlusion* (VDO) refers to the distance from the nose to the chin with the teeth in the MIP. It, too, is a structurally determined dental relationship that is unaffected by anything other than occlusion. The dental profession alone has exclusive rights by virtue of their training and expertise to manage pathology, impairment, functional limitation, and disability related to MIP and VDO. Having said that, there are other dental concepts that are influenced by functional factors, including head-neck posture, that clearly fall within the domain of the physical therapy profession. Five such concepts that are related and that clearly fall within the functional realm are mandibular rest position, interocclusal or freeway space, the habitual pathway of closure, initial tooth contact position, and the vertical dimension of rest (VDR). Though many would argue that these concepts are also dental in nature, there is no doubt that extradental factors (eg, head-neck posture) also play a role. For example, it has been established that head-neck extension exerts a posterior force on the mandible, which changes the pathway of mandibular closure and shifts the initial tooth contacts posteriorly.[1] With regard to head-neck posture, it has been demonstrated that forward head posture (FHP) exerts a superiorly directed force on the mandible that alters the rest position of the mandible and decreases freeway space as well as VDR.[2] Consequently, the basic examination of mandibular posture must include an inspection of the influences from below, namely an examination of the cervical and scapulothoracic region as previously covered.

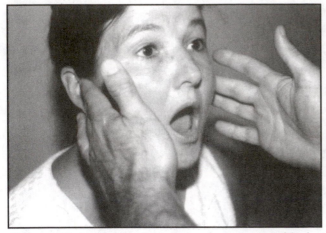

Figure 13-1a. TMJ palpatation during mandibular depression.

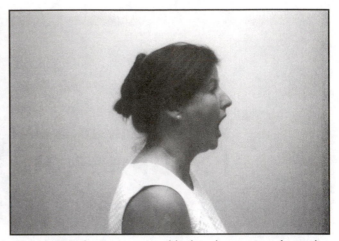

Figure 13-1b. Active mandibular depression from the side.

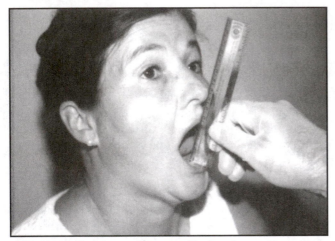

Figure 13-1c. Measuring mandibular depression.

Active Mandibular Movements

There are four active movements of the mandible that will be assessed. They include mandibular depression (opening), lateral excursion to the right and left, and protrusion.

When assessing depression of the mandible, the examiner must do the following:

1. Palpate the lateral poles of the mandibular condyles for joint sounds (Figure13-1a).
2. Observe for mandibular deflections and deviations (see Figure13-1a) from the front.
3. Observe for premature and/or excessive anterior mandibular translation from the side (Figure 13-1b).
4. Measure (Figure 13-1c) the maximal interincisal opening (MIO).

The normal TMJ (Figure 13-2) is freely moveable, friction-free, and noise-free.[3] However, in the impaired TMJ there are basically three types of joint sounds that can be palpated. They are clicking, crepitus, and a popping sound or "thud." Most clicks are single, short duration noises associated with a reducing disc displacement. They can be palpated during opening and/or closing and may occur at any point in the opening/closing cycle. When a TMJ demonstrates both opening and closing clicking, the term *reciprocal clicking* is used. This is a sign of an anterior disc displacement (ADD) with reduction (Figure 13-3a). The opening click is typically more pronounced than the closing click, which may require auscultation with a stethoscope in order to be heard. This is in contrast to an ADD without reduction (ie, a closed-lock of the TMJ) in which joint clicking is absent (Figure 13-3b). Reciprocal clicking must be distinguished from the clicking that occurs secondary to an articular surface defect. Whereas an articular surface defect click will occur at the same point in the opening and closing cycle, reciprocal clicking rarely occurs at the same point in both opening and closing. The opening click usually occurs beyond 20 mm and the closing click occurs just before the teeth meet in occlusion. Crepitus is a grating or gravelly noise associated with degenerative joint disease of which the TMJ is not excluded. A loud popping noise or thud palpated at the end of opening indicates TMJ hypermobility. This occurs as the disc and mandibular condyle, together, translate past the articular eminence of the temporal bone. This hypermobility can be confined to the TMJ or be a generalized state of increased motion throughout the body. When the disc/condyle complex translates anterior to the articular eminence and cannot return to its normal anatomic position, it is considered dislocated or an open-lock (Figure 13-4).

The second aspect of examining depression involves observing deflections and deviations of the mandible. The

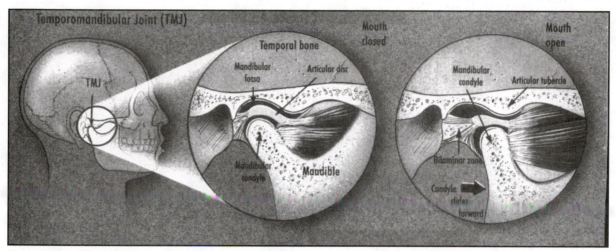

Figure 13-2. The TMJ at rest and in mouth opening (reprinted from Makofsky H, Morrone L. TMJ home exercise program. *Clinical Management in Physical Therapy.* 1991;11[2], with permission of the American Physical Therapy Association).

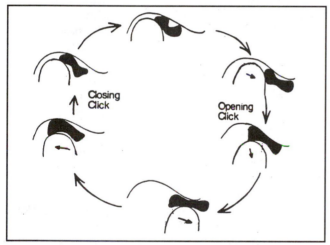

Figure 13-3a. Right TMJ anterior disc displacement with reduction.

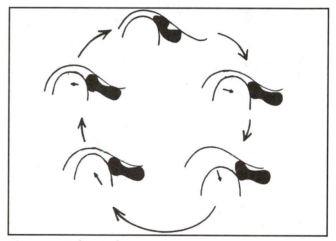

Figure 13-3b. Right TMJ anterior disc displacement without reduction (closed-lock).

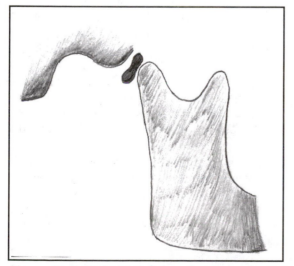

Figure 13-4. Right TMJ dislocation (open-lock).

mandible is said to deflect when it shifts from its midline position to either the right or the left side and fails to return to the midline. Deflections occur when the mandibular condyle has restricted anterior translation on the ipsilateral side and/or excessive translation on the contralateral side. For example, if translation is restricted on the right, a deflection will occur to the right; if excessive on the right, a deflection will occur to the left (usually toward the end of range).

The pathology leading to impairment of translation is most often due to either unilateral capsular tightness or an ADD without reduction. Although the underlying pathology is different (ie, capsular versus intracapsular), the deflection of the depressing mandible to the side of impairment is the same. The mandible is said to deviate when, it shifts to one side of midline during opening, but then returns as opening continues. Deviations during opening, when correlated to ipsilateral reciprocal clicking, are usually secondary to an ADD with reduction. Whereas the anteriorly displaced disc causes a shift of the lower jaw to the

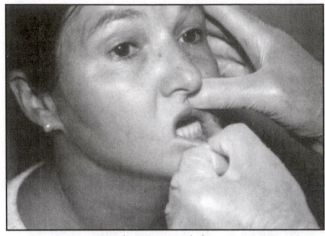

Figure 13-5a. Lateral excursion left.

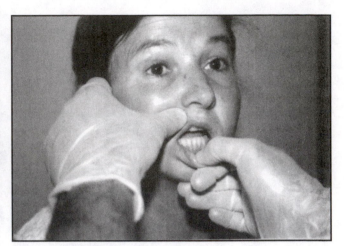

Figure 13-5b. Lateral excursion right.

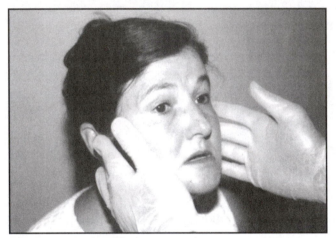

Figure 13-6. Mandibular protrusion.

(TMD) is premature and/or excessive translation. It is this premature and/or excessive translation that causes mechanical stress and strain within the tissues of the TMJ, leading to the common development of hypermobility.

The normal range of mandibular depression (MIO) is between 40 to 50 mm, as measured between the upper and lower anterior incisors (see Figure 13-1c). In the absence of a metric ruler, the patient is asked to place his or her knuckles between the upper and lower teeth in a sideways manner. One knuckle opening is hypomobile, two is low normal, three is high normal, and four tends toward hypermobility.

Normal range for mandibular lateral excursion is 8 mm to either side. A metric ruler can be used, but an easier method involves observing the lower lip frenulum as the lower jaw moves from side to side (Figures 13-5a and 13-5b). The therapist's gloved hand pulls the lower lip down to expose the frenulum. With the teeth slightly apart, the patient moves his or her mandible to the right and then to the left. Since the anterior upper incisor is approximately 8 mm in width, normal lateral excursion involves the lower lip frenulum clearing the upper anterior incisor on each respective side. Thus the patient's lateral excursions can be evaluated without the use of a ruler if desired. If impairment of motion is present, it can be described as minimal, moderate, or severe. Conversely, excessive motion should also be noted. For those patients who have difficulty coordinating lateral excursion of the mandible, placing the tongue on the upper, back molar will assist with lateral motion to that side. A distinction should be made between restricted mobility and incoordination.

The final active mandibular movement to assess is protrusion (Figure 13-6). The examination of mandibular protrusion includes palpating the lateral poles of the condyles for joint sounds, observing the motion for deflections and deviations, and measuring the quantity of motion present. Normal protrusion should obtain to 8 mm. A simple way of assessing this is to ask the patient to place his or her lower teeth anterior to the upper teeth. If this can be achieved,

affected side (due to a momentary interruption of mandibular translation), the return of the mandible to midline occurs when the displaced disc is reduced. This disc reduction (ie, normalization of position) produces the characteristic opening click. The closing click occurs when the condyle slips off the posterior aspect of the disc, usually at the end of closing.

Mandibular depression should also be assessed from the side (see Figure 13-1b). For simplicity's sake, depression of the mandible can be divided into three phases. The initial phase of opening consists of an X axis rotation. The middle phase consists of a combination of X axis rotation and translation of the mandible along the Z or anteroposterior axis, and the final phase of opening consists primarily of further translation along the Z axis. It is believed that rotational motion within the TMJ occurs in the inferior joint compartment between the head of the condyle and the articular disc, whereas translation or sliding motion occurs in the superior compartment of the TMJ, between the disc and articular eminence of the temporal bone. A common pattern seen in patients with temporomandibular disorders

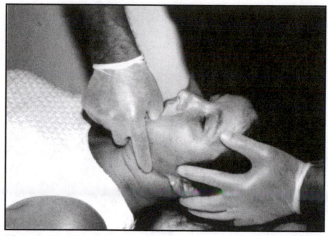

Figure 13-7.

then the motion has normal range. Abnormal motion can be described as minimal, moderate, or severe limitation or hypermobility. The clinical interpretation of joint sounds and deflections/deviations in protrusion is similar to the same findings in the opening/closing cycle of the mandible as discussed previously.

Intraoral Joint Play Motion

There are two indications for the use of intraoral joint play motion testing. One is suspected capsular hypomobility and the other is the likelihood of an ADD without reduction or a closed-lock (see Figure 13-3b). Because the TMJ is more often a disorder of hypermobility than hypomobility, manual therapists must be careful not to subject these tissues to unnecessary mechanical stress.

The indications of capsular hypomobility are as follows:

1. A history of macrotrauma to the jaw with subsequent inflammation and/or a history of jaw immobilization following surgery, infection, or as an intervention for TMD.

2. The presence of a capsular pattern when impairment is unilateral (ie, restricted depression associated with deflection to the affected side, restricted lateral excursion to the contralateral side, and restricted protrusion with mandibular deflection to the affected side).

In the presence of bilateral impairment, the mandible will not deflect nor deviate, but will demonstrate limitation in the normal range of depression, lateral excursion to either side, and protrusion.

The indications of an intracapsular closed-lock are a prior history of reciprocal clicking and intermittent closed locking and the presence of a capsular pattern as above (the term *capsular pattern* is used to describe the pattern of motion loss and is not a reflection of the structure(s) at fault). Though a closed-lock can occur following a single

macrotrauma, it usually occurs in response to cumulative microtrauma over a period of time and is associated with such parafunctional activities as bruxism, nail biting, gum chewing, and other nonessential activities that stress and strain the internal supportive structures of the TMJ.

Consequently, intraoral joint play testing of the TMJ is helpful in confirming the diagnosis of TMJ hypomobility and is useful in distinguishing a tight capsule from a nonreducing disc displacement (though a closed-lock results in hypomobility, its precursor, the ADD with reduction, is actually a form of hypermobility between the condyle and articular disc). Though an MRI examination is the gold standard for the diagnosis of a closed-lock, the MRI should not be ordered unless TMJ surgery is being considered. The difference between a tight capsule and a closed-lock relative to intraoral joint play testing is twofold. The trained manual therapist is usually able to detect a difference in the end-feel. Whereas the tight capsule has a slight degree of "creep" or "give" at the end-range, the nonreducing disc derangement is less yielding and is often associated with muscle splinting, which makes the end-feel even firmer. However, the more significant distinction between the two is found in the response to manipulation. Whereas the tight capsule gains millimeters, the closed-lock gains centimeters of increased motion. This distinction holds true whenever an internal derangement is reduced and a joint is "unlocked" (eg, the knee, spine, elbow).

There are three joint play motions of the TMJ that will be assessed intraorally. They are long axis distraction, lateral glide, and anterior glide. The therapist stands on the side opposite the joint to be mobilized and stabilizes the head while monitoring the affected joint with either the middle or index finger. The gloved thumb of the other hand is placed intraorally on the mandibular arch with the index finger alongside the body of the mandible extraorally. This examination technique is demonstrated with the patient in the supine position (Figure 13-7), but it can also be performed with the patient sitting.

For each of the intraoral movements tested, the quantity (a 0 to 6 scale), quality, tissue reactivity, and end-feel are assessed. Long axis distraction involves separation of the mandibular condyle away from the temporal fossa in a caudal direction, lateral glide involves translatoric motion in a straight lateral direction, and anterior glide consists of a translatoric motion in a forward or protrusive direction. Because of the potential for the cusps of the mandibular teeth to cause discomfort to the therapist's thumb, it is suggested that a sterile gauze pad be used as a cushion.

Soft Tissue Palpation

As with the palpation of other regions of the musculoskeletal system, the three markers of soft tissue impairment include an assessment of tenderness, tightness, and tone. Tightness involves an increase in myofascial density

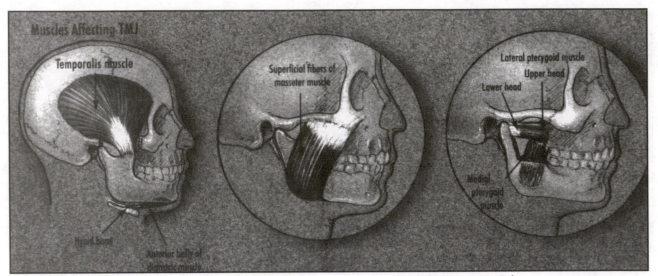

Figure 13-8. The muscles of mastication (reprinted from Makofsky H, Morrone L. *TMJ home exercise program. Clinical Management in Physical Therapy.* 1991;11[2], with permission of the American Physical Therapy Association).

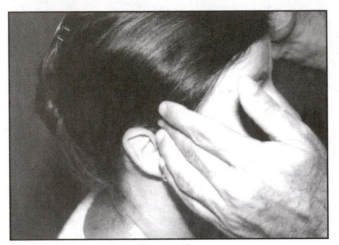

Figure 13-9a. Temporalis muscle.

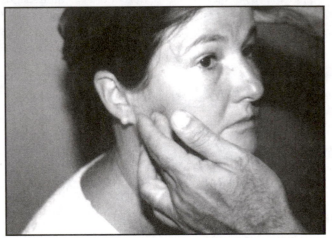

Figure 13-9b. Masseter muscle.

without associated hypertonicity, whereas an increase in tone (eg, splinting, guarding, bracing, etc) is neuroreflexive in nature and points to the presence of increased tissue reactivity as discussed previously in Chapter 3. Extracapsular impairment of the TMJ (ie, myofascial pain) is common in patients suffering from TMD. It can occur in conjunction with a capsular impairment, intracapsular derangement, or be found in the presence of a normal TMJ.

The basic evaluation of the TMJ soft tissues (Figure 13-8) consists of an extraoral examination (Figures 13-9a to 13-9e) of the following structures:

➡ Temporalis muscle (anterior, middle, and posterior fibers)

➡ Masseter muscle (no distinction made between superficial and deep fibers)

➡ Medial pterygoid muscle

➡ The soft tissues lateral and posterior to the mandibular condyle (ie, TMJ ligament, joint capsule laterally and posteriorly, and the lateral collateral ligament)

➡ The lateral pole of the condyle is palpated in the closed mouth position, but the mouth should be open to access the posterior aspect of the joint capsule, immediately behind the condyle. (Note: Some examiners perform this palpation through the external auditory meatus, but this can be unnecessarily painful for the patient.)

For an overview of the differential diagnosis of mechanical TMD, the reader is referred to Figure 13-10.

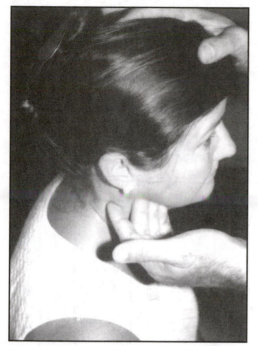

Figure 13-9c. Medial pterygoid muscle.

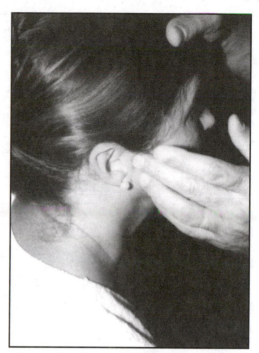

Figure 13-9d. Lateral pole in the closed mouth position (lateral structures).

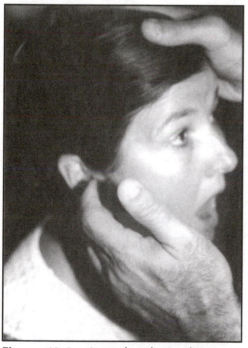

Figure 13-9e. Lateral pole in the open mouth position (posterior and lateral structures).

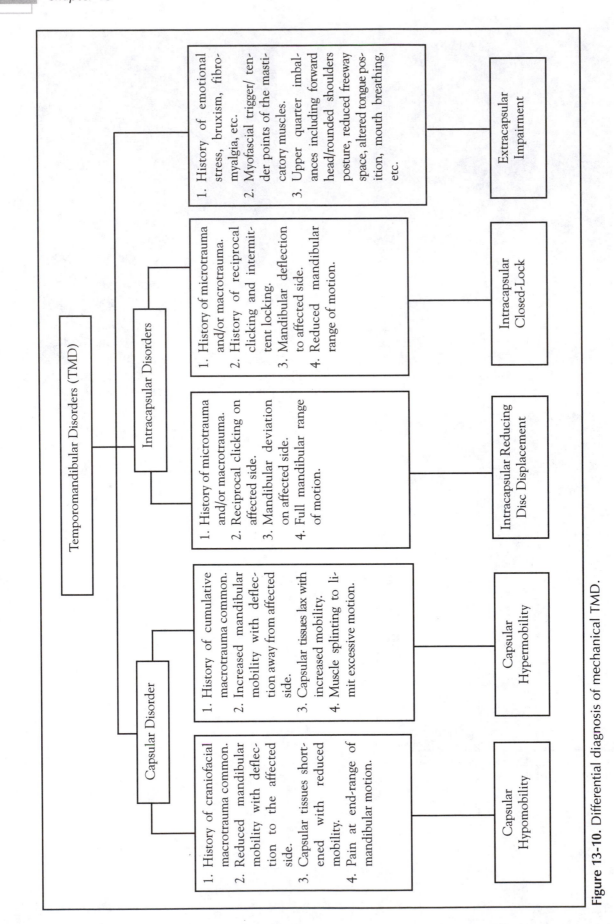

Figure 13-10. Differential diagnosis of mechanical TMD.

Connective Tissue Techniques for the Temporomandibular Joint/Facial Region

The utilization of direct fascial techniques for the purpose of achieving myofascial relaxation and relief of TMD symptoms is strongly recommended in conjunction with traditional physical therapy modalities (eg, ice, heat, electrical stimulation, ultrasound). Though intraoral soft tissue techniques are extremely useful as well, this chapter will concentrate on the more basic extraoral approach to treatment, which must be learned prior to delving into the sensitive tissues within the oral cavity. When performing myofascial massage to the TMJ/facial area, the therapist must be mindful of the emotions related to a patient's facial area. For those individuals with histories of physical abuse, touching the face may evoke unpleasant memories. The key to effective facial technique is a gentle and caring touch. Once the patient grows accustomed to having the soft tissues of the jaw and face massaged, the therapist is then able to explore the release of deep tissue tension, myofascial trigger points, and muscle holding states. For a review of the principles of direct fascial technique, the reader is referred to Chapter 5. A small amount of massage or hand cream is helpful when working in the craniofacial region.

Frontalis

The frontalis muscle, as with many of the TMJ/facial muscles, is overactive in many patients, often resulting in forehead wrinkles, frontal headache, and at times compression of the supraorbital nerve. Because the frontalis is contiguous with the occipitalis muscle (occipitofrontalis), this cutaneous muscle of the scalp will often require treatment of both components. Direct fascial technique of this epicranial muscle, along with the connecting temporoparietalis, can bring significant relief in patients suffering from chronic and episodic tension-type headache. Figure 14-1 illustrates a connective tissue technique that separates the muscle fibers of the frontalis in a medial to lateral direction. This approach can be extended posteriorly to include the occipitalis and laterally to include the temporoparietalis.

Corrugator, Orbicularis Oculi, and Procerus

The corrugator supercilii muscle (Figure 14-2) runs from the medial end of the superciliary arch to the deep surface of the skin above the middle of the orbital arch. It can be a source of pain at the medial and inferior aspect of the eyebrows and is overworked in patients who are habitual frowners. The orbicularis oculi is the closing muscle of the eye and is often tender and tight in patients who habitually squint. Proper eyeglasses and/or sunglasses will often remedy this problem. Direct fascial technique of these muscles must be performed with sensitivity, especially when releasing the taut fibers of the orbicularis oculi as they insert into the orbit and frontal bone above the eye. While in the upper nasal region, the procerus muscle should also be treated with gentle direct fascial technique, if necessary.

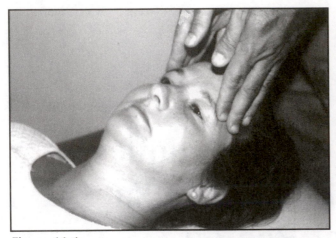

Figure 14-1.

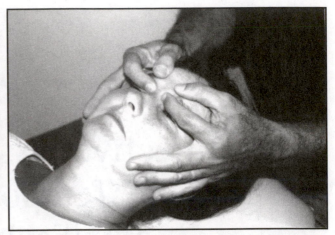

Figure 14-2.

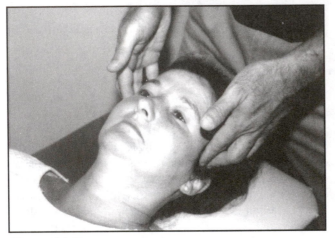

Figure 14-3.

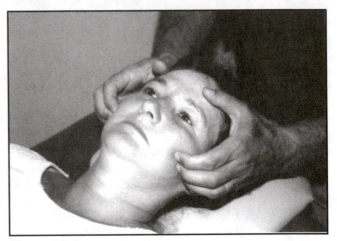

Figure 14-4.

It arises from either side of the nasal bone and runs upward to insert into the skin over the lower part of the forehead between the eyebrows. When the procerus muscles contract, the skin of the nose is pulled upward as the lower forehead is pulled down, forming horizontal wrinkles between the eyebrows and over the bridge of the nose. It is the facial muscle responsible for the expression of distaste.

Temporalis

The temporalis muscle (Figure 14-3) is commonly involved in patients with TMD, especially in those suffering from extracapsular/myofascial impairment associated with bruxism and emotional stress; it is also a source of symptoms in patients suffering from tension-type headache. In addition, there appears to be a correlation between forward head posture (FHP) and increased temporalis activity in which the mandible is displaced posterior and superior, thus reducing the interocclusal freeway space.[4] Consequently, treatment of the temporalis muscle with direct fascial technique is beneficial in a variety of musculoskeletal conditions.

The therapist works in a direction perpendicular to the fibers and addresses all aspects of the muscle, including the anterior, middle, and posterior fibers. As with all soft tissue mobilizations, the goal is to soften, relax, and improve local circulation to the area in hopes of relieving painful symptoms and restoring normal function. It is also important that the therapist identify and correct all related impairments (eg, posture, jaw parafunction, stress) so that temporalis tone can return to a normal level.

Masseter

The masseter muscle (Figure 14-4) is a powerful elevator of the mandible and is commonly involved in the presence of restricted jaw opening. Myofascial trigger points of the superficial fibers result in facial pain. Involvement of the deep layer can be a cause of TMJ and ear symptoms. In addition to ipsilateral ear pain, the deep fibers can also be a source of tinnitus.

There is no attempt to differentiate the superficial from the deep layer when performing direct fascial technique to the masseter muscle. The therapist will find the most

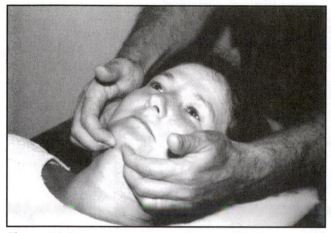

Figure 14-5.

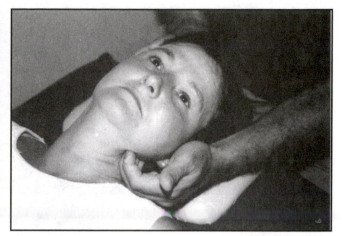

Figure 14-6.

myofascial impairment (ie, tenderness, tightness, and tone) along the inferior aspect of the zygomatic arch and all along the angle and ramus of the mandible. Digital oscillations along these bony landmarks is quite effective in achieving the desired release of tension in this area.

Suprahyoids

The suprahyoids (Figure 14-5) include the mylohyoid, stylohyoid, geniohyoid, and digastric muscles (anterior and posterior bellies). With FHP, the infrahyoids are under stretch but the suprahyoids tend to shorten as their origin and insertion approximate. This shortening will retrude the mandible and elevate the hyoid bone both of which can adversely affect swallowing and the rest position of the mandible. Whereas myofascial trigger points in the mylohyoid muscle can refer pain to the tongue, trigger points in the stylohyoid and posterior belly of the digastric can cause head and neck pain. In addition, dentists should be aware that myofascial dysfunction of the anterior belly of the digastric can refer pain into the lower incisors.[5]

Medial Pterygoid

The medial pterygoid (Figure 14-6) along with the masseter and temporalis muscles is an elevator of the mandible. In patients who clench and grind their teeth, these muscles are prone to developing myofascial pain. Because of the proximity to the tensor veli palatini muscle, hypertrophy of the medial pterygoid muscle may contribute to barohypoacusis (ie, ear stuffiness). Other myofascial symptoms include referred mouth, jaw, and ear pain.

Palpation for examination and intervention can be accomplished either intraorally or extraorally. Palpation extraorally is accomplished by having the patient tilt his or her head to the ipsilateral side in order to slacken the tis-

sues and permit greater access. The inner aspect of the angle of the mandible is explored with the palpating finger(s) as it presses in a superior and medial direction. The inferior fibers of the muscle's mandibular attachment are thereby accessed and treated with the appropriate direct fascial procedure. Strumming over taut fibers is especially useful in diminishing tone and restoring extensibility to the medial pterygoid muscle.

In addition to connective tissue techniques, electrotherapeutic modalities, heat or ice, biofeedback, spray and stretch with fluorimethane spray, acupuncture, and mandibular appliances are also useful nonmedicinal interventions when dealing with TMD of muscular origin. If indicated, the use of trigger point injections and short term muscle relaxants should be discussed with the patient's dentist and/or physician. With regard to the role of intraoral devices, the NTI-TSS (Nociceptive Trigeminal Inhibition Tension Suppression System) has shown promise for the management of nocturnal bruxism and may be an effective nonmedicinal intervention in the prevention of primary headache.[6] By disoccluding the posterior teeth, the clenching muscles are inhibited. Therefore, bruxism is also controlled, and the entire trigeminal afferent system is "defacilitated," explaining the therapeutic role of the NTI-TSS in both migraine and tension-type headaches.

Lateral Pole

There are several soft tissue attachments into the lateral pole of the mandibular condyle (Figure 14-7) that respond well to soft tissue mobilization. The author finds circular friction to be the intervention of choice in this region. The structures from superficial to deep include the TMJ ligament (outer-oblique and inner-horizontal fibers); the articular capsule, which is reinforced by the TMJ ligament; and the lateral collateral ligament, which secures the TMJ disc to the lateral pole. Circular friction around the lateral pole

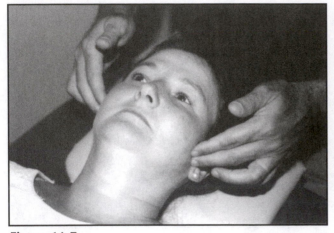

Figure 14-7.

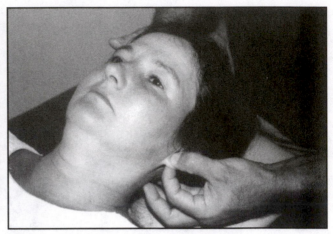

Figure 14-8.

assists with decongestion of venous and lymphatic stasis, an increase in arterial flow, and relief of painful symptoms through the stimulation of various mechanoreceptors.

Auricular Acupressure

The final manual soft tissue technique for the TMJ involves the use of ear acupressure, which is known as auriculotherapy. This system of therapy can be traced back to Ancient China but received modern day notoriety because of the work of the French neurologist, Dr. Paul Nogier. It was Nogier who developed the Somatotopic Map of the Ear, based upon an inverted fetus orientation, which was subsequently verified in modern China in the 1960s.

Practitioners of auriculotherapy[7] claim to make use of various ear points in both diagnosis and intervention. The use of needles or pressure at specific points is used by these practitioners to manage a plethora of musculoskeletal pain conditions, including headache and TMD. Neurologically, the auricle is differentially innervated by the trigeminal, facial, glossopharyngeal, vagus, and superior cervical plexus nerves, making it a rich sensory area of the body for the purpose of relieving painful symptoms. The analgesia attained in response to auriculotherapy is not well understood, but may be a function of the spinal "gating" mechanism, descending neural inhibition, and/or endorphin release.

To effect the relief of pain and muscle guarding in the TMJ/facial region, the therapist applies pressure to the lowermost aspect of the helix tail at its junction with the lobe for approximately 2 minutes (Figure 14-8). It is suggested that both ears be treated simultaneously. Even though specific points are assigned to various conditions, the author has found a generalized examination of the lobe, antitragus,

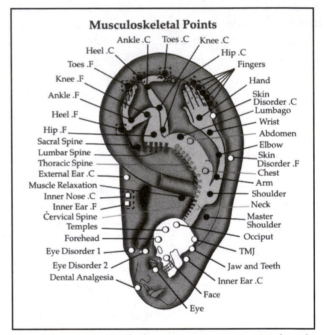

Figure 14-9. Auriculotherapy points (reprinted with permission from Oleson T. *Auriculotherapy Manual: Chinese and Western Systems of Ear Acupuncture.* Los Angeles, Calif: Health Care Alternatives; 1996).

and inferior helix tail to reveal heightened areas of sensitivity and soft tissue density that, when treated with digital pressure, give several hours of relief of head, jaw, and face pain (Figure 14-9).

The reader is encouraged to explore this exciting modality for the temporary relief of painful symptoms in other areas of the body as well.

Intraoral Manipulation of the Temporomandibular Joint

As discussed previously, there are two conditions under which the TMJ becomes hypomobile. They are capsular impairment and a closed-lock (ie, anterior disc displacement without reduction). In this chapter, both causes of TMJ hypomobility will be addressed with intraoral manipulation. In the case of a tight and restricted capsule, the purpose will be to restore normal extensibility to the dysfunctional connective tissues through a series of joint play movements. In the case of an internal derangement, the purpose is to reduce the disc displacement and return it to a more normal and functional position. The author's experience in the management of TMD patients is that manipulation is seldom required as the vast majority of patients are hypermobile and instead require neuromuscular stabilization. In fact, a closed-lock is the terminal stage of hypermobility and it must be followed by a stabilization regimen when reduction is accomplished. In this chapter, the patient is positioned in supine (Figure 15-1). The advantage of the supine position is greater relaxation of the masticatory muscles. However, manual intraoral mobilization of the TMJ can also be performed in the sitting position if necessary.

Long Axis Distraction

The therapist's gloved thumb is placed intraorally over the mandibular arch on the posterior molar region while the other hand stabilizes the cranium. As with all manipulative procedures, the joint being mobilized should be mon-

itored throughout the technique, in this case with the middle or index fingers at the lateral pole. As noted previously, the gloved thumb should be protected from the mandibular teeth with a sterile gauze pad.

Gentle long axis distraction involves separation of the mandibular condyle away from the mandibular fossa in a direction perpendicular to the fossa but parallel to the long axis of the mandibular ramus. Joint distraction is given a grade of 1 through 3 with 1 = joint unloading (Piccolo traction), 2 = the soft tissue slack is taken up, and 3 = the tissues are stretched beyond the slack to patient tolerance. As the therapist's thumb presses in an inferior direction, the other fingers simultaneously provide an upward force on the patient's chin.

Anterior Glide

Anterior glide or translation should be performed in conjunction with either grade 1, 2, or 3 distraction to avoid compression of the joint structures. The technique is performed as with long axis distraction with the addition of a pulling force on the mandible in an anterior direction. To enhance the stretch, the mandible can be mobilized anteriorly and slightly across midline, but only in those patients who show capsular impairment without signs of internal disc derangement.

Because the patient will be unable to speak during the intraoral procedure, he or she should indicate discomfort by raising his or her hand. The therapist should avoid exces-

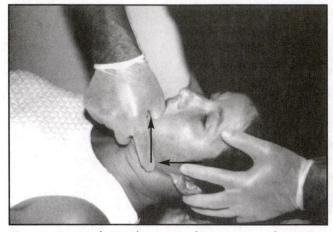

Figure 15-1. Left TMJ long axis distraction and anterior glide manipulation.

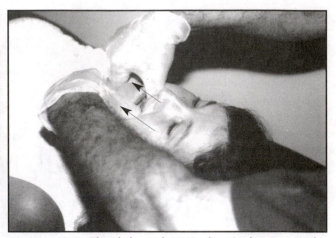

Figure 15-2. The bilateral TMJ disc reduction technique.

sive force on tissues that are prone to hypermobility and avoid working through pain except in rare cases of fibrous ankylosis in which some degree of discomfort is expected.

Lateral Glide

Lateral glide is achieved by applying a lateral force to the lingual surface of the posterior molar or to the lingual gum tissue on the side being treated. To avoid contralateral TMJ pain during this technique, the mandible should be slightly distracted and anteriorly glided.

With all the above joint play movements of the TMJ, graded mobilization is useful. As with other joints, grade 1 movements are used in the presence of high tissue reactivity, grade 2 and 3 movements are used in moderately reactive states, and grade 4 movements are indicated when tissue reactivity is low.

Manual Reduction of a Closed-Lock

The author has been comparing the efficacy of a unilateral manipulative technique to a bilateral approach for some time and has determined that patients with a closed-lock prefer and respond better to the bilateral approach. The muscles appear to "guard" less and the TMJ allows for more manipulative force when both joints are mobilized simultaneously. The goal in either method is to distract the TMJ enough to allow the disc to slide back over the head of the condyle so that condylar anterior translation can proceed without obstruction.

The bilateral reduction technique to unlock either the right and/or left TMJ will now be described (Figure 15-2). The patient must be assured that with the raising of a hand the manual reduction will be aborted immediately. At no time is the joint to be forcefully "unlocked." Rather, it should be coaxed open in a gentle manner without anything more than mild discomfort. With both hands gloved and gauze pads wrapped around the thumbs, the therapist makes contact with the posterior mandibular molars, bilaterally. While stabilizing the cranium through the abdominal region, the therapist distracts both TMJs slowly to the end of range (ie, grade 3) by pressing down on the molars and lifting up under the chin. The mandible is then translated anteriorly from the distracted position to the end of range at which time the patient is asked to open his or her mouth as wide as possible. The mandible is slowly returned to the rest position and re-examined. If the closed-lock persists, a slightly different approach is used. The TMJs are again distracted and anteriorly translated. However, instead of opening the mouth wide, the patient is asked to move the lower jaw from left to right several times. Again the mandible is returned to the rest position and re-examined.

Providing the nonreducing disc displacement has been successfully "recaptured," the patient should have cotton rolls placed between the posterior molars and go immediately to the dentist for fabrication of a TMJ intraoral appliance. A temporary splint can be used until the permanent device becomes available. In some cases, patients are able to remain reduced without the appliance, but in the majority of patients with chronic closed-lock, the reduction will not hold without it. As a general rule, the shorter the duration of the closed-lock, the better the likelihood of obtaining a manual reduction without the need for TMJ surgery. When considering a referral to a TMJ surgeon for a refractory closed-lock, the indications for either an arthroscopic or open joint procedure include intractable pain, failed conservative interventions (eg, physical therapy, TMJ occlusal splint therapy, pharmacologic measures, psychological therapy), and diagnostic confirmation of a nonreducing disc displacement with MRI, discography, etc. The author has only seen the need for surgical intervention on a few occasions and it has been the patient's intractable pain that has been the deciding factor. For those patients who choose to avoid TMJ surgery, the use of good physical therapy and dental splint therapy will enable the vast majority of patients to regain close to normal function despite the presence of a nonreducing disc displacement. The TMJ has a remarkable capacity to heal and should not be subjected to irreversible interventions unless absolutely necessary.

Therapeutic and Home Exercises
for the Temporomandibular Joint

When considering the various nonsurgical options available for the management of TMDs, the following exercises should rank high on the list. These exercises are based upon the prior works of Weisberg and Friedman,[8] Rocabado,[3] Kraus,[4,9] and Mannheimer,[10] who should all be recognized for their outstanding contribution to our current understanding of the role of physical therapy in dentistry and TMD. The exercises to follow in this chapter have been available to therapists and TMJ patients for several years based upon earlier publications by the author and his colleague, Lisa Morrone.[11] The feedback from across the country has been encouraging and with only a few modifications, they will be presented in their entirety at this time. With the exception of the tongue blade stretch, these exercises are geared toward the hypermobile TMJ, which represents the majority of TMDs seen clinically.

Balancing the
Upper Half with RPTTLB

The concept of balance in the upper half (ie, cervical/thoracic spine, craniofacial region, shoulder girdle, and upper extremities) is crucial in achieving the optimum neuromusculoskeletal rest position for the joints and tissues in this region of the body. With regard to the mandible and the temporomandibular joints, the rest position is critical. The physiologic rest position of the mandible has traditionally been described as a postural relation of the mandible to the maxilla in which the mandibular condyles are in a neutral, unstrained position in the glenoid fossae and the mandibular musculature is in a state of minimum tonic contraction.[4,9] Though this concept conveys the essence of the rest position, it is incomplete. Unless the influence of the head-neck region on mandibular position is appreciated, one can never discover the true rest or neutral position of the mandible and TMJs. Because of the neuromuscular and kinesiologic affects of head posture on the craniomandibular region, it is necessary to also place the head, neck, and back into physiologic rest or a neutral relationship at the same time. The author instructs his students and patients to liken the TMJs to a car's transmission. In this "transmission" there are three "gears," in addition to neutral, consisting of first, second, and third. In addition to achieving a physiologic rest position throughout the upper half, the use of the RPTTLB method ensures that the mandible is placed in its neutral "idling" state. It is this position that affords the greatest opportunity for relaxation, pain relief, and recovery of function to the resting tissues of the TMJ. We will now proceed to describe each component of this method in greater detail.

1. Relax: The first step in this process of balancing alignment and tension involves learning to completely relax. Patients are asked to perform a self-assessment of the muscle tension throughout the neck, shoulders, jaw and face, arms, legs, and trunk on an hourly basis. The key to "turning off" unnecessary muscle tension in the body is to understand the principle that only the muscles that are essential

to the task of the moment should be working while the other muscles should be relaxed. This is a good opportunity to take a deep breath and think about something positive. It may also be an opportunity to enjoy the present moment rather than stressing about things that haven't happened and probably never will! If the patient is unable to relax his or her muscles, EMG biofeedback may be indicated.

2. Postural adjustment: In order to achieve an optimal mandibular rest position and a normal "freeway" space of approximately 3 mm, the normal head-neck relationship must also be restored.[2] For example, an attempt to normalize mandibular rest position in the presence of forward head posture (FHP) is futile. This is because occipital extension will tend to displace the mandible in a posterior and superior direction. Unless the occiput is placed in its neutral position with the Frankfurt plane horizontally oriented, one cannot achieve neutrality in the TMJs. As discussed in a previous chapter, restoring balance and alignment to the head-neck region also lengthens and widens the torso. Consequently, according to Alexander,[12] the entire spine and all four extremities benefit when the head-neck-back relationship (ie, primary control) is restored to normal. In patients with somatic impairment, there is much requisite work to be done to allow for the optimal restoration of primary control. However, the entire process of moving toward "ideal" is contingent upon the patient's awareness of acceptable and unacceptable head-neck posture; that awareness can be inculcated with the following technique. Following the patient's hourly attempt at relaxing completely, he or she is asked to imagine a "rope" attached to a large balloon pulling the back of the head (Lambda) toward the ceiling. The imaginary rope serves to prevent occipital extension (ie, downward pull) as it retrains the patient's brain in the direction of primary control. Over time, patients actually sense the "upward pull" on the back of the skull. This improved kinesthetic perception is perhaps the single most important intervention that can be taught to patients!

3. Teeth apart: The patient must understand that, except for swallowing and chewing, the teeth should not be clenched together. In order to prevent masticatory muscle overuse, the patient should regularly ensure that the teeth are apart and that the elevator muscles of the jaw are relaxed. To do this, the patient is asked to pronounce the name Emma on an hourly basis following the performance of R and P. The cumulative effect of doing this will be to open the freeway space and to restore the postural vertical dimension (ie, vertical dimension of rest [VDR]). Patients presenting with tension-type headache, chronic cervical strain, masticatory myalgia, etc are often people who are doing just the opposite and that is why they experience symptoms.

4. Tongue up: Orthodontists and myofunctional therapists have long recognized the importance of establishing the physiologic rest position of the tongue on the rugae of the hard palate.[3] Just as mandibular rest position is dependent upon head-neck posture, it is also dependent on tongue position. On an hourly basis following the performance of R, P, and T, the patient is asked to make several "clucking sounds," which will automatically place the tip of the tongue on the hard palate just above the maxillary incisors. The result of this retraining can be significant. Clenching the teeth is now made less likely because the mandible will tend to assume a "down and forward" relationship as compared to an "up and back" relationship to the maxilla. For those patients, especially children, who have an anterior tongue thrust upon swallowing, this new position of the tongue may also assist in correcting malocclusion. One of the reasons for adjusting head-neck posture prior to addressing tongue position is that the upright position of the tongue is dependent on the support of the extrinsic tongue muscles, which in turn are dependent on head-neck posture.[4] In other words, as FHP slackens the extrinsic tongue muscles by bringing the two points of attachment (styloid process and anterior portion of the mandible) closer together, adjusting the occiput in a "forward and up" direction restores normal tension to this support mechanism by separating the attachments; thus, the tongue is able to assume its upright position on the palate.

5. Lips together: The next component of the RPTTLB system involves bringing the lips together while building on the previous steps. This may appear simple enough, but in patients with a short upper lip it may not be so easy. Normally, the upper lip should cover approximately 75% of the upper teeth.[3] However, when the upper lip is short and the upper teeth are exposed, the lower lip may compensate and work harder to provide teeth coverage. This results in hyperactivity of the mentalis muscle with elevation of the lower lip and sometimes of the lower jaw. If the upper lip is short due to inadequate length of the upper lip frenulum, stretching the upper lip between the thumbs and index fingers in an out and downward direction can sometimes help. If the upper lip remains short, the patient should learn to accept this situation and not attempt to overcompensate as described above. In severe cases of deformity, as in cleft palate and lip, oral, and maxillofacial surgery may be indicated.

6. Breathe nasodiaphragmatically: The final component of this system of retraining alignment, relaxation, and optimal use in the upper half of the body involves teaching the patient to breathe nasodiaphragmatically. A common finding in patients with poor structural alignment, abnormal muscle tension, and painful symptoms in the upper half is a tendency to be upper chest and mouth breathers. There are at least two detrimental effects on posture that result. The first adverse effect is related to mouth breathing. Mouth breathers tend to extend their head-neck region in order to maximally open the upper airway. Head-neck extension enhances airflow by drawing the hyoid bone up and forward off the pharyngeal airway and secondly, by tightening the pharyngeal musculature (ie, the stylopharyngeus, palatopharyngeus, and salpingopharyngeus muscles), which makes the upper airway more patent.[13] Conversely, normal nasal breathing facilitates physiologic alignment of the head-neck region. It is when nasal breathing is obstructed (eg, septal deviation, enlarged adenoids and tonsils) that mouth breathing ensues, resulting in the loss of normal head, neck, and mandibular alignment (ie, forward head posture). For this reason, chronic nasal obstruction may at times require surgical intervention so that balance and function can be restored to the upper half of the body. In other patients, mouth breathing may have developed because of transient nasal obstruction in early childhood, but persisted due to habitual use over time. In these cases, it is possible to retrain the patient in nasal breathing without the need for surgery.

The second adverse postural effect is related to upper chest breathing. Because the accessory muscles of respiration (eg, the scalenes, sternocleidomastoid, upper trapezius, pectoralis major/minor) are overly active in the upper chest breather, the head-neck region is forced to assume a position of upper cervical extension/lower cervical flexion consistent with FHP. Consequently, the importance of teaching diaphragmatic breathing becomes obvious, not only from a respiratory-efficiency perspective but also from the perspective of normalizing postural balance to the upper half. As long as an upper chest breathing pattern persists, normal alignment cannot be restored to the head, neck, jaw, and spine.

This brings us then to the final step of the RPTTLB system, which involves teaching the patient to breathe nasodiaphragmatically. The patient is instructed to place both hands over the lower lateral costal margins and to take a deep breath in through the nose such that lateral costal and abdominal expansion predominate followed by a longer exhalation through pursed lips out the mouth. If observing in a mirror, the patient should note that the sternum remains relatively quiescent as the lower ribs and abdomen expand with inhalation and recoil with exhalation. Two to three deep breaths per hour in this manner are recommended. Many patients prefer learning proper diaphragmatic breathing in supine before attempting it in the upright position.

In summary, the RPTTLB method of balancing the upper half is an effective adjunctive measure for the manual therapist. It is to be practiced on an hourly basis, each waking hour of the day. The patient must not deviate from the prescribed order of the system, as each step is dependent on the successful performance of the previous step(s). In the beginning, patients may need several minutes to complete all six steps. However, within a week or so it can be executed in less than 30 seconds. Patients should only concentrate on the method each hour. If the patient obsesses on changing prior habits too often, the system becomes a source of stress and that should not be the case. The short form of the system is as follows:

1. Relax: Turn unnecessary muscle tension off.
2. Posture: Imagine a rope attached to a large balloon pulling the back of the head up to the ceiling, preventing a backward tilt of the head on the neck.
3. Teeth apart: Say "Emma" and allow the teeth to separate.
4. Tongue: "Cluck" the tip of the tongue against the roof of the mouth and let it remain there just above the upper teeth.
5. Lips: If possible, bring the lips lightly together.
6. Breathe: In through the nose and out the mouth with lower rather than upper chest expansion, two to three times.

For those patients who have difficulty remembering the letters, RPTTLB, the following memory jogger is recommended: "Reflective Physical Therapists Treat Languishing Bodies." Go for it!

Temporomandibular Joint Rotation/Translation Control (Phases 1 to 4)

Now that the neutral position of the TMJ "transmission" has been restored, the "gears" must also be addressed. Consistent with normal TMJ arthrokinematics, the three "gears" encompass the three phases of the opening/closing cycle (ie, rotation, rotation/translation, and translation).

Phase 1 (Figure 16-1a) is performed in the RPTTLB state in front of a mirror. The patient places the index finger over the lateral pole of the condyle on the impaired side while the other index contact is placed on the chin. Phase 1 is an active-assisted rotational motion of the TMJ about

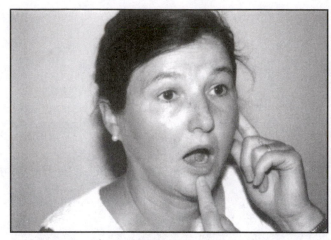

Figure 16-1a. Phase 1 opening.

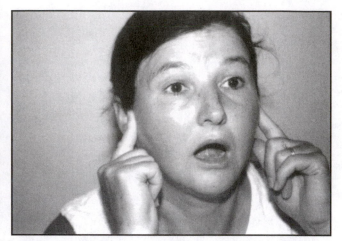

Figure 16-1b. Phase 2 opening.

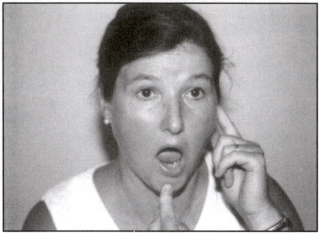

Figure 16-1c. Phase 3 opening.

the X axis. As a result of the tongue-on-palate position and the placement of the index finger on the chin, translation of the mandible is minimal to absent. Because of this, joint sounds in the TMJ are mitigated considerably. The patient is instructed to direct the chin "into the throat" with a hinge-type movement while maintaining proper head-neck posture at all times. This rotational movement is repeated five times and performed five times throughout the day. The problem with many TMJ patients is that they have premature and/or excessive translation of the mandible. The normalization of the first gear (ie, rotation only) will help to correct this problem and assist with the management of TMJ hypermobility.

Phase 2 (Figure 16-1b) is similar to phase 1 except that it is an active movement requiring a higher level of motor control. The patient is again positioned in front of a mirror in the RPTTLB state. The patient is instructed to open his or her mouth, directing the chin to the throat. The bilateral index finger contact over the condyles ensures rotational motion only without joint sounds. (Note: TMJ clicking is almost always eliminated when motion is confined to

rotation.) The mirror provides the necessary feedback to prevent deviations and deflections. Patients are progressed to phase 2 rotation once they have mastered phase 1. It replaces the previous phase and is again repeated five times and performed five times throughout the day. It, too, addresses the first gear but without the assistance of the finger-to-chin contact.

Phase 3 involves motion that includes both rotation and translation and therefore is directed toward the normalization of the second gear of the TMJ "transmission." Phase 3 begins as does phase 1 with a "rotation only" motion of the mandible. However, at the end of phase 1 opening, the patient is instructed to drop the tongue to the floor of the mouth and direct the lower jaw toward the throat. Thus, a combination of rotation/translation is introduced with the active assisted guidance of the index finger (Figure 16-1c). Phase 2 is now replaced by phase 3 and is repeated five times and performed five times per day.

Phase 4 opening addresses the third and last gear by restoring terminal translation to the disc/condyle complex. It begins as does phase 2 with the tongue on the hard palate in the RPTTLB state but proceeds from there with the patient continuing to open to the end of the active range with the tongue on the floor of the mouth (Figure 16-1d). The bilateral index contact on the TMJ ensures symmetrical joint motion with little if any joint sounds noted; the mirror continues to provide feedback in order to minimize deflections or deviations of the mandible. Phase 4 replaces phase 3 and is repeated five times and performed five times per day. Because phase 4 involves terminal translation, patients must not show signs of TMJ hypermobility when advanced to this final stage. The average patient takes 1 to 2 months of perfecting phases 1 to 3 before attempting phase 4. Consequently, the patient will often return to the clinic for a follow-up visit in order to advance to phase 4.

Having said that, patients are advised to resume phase 1 rotation immediately upon the first signs of an exacerbation of their TMJ symptoms (ie, phase 1 active assisted rotation

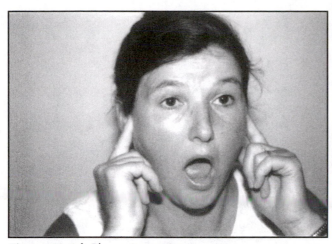

Figure 16-1d. Phase 4 opening.

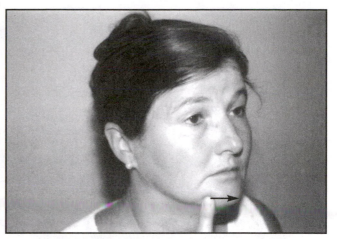

Figure 16-2a. Push to the left.

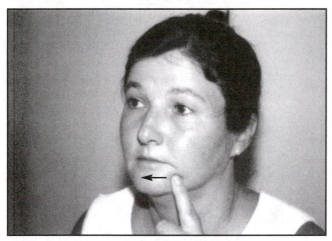

Figure 16-2b. Push to the right.

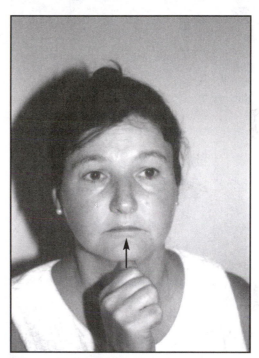

Figure 16-2c. Push upward.

has a "reducing" affect on TMJ disc derangements as well as a "relaxing" affect on muscle splinting).

TMJ Neuromusculoskeletal Stabilization (Phases 1 to 3)

The application of isometric muscle training has become popular as a means of achieving optimal neuromuscular control in many regions of the body. In the craniomandibular region, gentle isometric contractions help to reduce TMJ hypermobility as well as refine sensorimotor control of the mandible both statically and dynamically. In addition, neuromusculoskeletal stabilization training helps to alert the brain of potentially stressful postures and movements of the jaw so that the central nervous system can make the necessary adjustments to prevent injury and impairment from occurring. Although an increase in muscle strength may result from these exercises, their purpose is focused not on strength but on motor control.

As with the previous TMJ exercises, phase 1 stabilization is performed in the RPTTLB state in front of a mirror (Figures 16-2a to 16-2f). The patient is asked to apply a light pressure to the chin ("2" on a 0 to 10 scale), with his or her index finger in six different directions while maintaining the normal 3 mm freeway space between the upper and lower teeth. The mirror is used to ensure that the mandible remains stationary throughout the application of the gentle isometric force. The sequence is as follows:

1. Push to the left
2. Push to the right
3. Push upward
4. Push inward

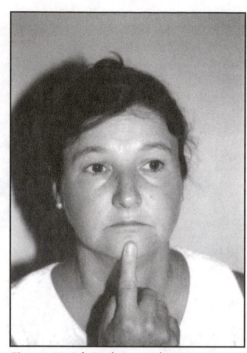

Figure 16-2d. Push inward.

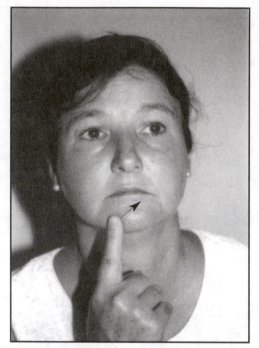

Figure 16-2e. Push to the left ear.

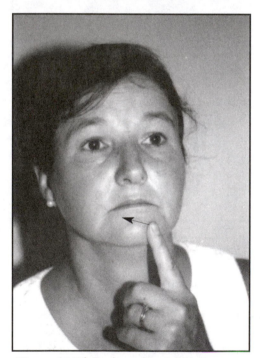

Figure 16-2f. Push to the right ear.

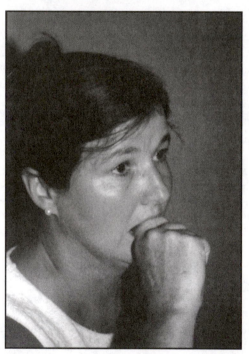

Figure 16-3. One-knuckle opening.

5. Push diagonally in the direction of the opposite ear to the left

6. Repeat step five toward the right ear

Each gentle isometric force is held for 2 seconds, repeated five times, and performed five times through the day.

Phase 2 and 3 stabilizations are similar to phase 1, except for the amount of space between the teeth. In phase 2 (Figure 16-3), the patient is asked to open to one knuckle's width; in phase 3 (Figure 16-4) to two knuckles' width. Once the desired opening is achieved, the knuckle(s) are removed and the stabilization exercises commenced. Unlike the TMJ rotation/translation control exercises in

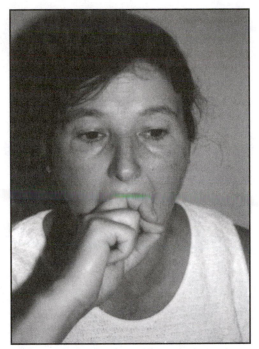

Figure 16-4. Two-knuckle opening.

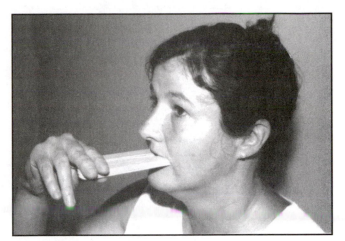

Figure 16-5.

which the subsequent phase replaced the previous one, the subsequent phase of the stabilization program is added onto the previous one. This is because the benefit of isometric exercise occurs in the specific joint position in which it is performed. Consequently, patients are progressed through all three phases over a period of weeks or months, depending upon exercise mastery and the state of tissue healing.

In the management of TMJ hypermobility, it is recommended that the above exercises (ie, RPTTLB, TMJ rotation/translation control, and TMJ stabilization) be integrated with other therapies, including pain-relieving modalities, manual therapy of hypomobile spinal joints, TMJ occlusal splint therapy, stress management/biofeedback, etc.[14] Patient compliance, however, is crucial to the overall success of the program; for this reason, a patient's willingness to commit to the exercises must be assessed early in the process.

Tongue Blade Stretch

Until this point, all self-treatment has been geared toward the management of TMJ hypermobility. However, there is a small percentage of patients who present with true capsular impairment and thus require a home program of stretching and joint mobilization. These include postsurgical TMJ and orthognathic cases, as well as healed craniomandibular fractures, which may develop adhesions and joint contracture.

There are devices on the market such as the Therabite (Therabite Corp, Newtown Square, Pa) and the Jaw Helper (MedDev Corp, Palo Alto, Calif) that are used to assist patients with self-TMJ mobility. A more recent concept involves the use of continuous passive motion (CPM) to the TMJ with the E-Z Flex (Fluid Motion Biotechnologies Inc, New York, NY), which is especially useful postoperatively to prevent fibrous ankylosis.[15]

There is, however, a simple, cost-effective way (Figure 16-5) of having the patient perform self-TMJ mobilization/stretching that the author has successfully used with nonsurgical and postoperative patients alike. The patient is shown how to use tongue blades placed between the upper and lower molars as a means of achieving an effective mobilization/stretch of the TMJs and associated elevator muscles of the jaw. Because tissues that are preheated become more extensible, the patient should also be instructed in home heat application (dry or moist) prior to the self-stretch.[16] The appropriate number of tongue blades is determined by the degree of mandibular depression. Given that the anterior incisor to posterior molar opening is in a 3-to-1 ratio and that a tongue blade is 1 mm thick, the number of blades begins with the maximal interincisal opening (MIO) divided by three. For example, a patient with an MIO of 30 mm should start with 10 tongue blades, which open the mouth 10 mm posteriorly and 30 mm anteriorly. The patient should maintain this position for 30 seconds and repeat this stretch three times every 2 hours. The therapist should progress the stretch by slowly adding tongue blades over time as determined by tissue reactivity, patient compliance, and the functional needs of the patient. When postoperative protocols are involved, there should be strict adherence to the guidelines; if questions arise, the surgeon should be consulted. In most cases, 40 mm of opening is functional; more than that puts the patient at risk for developing hypermobility and/or internal disc derangement.

References and Bibliography

References

1. Makofsky HW, Sexton TR, Diamond DZ, Sexton MT. The effect of head posture on muscle contact position using the T-scan system of occlusal analysis. *J Craniomandibular Pract.* 1991;9(4):316-321.

2. Darling DW, Kraus SL, Glasheen-Wray MB. Relationship of head posture and the rest position of the mandible. *J Prosthet Dent.* 1984;52:111-115.

3. Rocabado M, Iglarsh ZA. *Musculoskeletal Approach to Maxillofacial Pain.* New York, NY: JB Lippincott; 1991.

4. Kraus SL. Influences of the cervical spine on the stomatognathic system. In: Donatelli R, Wooden MJ, eds. *Orthopaedic Physical Therapy.* 3rd ed. New York, NY: Churchill Livingstone; 2001.

5. Simons DG, Travell JG, Simons LS. *Travell & Simons' Myofascial Pain and Dysfunction, The Trigger Point Manual. Vol 1. Upper Half of Body.* Baltimore, Md: Williams & Wilkins; 1999.

6. Shankland WE. Migraine and tension-type headache reduction through pericranial muscular suppression: a preliminary report. *J Craniomandibular Pract.* 2001;19(4):269-278.

7. Oleson TD. *Auriculotherapy Manual: Chinese and Western Systems of Ear Acupuncture.* Los Angeles, Calif: Health Care Alternatives; 1992.

8. Weisberg J, Friedman MH. Displaced disc preventing mandibular condyle translation: mobilization technique. *J Orthop Sports Phys Ther.* 1981;3(2):62-66.

9. Kraus SL, ed. *TMJ Disorders: Management of the Craniomandibular Complex.* New York, NY: Churchill Livingstone; 1988.

10. Mannheimer JS. Overview of physical therapy modalities and procedures. In: Pertes RA, Gross SG, eds. *Clinical Management of Temporomandibular Disorders and Orofacial Pain.* Chicago, Ill: Quintessence Publishing; 1995.

11. Morrone L, Makofsky HW. TMJ home exercise program. *Clin Manag.* 1991;11(2):20-26.

12. Alexander FM. *The Use of Self.* Long Beach, Calif: Centerline Press; 1989.

13. Makofsky HW. Snoring and obstructive sleep apnea: does head posture play a role? *J Craniomandibular Pract.* 1997;15(1):68-73.

14. Makofsky HW, August BF, Ellis JJ. A multidisciplinary approach to the evaluation and treatment of temporomandibular joint and cervical spine dysfunction. *J Craniomandibular Pract.* 1989;7(3):205-213.

15. Israel HA, Syrop SB. The important role of motion in the rehabilitation of patients with mandibular hypomobility: a review of the literature. *J Craniomandibular Pract.* 1997;15(1):74-83.

16. Poindexter RH, Wright EF, Murchison DF. Comparison of moist and dry heat penetration through orofacial tissues. *J Craniomandibular Pract.* 2002;20(1):28-33.

Bibliography

Darnell MW. A proposed chronology of events for forward head posture. *J Craniomandibular Pract.* 1983;1(4):49-54.

Ellis J, Makofsky H. Balancing the upper quarter through awareness of RTTPB. *Clin Manag Phys Ther.* 1987;7(6):20-23.

Friedman MH, Weisberg J. *Temporomandibular Joint Disorders: Diagnosis and Treatment.* Chicago, Ill: Quintessence Publishing; 1985.

Friedman MH, Weisberg J. The craniocervical connection: a retrospective analysis of 300 whiplash patients with cervical and temporomandibular disorders. *J Craniomandibular Pract.* 2000;18(3):163-167.

Hansson TL, Christensen CA, Wagnon Taylor DL. *Physical Therapy in Craniomandibular Disorders.* Chicago, Ill: Quintessence Publishing; 1992.

Hesse JR. *Craniomandibular Border Characteristics and Orofacial Pain.* Amsterdam: JR Hesse; 1996.

Langton DP, Eggleton TM. *Functional Anatomy of the Temporomandibular Joint Complex.* Tucson, Ariz: INFORC Publications; 1992.

Makofsky HW. The effect of head posture on muscle contact position: the sliding cranium theory. *J Craniomandibular Pract.* 1989;7(4):286-292.

Maloney GE, Mehta N, Forgione AG, Zawawi KH, Al-Badawi EA, Driscoll SE. Effect of a passive jaw motion device on pain and range of motion in patients not responding to flat plane intraoral appliances. *J Craniomandibular Pract.* 2002;20(1):55-66.

Mannheimer JS, Rosenthal RM. Acute and chronic postural abnormalities as related to craniofacial pain and temporomandibular disorders. *Dent Clin North Am.* 1991;35(1):185-208.

McNeill C, ed. *Temporomandibular Disorders: Guidelines for Classification, Assessment, and Management.* Chicago, Ill: Quintessence Publishing; 1993.

Nicolakis P, Burak EC, Kollmitzer J, et al. An investigation of the effectiveness of exercise and manual therapy in treating symptoms of TMJ osteoarthritis. *J Craniomandibular Pract.* 2001;19(1):26-32.

Okeson JP, ed. *Orofacial Pain: Guidelines for Assessment, Diagnosis, and Management.* Chicago, Ill: Quintessence Publishing; 1996.

Perrini F, Tallents RH, Katzberg RW, Ribeiro RF, Kyrkanides S, Moss ME. Generalized joint laxity and temporomandibular disorders. *J Orofac Pain.* 1997;11(3):215-220.

Solberg WK, Clark GT. *Abnormal Jaw Mechanics: Diagnosis and Treatment.* Chicago, Ill: Quintessence Publishing; 1984.

Wilk BR, Stenback JT, McCain JP. Postarthroscopy physical therapy management of a patient with temporomandibular joint dysfunction. *J Orthop Sports Phys Ther.* 1993;18(3):473-478.

Zeno E, Griffin J, Boyd C, Oladchin A, Kasser R. The effects of a home exercise program on pain and perceived dysfunction in a woman with TMD: a case study. *J Craniomandibular Pract.* 2001;19(4):279-288.

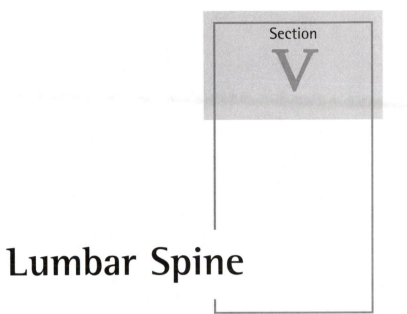

Section

V

Lumbar Spine

Examination and Evaluation of the Lumbar Spine

As alluded to in the beginning of Chapter 8, the divisions according to anatomic region in this textbook are necessary for instructional purposes. However, in the actual clinical application of the examination and intervention techniques, there is less separation and more integration. For example, the assessment of postural alignment of the entire lumbar-pelvic-hip complex can be approached as one functional unit and examined concurrently. Why then the didactic separation as per the anatomy? The author realizes that the trend in physical therapy education is toward integration, and there is no argument on that point. There is, however, disagreement as to when that integration process should begin. It is the author's philosophy that students, not unlike developing children, must "crawl before walking." Once the basic principles of examination/evaluation and intervention are learned for each of the various regions of the body, the student is then taken to the next step of integration. The venue for this progression can occur in the classroom with patient demonstrations, case studies, etc, as well as at the clinical site with patient rounds (as is performed in the clinical education of medical students and residents).

Posture

An important aspect of postural alignment is an understanding of clinical stability. Joints move through a physiologic range of motion consisting of the neutral zone, which is characterized by high flexibility, and the elastic zone, which is the region of high stiffness at the end of range.

Clinical instability of the spine occurs when the neutral zone increases relative to the total range of motion and the structures responsible for restraining such excessive mobility (primarily neuromuscular) are unable to do so.[1,2] This results in motion that is not only excessive and uncontrolled (ie, aberrant), but which ultimately undermines tissue adaptive potential, leading to the development of painful symptoms. The assessment of lumbar spine posture provides evidence for either stability or instability. If it is determined that the lumbar joints are not positioned in their neutral lordotic curve, but rather toward the end of range in the elastic zone, then there is reason to suspect that clinical instability is either present or developing. In severe cases of instability, the passive restraints (ie, osteo-oligamentous structures) may also be deficient, resulting in joint laxity at the end of range. Though poor posture may suggest the possibility of clinical instability, the final determination is always based upon motion testing, which will be covered subsequently.

As with previous assessments of posture, the standing patient is viewed laterally, posteriorly, and anteriorly. The lateral view of the lumbar spine (Figure 17-1) includes an evaluation of the following structures for misalignment:

1. The lumbar curve between the thoracolumbar and lumbosacral junctions should demonstrate a smooth posterior concavity (ie, lordosis) from top to bottom. As with all spinal segments, the balanced state is represented by a "tripod" consisting of the vertebral body/intervertebral disc in the front and the two apophyseal joints in the back. Unlike the lower cervical spine, where all three components bear

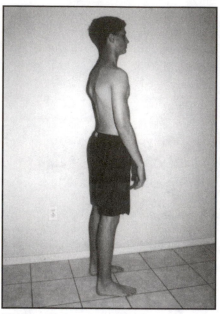

Figure 17-1.

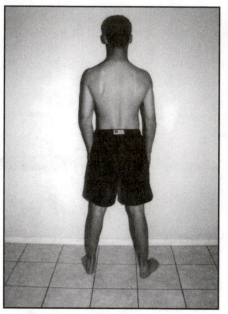

Figure 17-2.

equal weight, the typical lumbar segment bears approximately 85% of the weight anteriorly and 15% posteriorly. In states of increased lumbar extension (ie, hyperlordosis) the tripod shifts posteriorly onto the facets. When there is a decreased lordosis (ie, flat back), the tripod shifts onto the vertebral body/disc complex. Over time the hyperlordotic spine may accelerate degenerative changes in the posterior facet joints, whereas the flattened lumbar curve is often associated with discogenic conditions. If poor postural alignment persists into adulthood, impairment of mobility usually occurs with the flattened spine becoming restricted in extension; the hyperlordotic spine becoming limited in flexion. The sway-back posture is sometimes mistaken for hyperlordosis but is actually quite different. Its components include forward displacement of the hips, posterior rotation of the pelvis, a flat lumbar spine, and an increased thoracic kyphosis. Postural deviations can be quantified with an inclinometer or flexible ruler or be described as minimal, moderate, and severe.

2. The therapist should examine each of the lumbar spinous processes for a palpable "shelf" consistent with spondylolisthesis. These shelves or "steps" are most common in the lower lumbar region and tend to become prominent in the standing position. Paris[3] suggests that a palpable "step" in stance that normalizes in prone is less stable than a "step" that is palpated in both standing and prone; it is the unstable spondylolisthesis that is "the most likely to progress." According to Macnab,[4] the presence of a

spondylolisthesis is more likely to produce low back symptoms in younger patients; rarely, if ever, is it the sole cause of pain in those over 40.

3. The abdominal region should be observed for excessive protrusion, which is often associated with a hyperlordotic posture (this appears to be the case with pregnant women).

The patient is now observed posteriorly (Figure 17-2). Common misalignments include the following:

1. Asymmetrical fullness of the paravertebral muscles, which suggests spinal rotation toward the prominent side consistent with a neutral type 1 rotoscoliosis.

2. Segmental hypertonicity: A taut band of musculature at one level bilaterally suggests spinal instability at that level.

3. Lateral trunk shift (named for the direction the shoulders move and not the hips). Some authors refer to this antalgic posture of the lumbar spine as *acute sciatic*, or *protective scoliosis* (Figure 17-3). Regardless of the term used, most patients shift away from the side of the pain. When it occurs over a period of minutes to hours, it is highly suggestive of a lumbar derangement, usually at either L4,5 or L5,S1. More often than not, the lateral trunk shift is associated with an acute lumbar kyphosis. As discussed in Chapter 2, McKenzie's derangement syndrome[5] has traditionally been attributed to disc displacement. However, other possibilities include facet joint impingement, nonarticular reflex-induced muscle splinting (ie, hypertonicity from

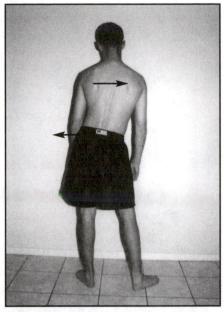

Figure 17-3.

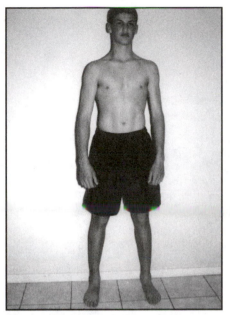

Figure 17-4.

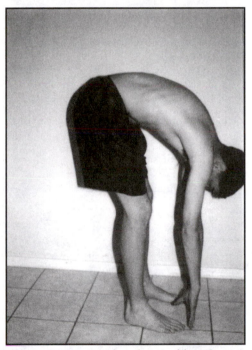

Figure 17-5a. Lumbar forward bending.

either nociceptive and/or hyperactive muscle spindle responses), pelvic girdle impairment (ie, sacral torsions), etc.

4. Asymmetrical waist angles.
5. Thoracolumbar scoliosis.

The patient is finally observed anteriorly (Figure 17-4). Asymmetries to note include the following:

1. Abdominal scars, which through the superficial fascia, exert asymmetric stress patterns with resultant skeletal misalignment.

2. Deviation of the linea alba, suggestive of a rotoscoliosis posteriorly.

3. An anterior perspective of a lateral trunk shift. In addition to observing the shift from the anterior aspect, this view also allows observation of the patient's face for signs of distress.

Active Movements

The examination of active lumbar movements consists of an analysis of the same six spinal motions observed in the scapulothoracic region (ie, forward bending, backward bending, side bending right and left, and rotation right and left) with the addition of side gliding to the right and left, which is named by the direction of the shoulder motion and not the hips (Figure 17-5a to 17-5h). This translational movement of the trunk may necessitate an explanation as well as a few tactile cues. The key to proper trunk side gliding is to keep the shoulders level as the hips and trunk move in opposite directions. Impairment of side gliding is useful in the detection of mild lateral trunk shifts that are not easily identified.

As with the previous examination of active motion in the cervical and thoracic spine, the visual estimation method is again employed. With training and experience, manually trained therapists can obtain significant information from observing active spinal motion. Although determining the quantity of motion available through the use of a tape measure, various range of motion devices, computerized technologies, etc is certainly useful, it is no substitute for the skillful observation of human motion. How else can it be determined that a patient's ability to place both hands on the floor is accomplished because of flexible hamstrings

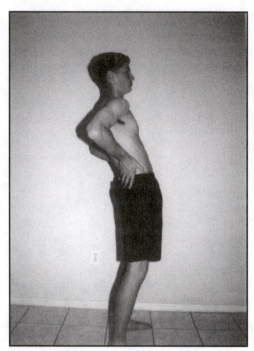

Figure 17-5b. Lumbar backward bending.

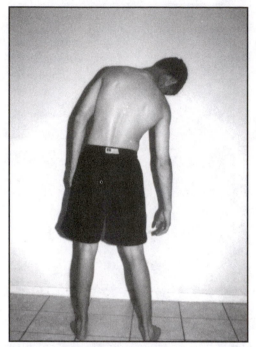

Figure 17-5c. Lumbar side bending right.

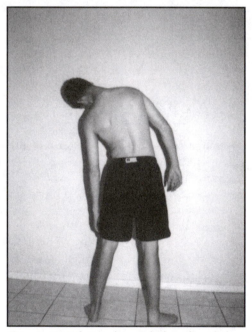

Figure 17-5d. Lumbar side bending left.

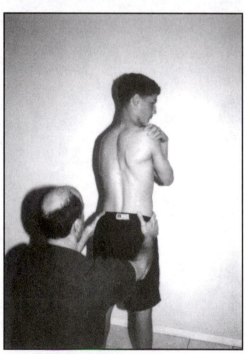

Figure 17-5e. Lumbar rotation right.

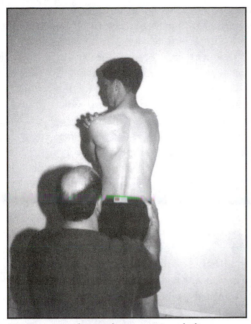

Figure 17-5f. Lumbar rotation left.

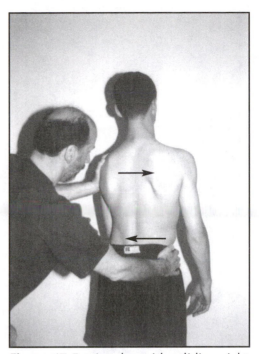

Figure 17-5g. Lumbar side gliding right with therapist assist.

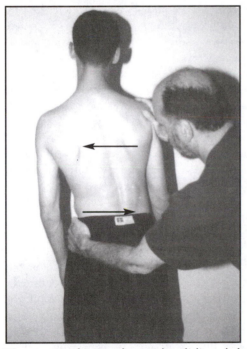

Figure 17-5h. Lumbar side sliding left with therapist assist.

while the lumbar lordosis fails to reverse its curvature? Instructors of manual therapy need to continue to teach this and other valuable assessment techniques even though they may lean more toward the art than the science of physical therapy.

Concepts worth remembering when observing spinal motion include balance, poise, coordination, distal mobility on proximal stability, segmental recruitment, roll-glid-ing, functionality, hypo/hypermobility, muscle splinting, tissue reactivity, etc. According to Paris,[3] sharp angulation at one or more levels suggests hypermobility, whereas a sudden "shake, catch, or hitch," especially in forward bending, indicates instability. The importance of this aspect of the spinal examination cannot be emphasized enough!

Repeated Movements Exam for Lumbar Derangement (Phases 1 to 3)

As discussed in Chapter 8, McKenzie's derangement syndrome[5] is suspected when certain symptom behaviors are present. They are symptoms occurring during movement, as compared to a dysfunction (ie, at end-range); symptoms that may be constant and severe, as compared to being intermittent and mild to moderate; symptoms that start proximal but with time become more distal (ie, below the knee); and symptoms that have neurologic features (eg, burning, tingling, shooting, sharp, piercing). Whereas it was previously believed that the intervertebral disc was insensitive to pain, it has been established that the outer annulus fibrosus is well supplied with nociceptive innervation[6,7] and is a common source of backache.[8] The majority of lumbar spine disc derangements occur at the L4,5 and L5,S1 levels and are most prevalent between the ages of 25 and 50, affecting more men than women.[4,9]

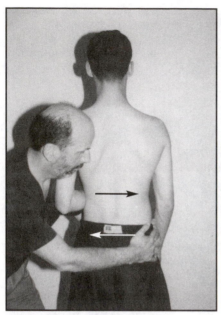

Figure 17-6.

In addition, the presence of an acute deformity (ie, lumbar kyphosis with or without a lateral trunk shift) is highly suggestive of a derangement. When patients use the phrase, "My back is out," think derangement!

When a McKenzie lumbar derangement is suspected, the therapist should proceed to placing the patient in one of seven categories. They are as follows:

- Derangement one: Central or symmetrical pain across L4,5. Rarely buttock or thigh pain. No deformity.

- Derangement two: Central or symmetrical pain across L4,5. With or without buttock and/or thigh pain. With deformity of lumbar kyphosis.

- Derangement three: Unilateral or asymmetrical pain across L4,5. With or without buttock and/or thigh pain. No deformity.

- Derangement four: Unilateral or asymmetrical pain across L4,5. With or without buttock and/or thigh pain. With deformity of lateral trunk shift.

- Derangement five: Unilateral or asymmetrical pain across L4,5. With or without buttock and/or thigh pain. With leg pain extending below the knee. No deformity.

- Derangement six: Unilateral or asymmetrical pain across L4,5. With or without buttock and/or thigh pain. With leg pain extending below the knee. With deformity of lateral trunk shift.

- Derangement seven: Symmetrical or asymmetrical pain across L4,5. With or without buttock and/or thigh pain. With deformity of accentuated lumbar lordosis.

McKenzie postulates that derangements one to six are progressions of the same disturbance within the intervertebral disc. The principle aim of treatment is to centralize pain and reduce deformity in order to reverse all derangements to derangement one. Derangements one to six are generally made worse by sitting and lumbar flexion and improved by standing and walking, which tend to restore the lumbar lordosis to normal. Although the McKenzie approach to the management of derangements is explained quite well with a nuclear displacement model,[10,11] there are other researchers who challenge the notion of nuclear "repositioning."[12,13] Perhaps one day our understanding of the true anatomic basis of lumbar derangement will become clearer. In the meantime, our focus as clinicians should be on the bedrock principles of intervention, which include reduction of the derangement based on signs and symptoms, stabilization of the reduction, recovery of function, and prevention of recurrence. As stressed so often to students, "Treat the patient's signs and symptoms and not the diagnosis." If at any time the derangement patient presents with frank neurologic signs (eg, muscle atrophy, weakness, hyporeflexia, sensory loss), the patient is not a candidate for mechanical therapy and should be referred to his or her physician for consultation. If at any time the patient reports a loss of bowel and/or bladder control, the patient requires an emergency referral to the physician.

The next step in the evaluation process is to determine the patient's response to the repeated movements examination using extension and flexion. However, for patients presenting with a lateral trunk shift (ie, derangements four and six), the lateral shift correction (Figure 17-6) should be performed prior to the initiation of these test movements. Depending on the severity of the shift and the associated symptoms, the technique should be performed slowly and gently, avoiding the excessive use of force. The patient's hips are rhythmically pulled under the trunk in and "on/off" fashion. Because the patient's legs may "give way," the patient should be positioned in front of a treatment table for support if needed. In addition to the improvement in trunk alignment, the patient's symptoms should be monitored throughout the lateral shift correction. As with cervical derangements, this is done by identifying the distal-most symptom and giving it a number from 0 to 10, with 0 being the absence of discomfort and 10 being the worst pain the patient has ever experienced. As the deformity improves, the symptoms should centralize in toward the center of the low back and eventually diminish in intensity.

For derangements one through six, the patient will be examined with an extension regimen; for derangement seven, repeated lumbar flexion is recommended. The main advantage of McKenzie over other manually-oriented systems, in the author's opinion, is the use of repeated movements. Derangements cannot be "forced into submission" but require a coaxing or "milking" force that often takes between 20 to 100 repetitions to respond. Though the

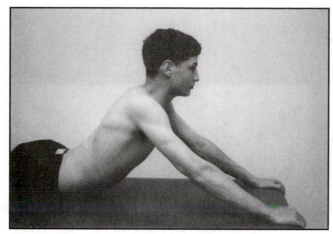

Figure 17-7.

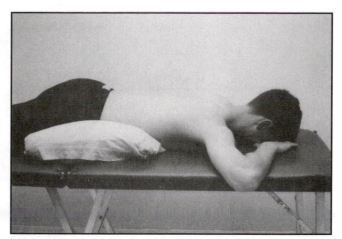

Figure 17-8.

reduction of a derangement is more of an art than a science, there are guidelines that may be helpful. The author uses a three-phase approach to guide the mechanical reduction of derangements one through six. The patient begins with phase one and is only progressed to phases two and three if necessary. Because derangement seven is so rare, it will not be covered in this text.

Phase 1: Self-Examination Prone Press-Ups

The patient must be instructed in the proper execution of the press-up (Figure 17-7). Simple instructions include the following:

1. Place the hands out in front far enough to permit the elbows to attain full extension without causing strain to the lower back upon pressing up.

2. The back muscles should not be working when performing the press-up. The work is done solely through the arms.

3. The hips are not permitted to leave the table (this ensures lumbar rather that hip extension).

4. When the arms are fully extended, there should be a slight pause before returning to the start position.

5. After each set of 10 repetitions, the distal-most symptom should be reassessed regarding its position and intensity. If there is no change or centralization has occurred, the patient should continue with Phase 1. If peripheralization has occurred and/or the pain becomes intolerable, the prone press-ups should be stopped.

6. When an increase in the extension effort is indicated by a good response, this can be achieved by bringing the hands closer to the shoulders prior to pressing upward. The goal is still to achieve full extension of the elbows so that the back muscles

remain relaxed. Once the elbows are fully extended, lumbar extension can be further enhanced by having the patient fully exhale through pursed lips after taking a deep breath through the nose. This progression continues until full reduction of the derangement has been attained.

The phase 1 self-exam is the basis for the intervention when the desired response is achieved. It is the starting point for derangements one, three, and five. For derangements four and six, the lateral trunk shift must be corrected prior to initiating phase 1 as mentioned above. Regarding derangement two, the patient may require a prone lying progression commencing with one or two pillows placed under the abdomen to accommodate the acute lumbar kyphosis (Figure 17-8). After a few minutes, the pillow should be withdrawn and the patient remain in the prone lying position for another few minutes, or longer if necessary, before commencing the phase 1 prone press-up.

Phase 2: Self-Examination Shifted-Hips Press-Ups

Patients are begun on shifted-hips press-ups when an additional lateral force is needed to reduce the derangement. Many posterolateral disc derangements respond well to straight press-ups, but others require a "wedge effect" in order to obtain complete reduction. The patient is instructed to shift his or her hips away from the side of pain and press-up from this position (Figure 17-9). Again, the patient's distal symptom and its intensity are reassessed following 10 repetitions for signs of centralization. As long as the desired response is obtained, the patient continues with the shifted press-ups in sets of 10. If at any time the patient's symptoms peripheralize, the exercises should be stopped. When the symptoms have settled in the center of the patient's low back, phase 1 press-ups may be resumed in hopes of obtaining a full reduction of the derangement.

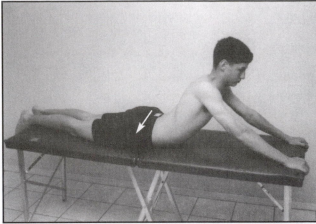

Figure 17-9.

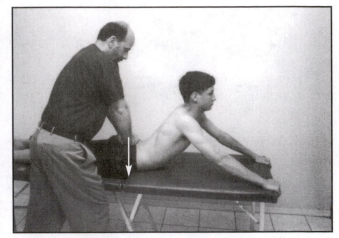

Figure 17-10a.

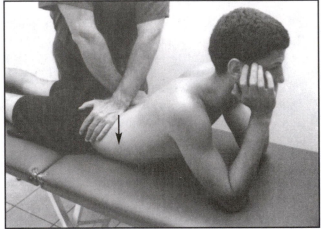

Figure 17-10b.

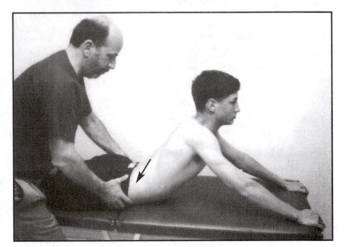

Figure 17-10c.

Phase 3: Therapist-Assisted Reduction

One of the main strengths of the McKenzie approach is the emphasis on self-treatment. However, there comes a point when therapist-assisted intervention is necessary. If the derangement persists following the application of phase 1 and 2 attempts at reduction, the patient is progressed to phase 3. Those who have poor success with the extension principle usually do so not because extension is inappropriate but because the amount of extension at the deranged segment is inadequate. If the patient is unable to "close down" with sufficient force independently, it is up to the therapist to ensure that the necessary extension takes place. When the extension force at the deranged segment is increased, the previously recalcitrant derangement often responds favorably.

Phase 3 intervention includes the following measures:

1. Manual stabilization of the inferior component (Figure 17-10a) of the involved segment (ie, sacrum for L5,S1 derangement, over the transverse processes [TP] of L5 for an L4,5 derangement).

2. Posteroanterior (PA) mobilizations over the TP of the lumbar vertebrae (unilaterally or bilaterally) and sacral base in neutral, prone on elbows (Figure 17-10b), and in the prone press-up position.

3. Manual stabilization of the hips and pelvis away from the side of pain during the performance of the prone press-up (Figure 17-10c).

Phase 3 intervention is the therapist's final attempt at coaxing a "stubborn" derangement back into place before determining that it is nonreducible. It is a manual skill that can be improved with practice.

Passive Physiologic Intervertebral Movements

As discussed in Chapter 4, PPIVMs are a means of evaluating physiologic motion in the spine, segment by segment, as it occurs during active movement with the exception of muscle contraction. As in the thoracic spine, the

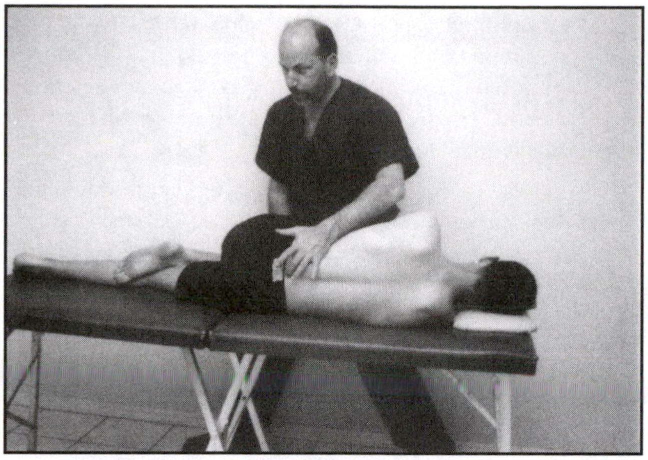

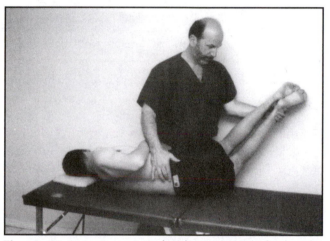

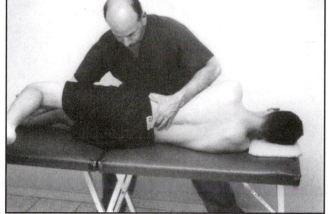

Figure 17-11a. Assessing lumbar intervertebral forward bending.

Figure 17-11b. Assessing lumbar intervertebral backward bending.

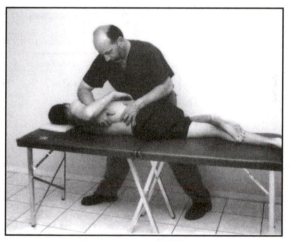

Figure 17-11c. Assessing lumbar intervertebral side bending right.

Figure 17-11d. Assessing lumbar intervertebral rotation right.

quantity, quality, and end-feel for each motion segment is assessed. Gonnella et al[14] demonstrated dependable intratherapist reliability using the 0 to 6 mobility scale, whereas intertherapist reliability was not dependable. The motions of forward and backward bending, side bending right and left, and rotation right and left will be assessed as the palpating finger (usually the index or middle finger) examines motion in the interspinous space from L1 to L5. Although these motions can be induced and assessed in both weight-bearing and nonweight-bearing positions, the recumbent position will be utilized for the basic, introductory approach (Figures 17-11a to 17-11d).

For forward bending, the palpating finger assesses the separation of the spinous processes starting at L5,S1, whereas for backward bending, the approximation of the spinous processes is examined. When assessing side bending, the ipsilateral aspect of the interspinous space is palpated. However, for rotation the contralateral aspect of the interspinous space is preferable. To determine segmental levels

in the lumbar spine, the L4,5 interspinous space is usually at the level of the iliac crest. However, it is better to identify the last mobile segment (L5,S1) in extension and work up from there.

Soft Tissue Palpation

As with other regions of the musculoskeletal system, the examiner is seeking to identify areas of tenderness (myofascial trigger points and/or tender points), tightness, and increased tone. The important structures of the lumbar region amenable to palpation include the following:

1. Abdominal muscles: Consisting of the rectus abdominis, external and internal obliques, and transversus abdominis.

2. Psoas muscle: Palpated anteriorly, approximately 2 inches lateral to the umbilicus at the lateral border of the rectus abdominis.

3. Skin and superficial fascia: Note temperature changes, erythema, moist or dry areas, edema, scar tissue/adherences, skin lesions, nodules, trigger points, etc. A tuft of hair ("faun's beard") may indicate a spina bifida occulta or diastematomyelia; café au lait spots may indicate neurofibromatosis or collagen disease.

4. Supraspinous ligament: Felt in the interspinous spaces.

5. Thoracolumbar fascia: Anterior, middle, and posterior layers (posterior layer is reinforced by the latissimus dorsi superficially).

6. Erector spinae muscles: Spinalis, longissimus, and iliocostalis. Palpate for signs of somatic impairment (ie, ropey, stringy, or boggy feel to the tissues).

7. Quadratus lumborum: Between the rib cage and the iliac crest. By having the patient lift the pelvis toward the thorax, the muscle can be felt to contract.

8. Transversospinalis muscles: Semispinalis, multifidi, and rotatores (deep to the erector spinae between the spinous and transverse processes).

In addition to the inspection for tenderness, tightness, and tone, the myofascial tissues of the lumbar spine and abdominal region can also be examined for extensibility and length. If during the soft tissue examination, findings of a medical nature emerge (eg, masses, large palpable pulsations, painful nodes, abdominal rigidity, suspicious skin lesions), the patient's physician should be notified immediately.

Special Tests

This section will be organized into three categories. They are neurologic, orthopaedic, and physician-based special tests. The reader is referred to other specialized textbooks and articles listed at the end of this section for a complete description of all the special tests mentioned below.

Under the neurologic tests, the following examination procedures should be included:

a. Myotomes (L1 to S2).

b. Dermatomes (L1 to S2): Light touch, pin prick, etc.

c. Deep tendon reflexes (knee and ankle jerk).

d. Neurodynamic testing (straight leg raise test, well-leg raise, Braggard's test, bowstring sign, femoral stretch test, slump test, and variations of the straight leg raise for the proximal sciatic, tibial, common peroneal, and sural nerves). These tests are performed to assess the mechanical movement of neural tissues and to test their sensitivity to mechanical stress and/or compression.

e. Upper motor neuron lesion (upper, middle, and lower abdominal skin reflexes, and Babinski's sign).

f. Valsalva's test (used to test for intrathecal pathology, such as tumor or disc herniation).

g. Waddell's signs (non-physiologic pain symptoms).

The following orthopaedic test procedures are recommended:

a. Kemp's compression or quadrant test (seated or standing).

b. Spondylolysis test (extension in one-leg standing).

c. Schober test (range of lumbar flexion).

d. Johnson's lumbar stability tests (vertical compression test, elbow flexion test, lumbar protective mechanism-flexion, and lumbar protective mechanism-extension).

e. Nine-point Brighton scale for generalized hypermobility.

f. Hoover test (assists in identifying the malingering patient).

g. Functional assessment (Oswestry Disability Index, Dallas Pain Questionnaire, Hendler 10-Minute Screening Test for Chronic Back Pain Patients, Functional Capacity Evaluation, etc).

Regarding physician-based special tests, the following tests and procedures are performed as indicated:

a. Examination (S3 and S4 sensation and sphincter ani control should be tested by the physician when cauda equina syndrome is suspected; the cremasteric, along with the other superficial reflexes, are performed to rule out upper motor neuron disease).

b. Radiologic (x-rays, CAT scan, MRI, myelogram, discography, bone scan, etc).

c. Electrodiagnosis (EMG, conduction velocity, etc).

d. Lab work (CBC, ESR, rheumatoid factors, HLA-B27 antigen, Lyme, Epstein-Barr virus, antinuclear antibodies, etc).

e. Tissue biopsy.

f. Sleep studies (sleep apnea, fibromyalgia/chronic fatigue, etc).

g. Psychiatric/psychological evaluation.

Connective Tissue Techniques
and Stretching Procedures
for the Lumbar Spine

Thoracolumbar Junction Release

This release (Figure 18-1) is an important myofascial release technique for both the thoracolumbar junction and the posterior diaphragm. The therapist's hands are placed lightly on either side of the prone patient's thoracolumbar junction with the thumbs close to the spinous processes and the fingers pointing cephalward. The "shear-clock" method is again utilized to identify impairment in mobility of the skin and superficial fascia (indirectly, the deep fascia as well through its connection to the basement membrane of the dermis). Once the area of greatest restriction (AGR) is located, the therapist uses either indirect or direct treatment technique to obtain the desired "release" (the 4 Ms procedure described in Chapter 5 is applicable to either approach).

Ward[15] describes a direct myofascial release technique in which he employs tension, traction, and twist to the tissues between the right and left hands for 10 to 30 seconds. As softening and elongation occur (ie, myofascial "release"), the therapist follows behind in search of new motion barriers. Tension is achieved through light compression, traction involves a perpendicular stretch of the paraspinal tissues, and twisting is achieved through a clockwise/counterclockwise rotation of the hands. These three "prerelease" forces cause a "winding up" of the tissues, which sets the stage for myofascial "unwinding." The Ward approach is actually a combination technique that begins direct and ends indirect.

Quadratus Lumborum Release

This connective tissue technique (Figure 18-2) employs a combination of muscle stretching, hold-relax or postisometric relaxation, direct fascial technique, and myofascial release. With the patient in the side lying position, the therapist prestretches the soft tissues by separating the iliac crest from the rib cage, while simultaneously grasping and lifting the soft tissues upward. This is followed by a longitudinal stretch of the quadratus lumborum muscle. To enhance the stretch, several hold-relax contractions/relaxations are added. At any time during the stretch, direct fascial technique can be integrated (eg, perpendicular strumming, muscle play, myotherapy, progressive pressure technique).

The clinical importance of eradicating trigger points and restoring length and myofascial extensibility to the quadratus lumborum muscle cannot be emphasized enough. The quadratus has been identified as a source of backache and lumbar myalgia. It is also a source of referred pain into the sacroiliac region, hip, buttock, greater trochanter, abdominal region, and groin.[16]

Iliopsoas Fascial Technique

Understanding the actions of the iliopsoas muscle serves as a useful guide in both the evaluation and intervention of patients with lumbar-pelvic-hip impairment. The actions are as follows:

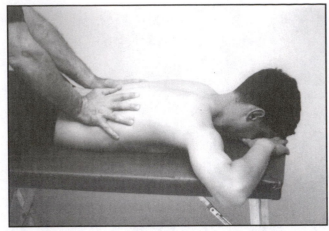

Figure 18-1.

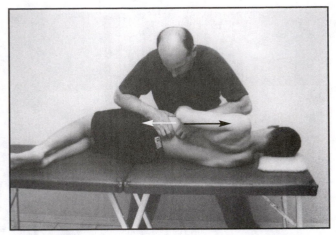

Figure 18-2.

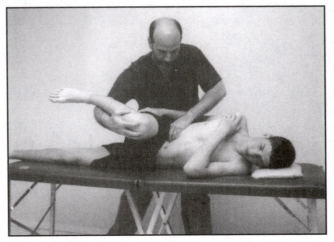

Figure 18-3a.

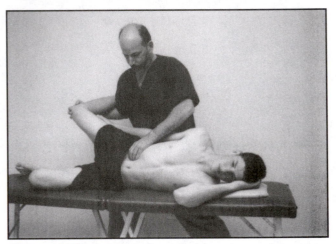

Figure 18-3b.

1. Hip flexion with a secondary role in external rotation and abduction.

2. In erect posture, upper lumbar extension with lower lumbar flexion (ie, exaggerated lumbar lordosis with anterior pelvic tilt).

3. In the forward bent position, the iliopsoas contributes to lumbar flexion.

4. A unilateral contraction laterally flexes the lumbar spine to the ipsilateral side and by compression, contributes to spinal stability.

5. Unilateral tightness may also contribute to a type 2 impairment such that the inferior component of the motion segment is laterally translated to the ipsilateral side. For example, left-sided tightness at L3,4 causes lateral translation of L4 to the left with overturning of L3 into flexion, rotation, and side bending to the right (ie, FRS right at L3,4).

In the author's opinion, it is imperative that the status of the iliopsoas muscle be assessed in all low back patients. In the pelvic girdle section of this textbook, the length of the iliopsoas will be assessed and treated as one component of the TRI muscle stretch (tensor fascia latae, rectus femoris, and iliopsoas). At this point, however, our focus will be on the application of a direct fascial technique with the muscle on slack and under stretch.

As illustrated, the patient is positioned in side lying with the involved side up. The initial phase of this technique (Figure 18-3a), involves passively placing the upper-most hip in flexion and external rotation in order to relax the iliopsoas for greater access. While adjusting the lower limb for maximal relaxation, the other hand monitors the psoas approximately 2 inches lateral to the umbilicus. In this position, an isometric contraction of the hip flexors ensures that the iliopsoas has been located. Following deep tissue massage in the muscle's slackened state, the iliopsoas is then placed under stretch by extending the lower limb at the hip (Figure 18-3b). In this position, the therapist again applies deep tissue massage in conjunction with postisometric relaxation, which helps to decrease the resting tone of the iliopsoas muscle (the therapist may have the patient hold the bottom leg in hip and knee flexion for enhanced counter stability of the pelvis).

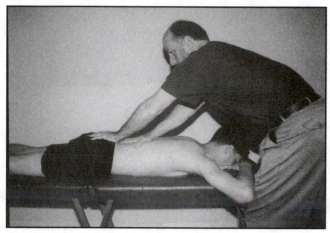

Figure 18-4.

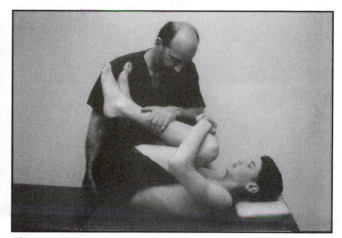

Figure 18-5.

Treating the muscle in both positions (ie, slackened or stretched) allows either an indirect or direct approach to intervention, depending on the state of tissue reactivity present (see Chapter 3 for a description of direct and indirect treatment methods).

Lumbosacral Junction Release

In order to "disengage" the lumbosacral junction and release abnormal soft tissue tension (Figure 18-4), the therapist's cephalic hand is placed over the lower lumbar spine, while the caudal hand is placed over the sacrum with the heel of the hand on the sacral base. The therapist can approximate the two hands to perform an indirect myofascial "unwind" or place the tissues of the lumbosacral junction on maximal stretch and perform a direct technique against the restrictive barrier(s). A pillow can be placed under the patient's abdomen to further decompress the region.

Sacrospinalis Stretch

Patients with McKenzie's flexion dysfunction respond well to the sacrospinalis stretch (Figure 18-5). However, it is contraindicated in patients with posterior derangement of the lumbar spine.

With the patient placed in the "knees to chest" position, the therapist places his or her other hand under the patient's sacrum with the fingers on the base and the heel of the hand over the apex. The stretch is accomplished by directing the lumbar spine into further flexion through the lower limbs as the sacrum is counternutated. A gentle postisometric relaxation often enhances the technique's efficacy, providing that the patient's symptoms are not exacerbated by this procedure.

Neural Mobilization

Butler[17,18] recommends that neural mobilization be viewed as another form of manual therapy similar to joint mobilization. In this regard, the treatment of signs and symptoms based on the severity, irritability, and nature of the impairment must be kept in mind at all times. The danger in presenting this material outside the context of the entire art and science of neural mobilization is that it be seen as a technique rather than as a comprehensive system involving clinical reasoning, problem solving, and a thorough understanding of the anatomy, physiology, and pathophysiology of neurobiologic structures. Having said that, we will proceed to using manual methods in order to restore the mechanical function of impaired neural tissues (intra- and extraneural impairment) in the lumbar-pelvic-lower limb complex. As with all manual therapy procedures, the goal remains the same (ie, "to restore maximal pain-free movement within postural balance"). Contraindications include irritable conditions, inflammation, spinal cord signs, malignancy, nerve root compression, peripheral neuropathy, and complex regional pain syndromes I and II.

Proximal Sciatic Nerve

The sciatic nerve is the largest nerve in the body, but actually consists of two nerves: the common peroneal and tibial, which are tightly bound together by connective tissue. The common peroneal nerve is a posterior branch of the sacral plexus originating from the lumbosacral trunk (L4 to S2); the tibial nerve is an anterior branch of the sacral plexus originating from the ventral rami of L4 to S3. Sites of potential proximal compression include the lower lumbar spine (eg, intervertebral disc, spinal canal, lateral recess, intervertebral foramina, etc), the piriformis muscle, and hamstrings. Because the sciatic nerve runs posterior to the hip and knee joints, the optimal means of inducing lon-

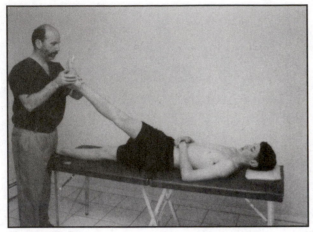

Figure 18-6.

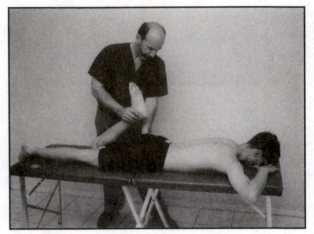

Figure 18-7.

gitudinal tension is through the straight leg raise first described by Leseague in 1864.[17] The leg is lifted upward, as a solid lever, while maintaining extension at the knee. To induce dural motion through the sciatic nerve, the leg must be raised past 35 degrees in order to take up slack in the nerve. Since the sciatic nerve is completely stretched at 70 degrees, pain beyond that point is usually of hip, sacroiliac, or lumbar spine origin. The unilateral straight leg raise causes traction on the sciatic nerve, lumbosacral nerve roots, and dura mater. Adverse neural tension produces symptoms from the low back area extending into the sciatic nerve distribution of the affected lower limb. To introduce additional traction (ie, sensitization) into the proximal aspect of the sciatic nerve, hip adduction is added to the straight leg raise (Figure 18-6). This is because the sciatic tract is lateral to the ischial tuberosity; therefore, adduction causes further tensing of its proximal aspect.

Prior to commencing neural mobilization, McKenzie's derangement syndrome must be ruled out. Stretching nerve roots that are reacting to local compression is only indicated for examination purposes. Cyriax[19] described the straight leg raise "painful arc" sign, which usually appears from 45 to 60 degrees. This sign, in which there is no pain above and below the point of adverse neural tension, implies that the nerve root momentarily "catches" against a small protrusion and then slips over it. In the presence of this finding or other indications of disc herniation, neural mobilization should not be performed. The purpose of neural mobilization is to restore normal function to impaired neural structures that were previously compressed, irritated, and inflamed. The intervention recommended is a "flossing" of the nerve in which gentle, short duration (1 second) and large amplitude passive movements are performed at the "feather edge" of the patient's neural symptoms in an "on/off" fashion. In other words, a mild degree of discomfort is permitted during the momentary stretch (ie, "on" phase), which must completely abate when the tension is withdrawn (ie, "off" phase). The patient's symptoms must be monitored at all times, and it is suggested that the patient be initially undertreated until the irritability of the impairment becomes apparent. Thirty to 60 seconds of on/off mobilization is a useful guideline for intervention.

Femoral Nerve

The femoral nerve is a branch of the lumbar plexus, which is formed by the ventral primary rami of L1, L2, L3, part of L4, and possibly T12. The femoral nerve continues medial to the knee as the saphenous nerve. The femoral nerve stretch was first described by Wasserman[17] in 1919, who proposed it as a physical sign to explain anterior thigh and shin pain in soldiers. In 1946, O'Connell recommended the inclusion of hip extension.[17]

As with other nerve stretching maneuvers, the femoral nerve stretch (prone knee bend or Nachla's test) can be used for both examination and intervention. There are two components to the nerve stretch:

1. The uppermost part of the thigh is passively extended just short of producing lumbar spine extension. By creating tension in the iliopsoas, the upper lumbar nerve roots are put under traction

2. The knee is then progressively flexed to increase femoral nerve tension by stretching the quadriceps femoris muscle. Pain in the anterior thigh may be of muscular or nerve origin. A careful history should help to delineate the problem.

Again, the neural flossing technique in an on/off fashion is recommended for adverse neural tension (Figure 18-7). The pelvis should be properly stabilized to prevent stress from being placed on the sacroiliac joint and lumbar spine (Yeoman's test). The lateral femoral cutaneous nerve can be stretched by adding hip adduction to the extended hip and flexed knee. The saphenous nerve is stretched by placing the hip in extension, abduction, and lateral rotation while extending the knee and dorsiflexing/everting the ankle.

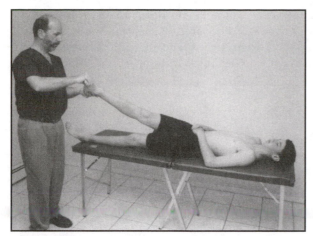

Figure 18-8.

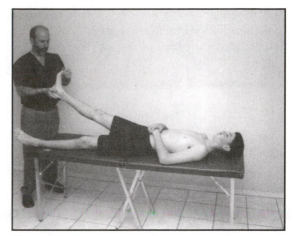

Figure 18-9.

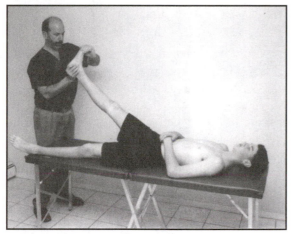

Figure 18-10.

Common Peroneal Nerve

The common peroneal nerve (L4,5; S1,2) lies directly posterior to the proximal fibular head and, therefore, can be injured with posterior fibular head displacement and/or fracture of the fibula. Since supination of the ankle causes a posterior glide of the fibular head, a lateral ankle sprain can be a contributing factor to injury of the nerve.

To place the common peroneal nerve under tension, the hip is flexed and medially rotated, the knee is extended, and the ankle is plantar flexed and inverted (Figure 18-8). According to Butler,[17] plantar flexion/inversion may be added before the straight leg raise (SLR), or at the completion of the SLR. Once again, the management of adverse neural tension involves a gentle on/off stretch of large amplitude at the onset of symptoms. The goal is to achieve functional gliding of the common peroneal nerve along its complete course from proximal to distal.

Tibial Nerve

The tibial nerve (L4,5; S1 to S3) is brought under tension with the addition of ankle dorsiflexion. This is because

its terminal branches, the medial and lateral plantar nerves, course along the plantar surface of the foot and are therefore stretched by dorsiflexing the ankle. In addition to hip flexion, knee extension, and ankle dorsiflexion, the tibial tract can be further sensitized by everting the ankle, extending the toes, and stretching the plantar fascia (Figure 18-9). Butler states that ankle dorsiflexion may be added first and then the limb lifted, or performed at the limit of the SLR. The tibial nerve forms the largest component of the sciatic nerve in the thigh. Inferiorly, it descends through the popliteal space, passing between the heads of the gastrocnemius muscle to the dorsum of the leg, as the posterior tibial nerve, and into the ankle and foot. As the posterior tibial nerve traverses under the flexor retinaculum at the tarsal tunnel, it is subject to possible compression (ie, tarsal tunnel syndrome). As mentioned above, it then divides into the medial and lateral plantar nerves, which supply sensation to the sole of the foot and toes as well as supplying sensation to the foot joints and efferent fibers to the small muscles of the foot. When adverse neural tension is present, neural mobilization is gently performed for 30 to 60 seconds.

Sural Nerve

The medial sural cutaneous nerve, a branch of the tibial nerve, joins the lateral sural cutaneous nerve, a branch of the common peroneal nerve, to form the sural nerve (L5, S1, S2), which supplies the skin of the posterolateral part of the leg and the lateral side of the foot. According to Butler,[17] "The sural nerve is a forgotten nerve and is responsible for far more symptoms than it is given credit for." With practice, the sural nerve can be palpated along the lateral aspect of the foot, behind the lateral malleolus, and lateral to the Achilles' tendon. The position of maximal sural nerve tension consists of hip flexion, knee extension, and ankle dorsiflexion followed by ankle inversion (Figure 18-10). Butler refers to this combination of movements as the sural nerve tension test. As with the other nerve tension tests, the same limb position is then transformed into a neural mobilization in the presence of impairment.

To further sensitize the tibial, common peroneal, and sural nerves, additional loading is made possible by adding cervical flexion, lumbar and thoracic side bending to the contralateral side, hip adduction, and medial rotation.

Lumbar Spine Manipulation

As with manual therapy of the thoracic spine (see Chapter 6), PPIVMs can be easily transformed into interventional manipulations. This is done by identifying the AGR and then proceeding with either the "hold one/move one" approach (ie, stabilize the bottom and mobilize the top vertebra of the motion segment into its restricted range) or the "roll-glide" technique. The specific grade (1 to 4) is, of course, determined by the level of reactivity present.

Having said that, this chapter will not cover manipulation of the lumbar spine in each of six possible directions (ie, flexion, extension, side bending right and left, and rotation right and left). Instead, an apophyseal distraction (ie, gapping) maneuver will be described as a means of introducing a simple, efficient, and effective way of mobilizing any of the impaired 10 lumbar spine facet joints when necessary. A hypomobile lumbar facet joint demonstrates restriction in the capsular pattern as follows: limited contralateral side bending/ipsilateral rotation and flexion associated with trunk deflection to the affected side. Because it is a joint distraction technique, grades 1 to 3 will be utilized as with cervical distraction: grade 1 (support of the joint to neutralize negative pressure), grade 2 (to the end of the tissue slack), and grade 3 (beyond the tissue slack to patient tolerance).

Apophyseal Joint Gapping

A manipulative distraction of the right L4,5 facet joint will described. The patient is placed in the left lateral decubitus position (ie, side lying on the left side) with the affected joint uppermost. In order to "gap" the right L4,5 facet, a combination of flexion, left side bending, and right rotation is introduced. In this position, the inferior articular process of L4 separates from the superior articular process of L5 in a perpendicular direction (Figure 19-1). In females, the width of the pelvis may necessitate placing a towel roll under the waist in order to enhance lumbar side bending to the left.

The components of proper manipulative technique include localization, balance, and control. The therapist must properly localize the forces of X axis flexion, Y axis rotation, and Z axis side bending to the "feather edge" of the restrictive barrier prior to performing the graded distraction. The L4,5 level can be located by first identifying the last mobile segment (ie, L5, S1) in extension and then coming up one level. The L4,5 interspinous space is usually at the level of the iliac crest as well. With the right middle finger between L4 and L5, the patient's right lower limb is flexed at the knee and hip with the therapist's left hand until flexion first arrives at L4,5. The patient's right foot is then placed on top of his or her left knee and kept there (Figure 19-2).

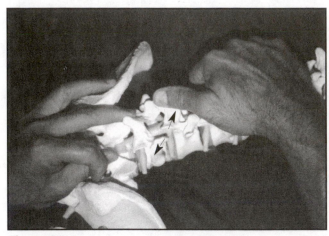

Figure 19-1.

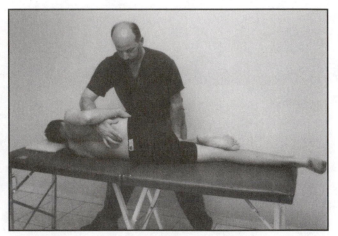

Figure 19-2.

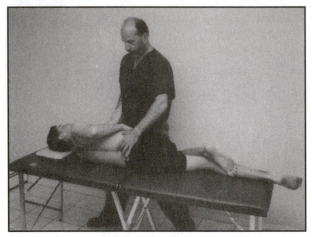

Figure 19-3.

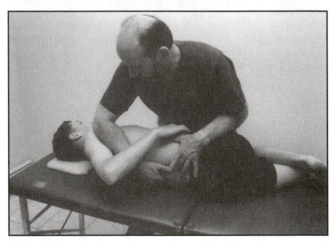

Figure 19-4.

At this point, the movement of right rotation of the trunk is introduced from above until motion is first detected at L4,5 with the left middle finger. This can be achieved by pulling the left upper arm up and forward with the "lawn mower" maneuver (Figure 19-3). The patient's right arm is then placed on his or her flank with the elbow flexed.

The final phase of the set-up involves the localization of L4,5 side bending left. The therapist does this by separating the patient's pelvis from his or her shoulder girdle with a pushing force in opposite directions (Figure 19-4). When the side-bending left motion is felt to arrive at L4,5, the position is maintained.

Now that the motions of flexion, right rotation, and left side bending have been localized to the restrictive barrier at the right L4,5 apophyseal joint, the manipulative force can be introduced. As with any of the mobilizations performed thus far, a postisometric relaxation technique can be utilized to reduce muscle hypertonus.[20] Following two to three cycles, the patient can be relocalized to the new barrier in preparation for graded distraction (recall that postisometric relaxation is synonomous with muscle energy technique).

The manual distraction of the right L4,5 apophyseal joint involves a "gapping" of the joint such that the facet surfaces are separated in a perpendicular fashion. The best way to accomplish this without causing undue stress on the intervertebral disc is by emphasizing additional left side bending by gently pushing the patient's pelvis and shoulder girdle in opposite directions. However, in order to maintain the right rotation component, the therapist's right thumb maintains contact on the right side of the L4 spinous process as the therapist's left middle finger provides pressure on the L5 spinous process from below (Figure 19-5). The specific grade selected (ie, 1 through 3) is dependent upon the reactivity and the degree of facet impairment present. In addition to the effects of mobilization on the articular tissues, this manipulative distraction will also widen the intervertebral foramina between L4 and L5, and consequently is useful when there is nerve root compression (ie, pinched nerve) at the foramina and/or the lateral recess. Because the female pelvis is wider, as mentioned previously, it may be necessary to place a towel roll under the female patient's waist in order to achieve the desired side bending on the inferior side.

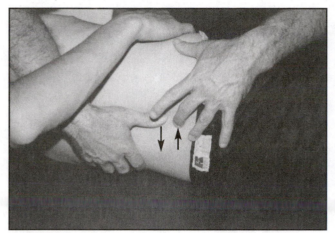

Figure 19-5.

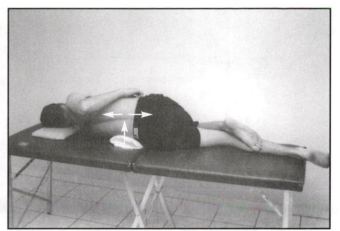

Figure 19-6.

The towel roll can also be used as a means of achieving positional distraction, which can be taught to the patient for home use. It is an excellent way of decompressing irritated nerve roots in the lumbar spine in a safe and effective manner (Figure 19-6).

As mentioned previously, the "gapping" maneuver described in this chapter can be used for any of the 10 facet joints in the lumbar spine. For those who are trained in the correction of FRS impairment, it is useful to first distract the affected facet prior to closing it.

Therapeutic and Home Exercises for the Lumbar Spine

As with all regions of the vertebral column, there needs to be a balance between mobility and stability. In states of impairment, the thoracic spine tends toward hypomobility, whereas the cervical and lumbar regions tend toward hypermobility, especially at their lower levels. The Panjabi model[1,2] refers to this balance as clinical stability and the loss of balance in the direction of hypermobility as clinical instability. More specifically, spinal instability is a failure of the spinal stabilization system to restrict the neutral range or zone to the physiologic borders of a segment's range of motion. According to Panjabi, the three components of this spinal stabilization system are the passive, active, and neural control subsystems. The passive spinal subsystem consists of the osseous and articular structures of the vertebral column, the active spinal subsystem consists of the musculofascial structures that promote stability of the spine, and the neural control subsystem consists of the sensorimotor control process that regulates motion of the spinal joints. The purpose of spinal stabilization training, therefore, is to restore an optimal neutral range whereby all three subsystems are working together to prevent segmental hypermobility and to consequently reduce the problems associated with this condition (eg, recurrent pain, repetitive microtrauma, and degenerative changes).

In the lumbar spine specifically, Richardson et al[21] from the University Queensland and the Prince of Whales Medical Research Institute in Sydney, Australia, have introduced the concept of a deep local muscle system that is ideally suited for the control of neutral zone motion, including shear forces between spinal vertebrae. The deep muscles of this local system, being closer to the center of rotation with short muscle lengths, are ideal for controlling intersegmental motion. According to these Australian researchers, the functional unit of local stabilization consists of the respiratory diaphragm, the pelvic floor, the lumbar multifidus, and the transversus abdominis (Figure 20-1). Under normal conditions, the action of drawing the navel "in" toward the spine not only causes a deep contraction of the transversus abdominis, but also causes a cocontraction of the other components of the system. Consequently, this deep, local system cocontraction acts as an inner corset of musculofascial support that provides static and dynamic stability to each of the lumbar segments. To better understand the mechanism for spinal support, one needs to appreciate the concept of intra-abdominal pressure (IAP) and LaPlace's law, which states $T = Pr$, where T is circumferential tension, P is pressure, and r is radius. Theoretically, contraction of the transversus abdominis raises IAP by increasing abdominal wall tension (T) as well as by decreasing abdominal radius (r). This increase in IAP helps to convert the abdomen into a semirigid cylinder, which results in a stiffer and more stable structure. In addition, the transversus abdominis muscle exerts lateral tension on the middle and posterior layers of the thoracolumbar fascia through its attachment to the entire lateral raphae. Because the thoracolumbar fascia acts on the transverse and spinous processes of the lumbar spine, the transversus abdominis provides additional support and stability to the lumbar region.[21]

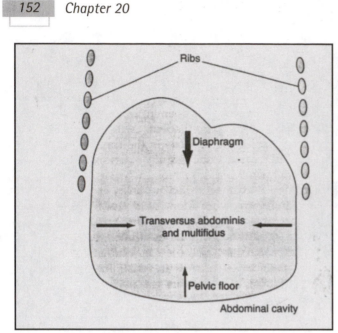

Figure 20-1. The functional unit of core stability (reprinted from Richardson C, Jull G, Hodges P, Hides J. *Therapeutic Exercise for Spinal Segmental Stabilization in Low Back Pain: Scientific Basis and Clinical Approach*. Edinburgh: Churchill Living-stone; 1999, by permission of the publisher Churchill Livingstone).

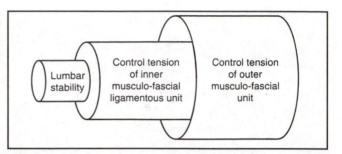

Figure 20-2. The inner "corset" concept of the core stabilizers (reprinted from Richardson C, Jull G, Hodges P, Hides J. *Therapeutic Exercise for Spinal Segmental Stabilization in Low Back Pain: Scientific Basis and Clinical Approach*. Edinburgh: Churchill Livingstone; 1999, by permission of the publisher Churchill Livingstone).

pain, the global system appears to overpower the local one, which has become inhibited and ineffective. This loss of core stability is what causes many of the problems found in low back pain patients and what practitioners of spinal stabilization therapy and Pilates[22] attempt to retrain.

In this chapter, we will address the issue of core stability, but first we must deal with the self-treatment of common lumbar derangements and dysfunctions in the lumbar region.

Management of Lumbar Derangement (Phases 1 to 3)

The patient's response to the repeated movements exam provides the foundation upon which the self-treatment model for lumbar disc derangement is based. Because the techniques used for intervention are the same as for the examination, the reader is advised to review phases 1 through 3 in section three of Chapter 17. Having said that, the patient must be taught one additional maneuver not yet covered: the McKenzie self-correction of a lateral shift for derangements four and six. For example, a patient with a right lateral shift stands with his or her right side against the wall (Figure 20-3). The right elbow is then flexed to 90 degrees with the right forearm placed against the lower ribs. With the feet approximately 12 in from the wall, the patient is advised to gently and rhythmically shift the hips to the right in an on/off fashion several times with the left hand. The patient is properly instructed in McKenzie's principles of derangement reduction (ie, centralization phenomenon) and advised to perform this self-treatment procedure as often as necessary. Once the lateral shift has been corrected, the patient can proceed with phases 1 through 3, as indicated, to obtain complete reduction of the posterior derangement.

Regarding the McKenzie management of derangement syndrome, the following guidelines must be kept in mind:

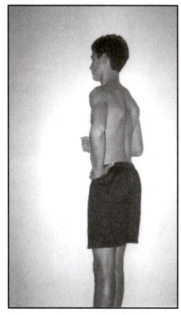

Figure 20-3.

The "global" muscles are those torque-producing muscles that attach the pelvis to the thoracic cage. Unlike the local system, which provides core stability, the global muscles provide a more general lumbopelvic stability function. In normal function, the local and global systems work together to provide trunk mobility on "core stability" (Figure 20-2). However, in patients with chronic low back

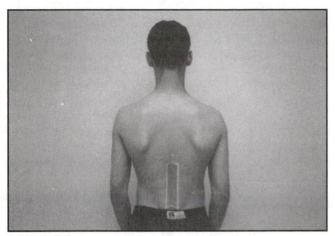

Figure 20-4.

1. The therapeutic movement is the one that yields the "most for the least" (ie, the least force for the most centralization).

2. Self-treatment is preferred to therapist-assisted technique because it empowers the patient to become independent.

3. The myth of not performing lumbar extension must be overcome. For those therapists trained in "flexion only," lumbar extension feels like the unpardonable sin! These therapists must remember that the McKenzie approach is not synonymous with extension. The approach taken is based upon what works for the patient. There are situations when flexion is indeed necessary (eg, derangement seven, flexion dysfunction). However, the efficacy of lumbar extension exercises for the management of certain posterior and posterolateral disc derangements is undisputed. As long as the patient possesses an intact nociceptive afferent system, there is minimal risk to the patient. When the intervention is working, the centralization phenomenon will be observed; when the lesion is not responding or becoming worse, the peripheralization phenomenon will reveal this and the exercise is stopped. Regarding the role of extension exercises in cases of clinical instability, the therapist is attempting to reduce the derangement that may be placing the patient in an unstable position. If, as just stated, the intervention is working, the patient's symptoms will centralize and improve, but if the patient is being made more unstable by extension, then the symptoms will worsen and the intervention stopped. This is why McKenzie stresses ongoing feedback from the patient at all times. In the presence of a stable spondylolisthesis (grade 1 or 2), extension is not contraindicated. However, in the presence of an unstable grade 3 or 4 spondylolisthesis, lumbar extension should be avoided because of anterior shearing of the inferior vertebra of the motion segment.

4. The patient is only escalated to the next phase when necessary (eg, prone press-ups before shifted-hips press ups, self-treatment before manual stabilization and mobilization).

5. It must be stressed to the patient that derangements require constant vigilance. If the patient is not committed to performing the derangement-reducing movements a minimum of three sets of 10 every 2 hours, results in most cases will be limited.

6. Following the repeated movement component of the McKenzie approach, the patient must be instructed in the proper maintenance of a neutral lumbar lordosis. In the case of derangements one through six, lumbar flexion must be avoided for at least 3 to 5 days to allow stabilization of the derangement to occur. The patient should avoid sitting, if possible, because of greater intradiscal pressure in this position.[23] However, if this is not possible, then the chair should be such that the knees are lower than the hips. There are several commercially available lumbar support pillows that are also helpful. In addition to their role in managing disc derangements, lumbar supports are useful in managing backache associated with McKenzie's postural and dysfunction syndromes. They are also used to prevent the postural problems associated with slump-sitting (eg, forward head, rounded shoulders). To maintain the lordosis, a beach towel around the waist at night is recommended. The author has also had good success with taping. Leukotape P is applied over the spinous processes, vertically spanning the thoracolumbar and lumbosacral junctions with the patient in standing while maintaining a neutral lordosis (Figure 20-4). The tape pulls on the patient's skin each time he or she flexes the lumbar spine and acts as a reminder to maintain the position of optimal healing.

Once the derangement has been reduced and properly stabilized, the final goals are to recover lost function and prevent recurrence. For derangements one and two, the recovery of lost function involves the use of lumbar flexion (ie, knees to chest), for derangements two through six it involves the use of combined flexion and contralateral side bending, and for derangement 7 the use of extension. The derangement must be healed and stable prior to the use of forces that stretch the tightened area. It is wise to follow all stretches with a prophylactic set of 10 prone press-ups to ensure that the discal tissue remains in proper alignment.

Regarding the prevention of recurrence of the derangement, the patient must be aware of proper body mechanics (ie, the 5 Ls of lifting, which will be covered subsequently),

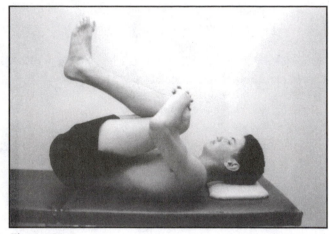

Figure 20-5.

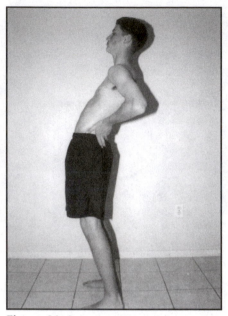

Figure 20-6.

ergonomic factors at home and in the workplace, the effect of emotional stress and tension, etc. Any persistent musculoskeletal impairments and/or imbalances must be addressed by the therapist (eg, impaired neurodynamic function, tight postural muscles, weak phasic muscles, poor postural alignment). If chronic pain (ie, symptoms lasting longer than 3 months) becomes an issue, a referral to a chronic pain clinic may be necessary.

As mentioned in the cervical section, there are times when disc derangements are not amenable to conservative measures. Spine surgeons are appreciative of patient referrals in whom nonsurgical interventions have been exhausted. This removes one of the criteria in their consideration of surgery as the next option. The remaining three criteria include intractable pain, neurologic signs of nerve root compression, and diagnostic confirmation of disc herniation with imaging. Some surgeons may add one or two additional criteria, but these four form the basis of whether to operate in most cases. The decision regarding the type of surgical intervention most appropriate for the patient lies within the realm of spinal surgery. A good working relationship between the surgeon and the therapist helps to reduce the incidence of unnecessary surgery, but ensures that surgery is performed when indicated. It also increases the likelihood of appropriate postoperative rehabilitation, which is often overlooked.

Self-Mobilization of the Lumbar Spine

The indications for flexion exercises include lumbar flexion dysfunction, healed posterior derangement, and anterior derangement (derangement seven). Although the supine "both knees to chest" exercise (Figure 20-5) is used for all three conditions, the manner in which the exercise is performed is dependent upon the type of underlying impairment. The self-mobilization of lumbar flexion in the presence of McKenzie's flexion dysfunction syndrome (see Chapter 2) can be performed as with other stretches (ie, 5-to-10-second stretch to begin, working up to a 30-second stretch, repeated three times every 2 hours if possible). However, in the case of an anterior disc derangement or status post healed posterior derangement, the knees to chest maneuver should be performed gingerly in an on/off manner. If they are introduced following a recently healed posterior derangement, it may be wise to begin with the "single knee to chest" maneuver until it can be demonstrated that lumbar flexion is tolerated by the patient. Regardless of the reason for performing flexion exercises, the patient should always end each session with prophylactic prone press-ups to guard against the possibility of developing a posterior derangement.

The indications for extension exercises include lumbar extension dysfunction, healed anterior derangement, prophylactic extension to follow all flexion exercises, and as discussed above, posterior derangements one through six. As with management of posterior derangements, prone press-ups are the method of choice. However, standing extension (Figure 20-6) is extremely useful because it is so easily performed in comparison to lying extension, which requires a carpeted floor, mat, or table.

It is imperative that patients be given instruction in the proper performance of extension exercises. For prone press-ups, the arms and not the back extensors should perform the movement. The spine should be sequentially extended from the thoracic region down to the lumbosacral junction with the hips on the table at all times. The hands should be positioned so that the elbows are able to fully extend; as extension range improves, the patient's hands should be

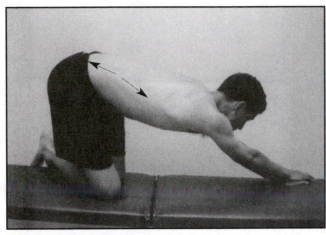

Figure 20-7.

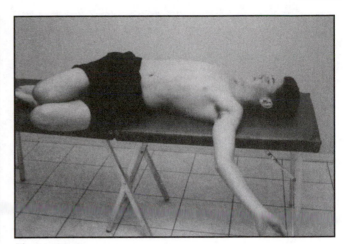

Figure 20-8.

moved closer to the trunk. As with the management of cervical derangements, at least three sets of 10 repetitions are recommended every 2 hours. Standing extension should be performed with the hands on the hips with the thumbs forward. This should be done 10 times whenever rising from the sitting position. The patient must not "cheat" by extending at the hips!

Lumbar side bending is achieved in quadruped as shown for the thoracic spine in Chapter 7. It has utility for stretching the quadratus lumborum and sacrospinalis muscles unilaterally, as well as self-mobilizing the lumbar spine in the presence of side-bending restriction. In addition, it is carefully used to recover lost function following a healed posterolateral disc derangement.

The patient is instructed to place the hands and feet away from the side of the stretch without tilting the shoulders or hips. By simply leaning into the convexity, the desired stretch is achieved (Figure 20-7). The patient must stop at the point of the initial stretch and, if possible, hold for 30 seconds. If this is uncomfortable for the patient, he or she should begin with a 5- to 10-second hold and escalate upward from there. As range improves, the hands and feet can be moved further apart to enhance the efficacy of the stretch. To mitigate any untoward effects of the stretch, the patient should perform 10 prophylactic prone press-ups before standing. If at any time symptoms peripheralize, the stretch should be stopped immediately.

The final lumbar spine self-mobilization is rotation. It can be argued that lumbar rotation be omitted from the list of therapeutic exercises for two reasons. First, there is minimal rotation in the lumbar spine because of the sagittal orientation of the apophyseal joints and second, unstable disc derangements may respond poorly to rotation, which places added mechanical stress on disc structures. Nevertheless, rotation is a physiologic movement of the lumbar spine that can be limited in states of impairment, which should be enhanced when possible. However, because of the shear forces placed on the disc during rotation, it should be avoided in the presence of acute derangements.

Unlike quadruped rotation in the thoracic spine, which occurs from top to bottom, lumbar rotation is performed in the hooklying position with the arms abducted to 90 degrees (Figure 20-8) and occurs from below upward. With practice, the patient can be trained to move segmentally upward from L5 to L1 on either side (ie, when moving the bent knees to the left, the motion involves L5 rotation to the left under L4, followed by L4 under L3, and L3 under L2, etc). The benefit of this type of movement is not only to improve the quantity of motion, but the quality as well. This self-mobilization/stretch should be monitored for possible peripheralization and followed by prophylactic prone press-ups.

Core Stability

There are two ways of effectively training patients to achieve an isolated contraction of the transversus abdominis muscle.[21] The first method involves placing the patient in the hooklying position with the index and middle fingers placed over the anterior superior iliac spines (ASISs). The patient is asked to draw the navel in toward the spine without moving the pelvis (Figure 20-9). If the patient performs a posterior pelvic tilt, then the global abdominal muscles are substituting for the local system. The patient may also inhale as an incorrect means of drawing the abdomen inward. Consequently, the drawing in of the navel must be performed without lumbopelvic motion and during exhalation. It is the motor control of an isolated transversus abdominis contraction that is crucial in obtaining core stability. Otherwise, the torque-producing superficial muscles (ie, the external obliques, the rectus abdominis, and all but the posterior fibers of the internal obliques, which insert into the lateral raphe in most peo-

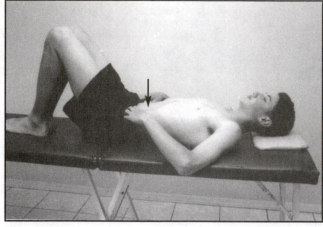

Figure 20-9.

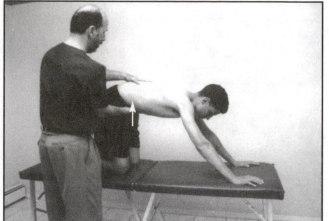

Figure 20-10.

ple) will dominate and inhibit one's ability to isolate the deeper core system.

The second way of achieving an isolated contraction of the transversus abdominis muscle is with the patient in the quadruped position. The therapist instructs the patient to relax the abdominal wall into the therapist's hand. The patient is then advised to lift the abdominal wall off the therapist's hand while exhaling through pursed lips. Again, the patient's trunk should be motionless throughout, indicating an isolated contraction of the transversus abdominis without global muscle substitution (Figure 20-10).

Once the patient has mastered the art of isolating the transversus abdominis, he or she is ready to activate the pelvic floor muscles (ie, the levator ani consisting of the puborectalis, pubococcygeus, levator prostatae or pubovaginalis, iliococcygeus muscles, and the coccygeus muscle, posteriorly). There is thought to be a synergistic relationship between the transversus abdominis and the pelvic floor muscles, especially the pubococcygeus muscle. Patients with stress incontinence have reported improvement following training of the transversus abdominis, while patients with low back pain have reported improvement with the use of pelvic floor exercises.[21] It is also believed that the core stabilizing function of the transversus abdominis is contingent upon the simultaneous contraction of the pelvic floor and respiratory diaphragm. In this way, a transversus abdominis contraction is able to generate an increase in intra-abdominal pressure.

To train the pelvic floor, males are instructed to draw the testicles upward, while females are instructed to stop the flow of urine or perform Kegel exercises. Pelvic floor training can be performed in isolation or in conjunction with a contraction of transversus abdominis. In either case, the contraction should be slow, gentle, and of low effort. Because of the synergistic relationship of the core musculature, pelvic floor activation assists in the facilitation of the multifidus as well as the transversus abdominis; therefore, it should be recruited first. As important as contraction of the pelvic floor is for core stability, the relaxation of these same muscles is equally as important. Tonic holding, especially of the coccygeus muscle, often results in "crampy" pain in the groin and/or tail bone region. In addition, tonic holding will weaken the urogenital diaphragm and may result in stress incontinence during coughing and sneezing.

Once the motor control aspect of core muscle activation is achieved, the patient is then instructed in functional neutral/lower abdominal exercises. However, throughout the performance of these exercises, the patient must maintain a tonic contraction of the local system. The most common mistake made in abdominal training is to neglect to recruit the core muscles first. If this core recruitment does not occur, the patient is only training the global torque producers and does not attain optimal improvement in lumbar stability.

A quantitative way of training the transversus abdominis and other core components is by placing the patient prone with a blood pressure cuff under the umbilicus. The cuff is then elevated to 70 mmHg and the patient is asked to lessen the pressure by 6 to 10 mmHg during exhalation by drawing the abdominal wall inward without performing a posterior pelvic tilt. Once this is achieved, the patient is instructed to maintain this pressure reduction for 10 to 30 seconds while breathing normally (Figure 20-11).

Functional Neutral/Lower Abdominal Training

The interest in spinal stabilization therapy peaked in the early 1990s with a wave of interest and enthusiasm that spread quickly from the west to the east coast. A new lexicon of words, including neutral, functional range, abdominal bracing, lower abdominals, instability, spinal stabilization, etc became the jargon of the times; new forms of exercise involving Swiss balls, foam rollers, rocker boards, and

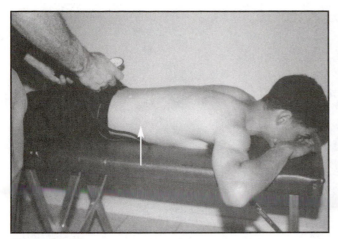

Figure 20-11.

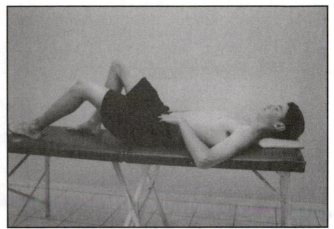

Figure 20-12.

sophisticated medical exercise equipment suddenly appeared in clinics across the country and around the globe. Some of the pioneers involved with this form of therapy include Biondi, Drinkwater-Kolk, Johnson, Saliba-Johnson, Parker, Morgan, Moore, Christensen, Irion, Liebenson, Posner-Mayer, Paris, Sahrmann, Holten, Grimsby, Rogers, Svendsen, Janda, Saunders, Bookhout, Ellis, Sarver, etc. The basic principles, however, can be traced back to the work of the Kendalls, the Bobaths, Knott, Voss, Pilates, Daniels, Worthingham, and others, to mention a few.

Training low back patients in this way begins by identifying the functional neutral range or what Panjabi[1,2] refers to as the neutral zone. This is the optimal position or range of position within which the lumbar spine is stable, the least symptomatic, and within which it functions the most efficiently. To borrow a term from Kaltenborn,[24] it is the loose-packed or resting position of the lumbar region. The author also uses the term *osteocentric* when describing a joint's neutral position. To find the neutral position or range, the hooklying patient is instructed to explore the extremes of an anterior pelvic tilt (ie, hyperlordosis) and posterior pelvic tilt (ie, lumbar kyphosis). The neutral position or range is approximately half-way between the two extremes of sagittal motion where the patient experiences maximal ease or comfort. It is what osteopathic physicians refer to as dynamic neutral. Some patients prefer a slight flexion bias, while others incorporate a slight bias toward extension in their neutral range. The basic philosophy of functional neutral/lower abdominal training is that patients can be made more stable and less symptomatic if they learn to function in the neutral range in which tissues are less apt to be mechanically stressed and strained. This is consistent with Panjabi's concept of training the active and neural control subsystems to enhance neutral zone function, while discouraging movements into the hypermobile and symptomatic elastic zone where the passive subsystem controls motion.

In retrospect, one of the shortcomings of the spinal stabilization revolution was the lack of recognition of the deep local system of core stability. By failing to first activate the core system, the torque-producing global system was strengthened instead. With the discovery of the role of the deep local muscle system in the late 1990s came the realization that the approach to functional neutral training needed modification. Consequently, the exercises covered below will integrate our newer understanding of core stability into many of the traditional spinal stabilization exercises. In this way, patients will benefit from local as well as global trunk stabilization training. The patient is progressed from stable to unstable positions; from less to more difficult exercise procedures requiring increased levels of strength, endurance, and motor control.

Exercise 1: Heel Slides

1. The patient is placed on a mat or table in the hook-lying position with the index/middle fingers on the ASIS, bilaterally.

2. The patient finds his or her neutral lumbopelvic position.

3. The deep local muscle system is activated by contracting the pelvic floor muscles (ie, "testicles pulled upward" for males and "stop the flow of urine" for females) first, followed by drawing in the abdominal wall.

4. Once the core muscles are set, the patient is now instructed to slide the right heel along the table in order to straighten the right knee (Figure 20-12). This is done during exhalation, counting backward slowly from 5 to 1 while maintaining both the neutral position and the activation of the core muscles. Once the leg is straight, the patient can relax completely and repeat this sequence 10 times. The entire procedure is then performed on the left side.

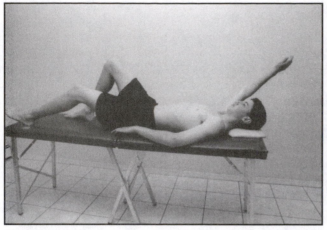

Figure 20-13.

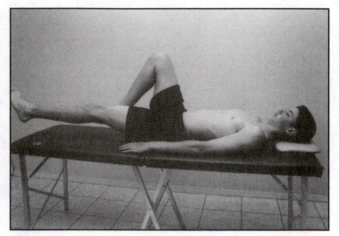

Figure 20-14.

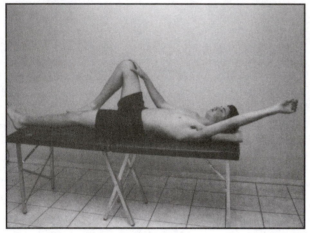

Figure 20-15.

Exercise 3: Unilateral Leg Lowering

1. The patient is now progressed to raising both feet off the table in supine.
2. Following core muscle setting in a neutral position, the patient lowers one leg at a time without touching either foot to the table or mat (Figure 20-14).
3. Ten repetitions per side is performed to a slow count of 5 to 1 on exhalation.
4. The leg must not be lowered beyond the point at which the pelvis anteriorly tilts, the lumbar spine hyperextends, and/or the local core muscles fail to maintain drawing in of the abdominal wall.

Exercise 4: Hand to Ipsilateral Knee (Figure 20-15)

1. The patient again begins by raising both feet off the table in supine as in exercise 3 with bilateral arm support.
2. Once the core muscles are set in the neutral lumbopelvic position, the patient brings one hand to the ipsilateral knee while the opposite arm and leg move away from each other (Figure 20-15). This maneuver is then repeated in an alternating fashion on the contralateral side for a total of 10 repetitions on each side.
3. It is essential that a neutral core contraction be maintained at all times while the patient inhales and exhales normally.

Exercise 5: Bilateral Leg Lowering

1. The supine patient begins by raising both feet off the table (Figure 20-16).

In order to progress the patient to the next level of difficulty, he or she must be able to maintain a decent core contraction (ie, abdominal drawing-in) and not allow the lumbar spine to hyperextend as the legs are lowered.

Exercise 2: Heel Slide With Opposite Arm Elevation

1. Steps 1 to 3 are repeated as in exercise 1.
2. While maintaining a core contraction in the neutral position, the patient performs the heel slide but now simultaneously raises the opposite arm overhead to a slow count of 5 to 1 on exhalation (Figure 20-13).
3. This sequence is repeated 10 times with the right heel slide/left arm combination and 10 times with the left heel slide/right arm combination. As with exercise 1, the patient must be able to maintain a decent contraction of the transversus abdominis and not allow the lumbar spine to hyperextend as the legs are lowered before moving on to exercise 3.

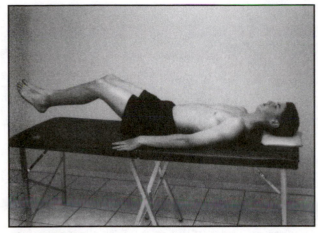

Figure 20-16.

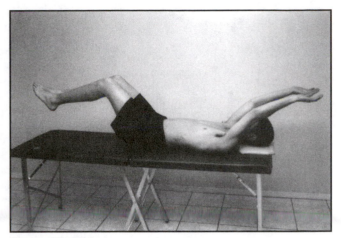

Figure 20-17.

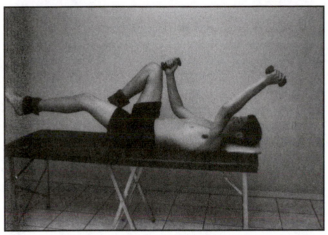

Figure 20-18.

Exercise 6: Bilateral Leg Lowering With Bilateral Arm Elevation

This is the most advanced of the exercises thus far. For those who master exercise 5, this next maneuver is attempted.

1. As the legs are lowered, the arms are simultaneously elevated on exhalation (Figure 20-17). The patient must not proceed to the point where the pelvis begins to anteriorly rotate and the lumbar spine hyperextend.

2. The core system must also be able to maintain the drawing in of the abdominal wall at all times.

3. Each of the 10 repetitions should be performed to a 5 count; the degree of leg lowering/arm elevation is based upon the patient's mastery in the early ranges of motion.

At any point in the performance of exercises 1 through 6, ankle weights and/or dumbbells can be added to enhance muscular effort (Figure 20-18). In order to maintain cervical spine stability, a chin tuck is performed with the occiput either making contact with the mat/table or elevated less than an inch off the surface for maximum recruitment of the deep neck/occipital flexors along with the core stabilizers/lower abdominals.

Exercise 7: Foam Roller Training

Foam rollers (Figure 20-19) are especially helpful in training core stability. Because they are inherently unstable, they provide sensorimotor challenges on a subcortical level, which is an efficient and effective way of training several muscle groups simultaneously.[25]

Exercises 1, 2, 3, and 5 are well-suited to the foam roller, whereas exercises 4 and 6 are not because of the tendency to fall off the roller without arm support. Ankle weights and/or dumbbells can be added at the appropriate time. In

2. Once the pelvic floor and other core muscles are set by drawing the abdominal wall inward in the neutral lumbopelvic position, the patient proceeds by lowering both legs simultaneously.

3. The objective of this more challenging exercise is to maintain core stability as the weight of the descending lower limbs are inducing an anterior pelvic tilt/lumbar spine hyperextension. It is the lower abdominals (primarily the external oblique muscles) that work with the local muscle system to prevent this from occurring.

4. The patient must be proficient with exercises 1 through 4 before attempting this more challenging maneuver; the degree of leg lowering must be commensurate with the patient's ability to maintain a neutral lumbopelvic position.

5. Ten repetitions are performed to a slow count of 5 to 1 on exhalation.

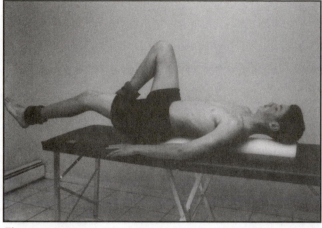

Figure 20-19.

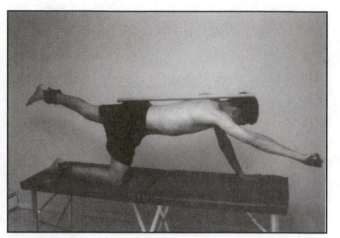

Figure 20-20.

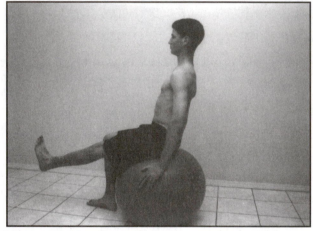

Figure 20-21.

3. To progress the patient, diagonal raises are performed such that the right arm and left leg are raised simultaneously, followed by the left arm and right leg (Figure 20-20). Care must be taken not to permit lumbar hyperextension during the raises. This exercise, like the others, is more about motor control than the generation of brute strength. There are many low back patients with "great looking abs." The key is not the appearance, but the functionality!

4. As with the other lower abdominal exercises, ankle weights and the use of dumbbells can be added when the patient has mastered the maneuver without weights.

Exercise 9: Sitting Swiss Ball Training (Figure 20-21)

The "Swiss Ball" originated in 1963 when an Italian manufacturer started manufacturing toys made of vinyl instead of rubber.[26] Some of the people responsible for the use of the Swiss ball in physical therapy clinics today include Kong, Quinton, Bobath, Klein-Vogelbach, Kucera, Carriere, Hanson, Schorn, Posner-Mayer, Corning-Creager, Irion, Christensen, Morgan, Johnson, Saliba-Johnson, Biondi, and Rocabado. The Swiss ball, also known as the Physio, Gymnic, Yoga, Opti, or Gym ball, is useful in promoting proper movement patterns using key muscle groups. The outcome involves safe and pain-free functional movement, which translates into reduced disability in one of our most challenging patient populations, namely chronic back pain sufferers.

The patient sits on the ball with knees and hips flexed to 90 degrees and the feet placed flat on the floor (Figure 20-21). To begin, the patient rocks back and forth into an anterior and posterior pelvic tilt. Once the neutral position

addition to the use of foam rollers mentioned above, there are many more exercise applications for a variety of patient conditions. For further information on the clinical use of foam rollers, the reader is referred to Corning-Creager's book listed in the bibliography.

Exercise 8: Quadruped Training

Patients with lumbar hypermobility/instability must be taught to maintain a stable, neutral core while involved with limb movements that threaten to undermine their spinal stability even further. Quadruped training enhances the concept of "distal mobility on proximal stability," which is hopefully carried over into a patient's activities of daily living.

1. In the quadruped position, the patient "sets" the core system in the neutral lumbopelvic region.

2. The patient starts by raising all four limbs, one at a time, while maintaining a neutral and stable core throughout.

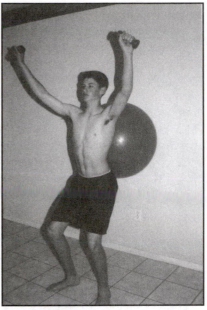

Figure 20-22.

Variations of the wall slide include unilateral or bilateral arm elevation during the knee bending phase as well as maintenance of the core contraction and chin tuck in both the up and down directions. The Swiss ball can be placed between the patient and the wall to facilitate the up and down movement of the spine; dumbbells can be used for added difficulty (Figure 20-22).

Sensorimotor Training (Feldenkrais)

The Feldenkrais method[27] is based upon the work of Moshe Feldenkrais (1904 to 1984), an Israeli physicist who devoted his career to the relationship between human movement, conscious thought, and sensorimotor learning. His findings led to the discovery of a new method of neuromuscular re-education that has had profound implications in the rehabilitation of patients with movement disorders. The Feldenkrais sensorimotor learning system is based upon the sciences of biomechanics, neurophysiology, stress reduction, and accelerated learning. When applied to patients with orthopaedic impairments, its purpose is to reduce or eliminate painful symptoms in the musculoskeletal system as a consequence of the rediscovery of the ease and flexibility of movement. In computer terminology, manual therapy is to the "hardware" what the Feldenkrais method is to the "software." Restoring the mechanical properties of human motion is what manual therapy proposes to accomplish. However, without restoring the sensorimotor control aspect of movement, it is only a matter of time before the mechanics once again become dysfunctional.

It is beyond the scope of this book to do more than introduce the topic to the reader. To that end, an "awareness through movement" lesson will be discussed as a means of introducing the therapist and his or her prospective patients to the Feldenkrais method. The lesson chosen here because of its great utility with low back patients, is known as the pelvic clock.

The hooklying patient (Figure 20-23) is asked to imagine a large "clock" placed over the lower abdominal region. To begin the patient is advised to move the pelvis from 12:00 to 6:00 (12:00 brings the pelvis into a posterior tilt whereas 6:00 brings the pelvis into an anterior tilt). The patient then proceeds in diagonal patterns of movement from 1:00 to 7:00, 2:00 to 8:00, 4:00 to 10:00, and 5:00 to 11:00. The patient also explores the horizontal 3:00 to 9:00 movement as well. Other options for gaining greater sensorimotor control of lumbopelvic movement include moving around the "clock" in a clockwise as well as counterclockwise fashion. When Feldenkrais practitioners are teaching new movements to a student, they often place their hands on the body to provide a manual assist with the acquisition of a new motor skill. This is referred to as functional integration.

is discovered, the core muscles are set as usual by contracting the pelvic diaphragm and drawing the abdominal wall inward on exhalation without pelvic motion. From here patients can perform such exercises as the basic bounce, the leg march, the kick out, march-arm and leg, etc with or without ankle weights and dumbbells while maintaining core muscle stability in the neutral lumbopelvic position. The reader is referred to Posner-Mayer's book[26] for a complete description of Swiss Ball options with emphasis on mobility, strength, cardiovascular training, sensory perceptual retraining, balance, postural relearning, as well as injury prevention and fitness.

Exercise 10: Standing Wall Slides

The final exercise in our series of functional neutral/lower abdominal exercises involves the wall slide. There are many variations of this exercise, but all claim to assist with lumbar stabilization and the dissociation of the hips from lumbar motion.

1. The patient stands with his or her back to the wall.
2. With a moderate bend of the knees (approximately 45 degrees), the patient sets the core muscles in the neutral lumbopelvic position.
3. A chin tuck is then performed to stabilize the cervical region and lengthen the spine.
4. The patient then straightens his or her knees while maintaining neutral core and cervical stability (ie, chin tuck) to a slow count of 5 to 1.
5. Once the patient has returned to normal stance, the core contraction and chin tuck can be released.
6. This sequence is repeated 10 times.

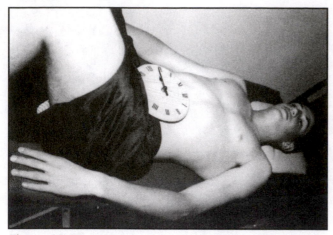

Figure 20-23.

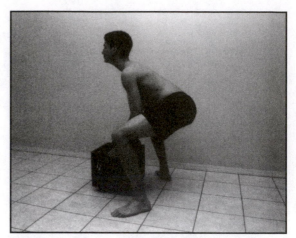

Figure 20-24.

Once the patient becomes more adept with these movements in hooklying, the patient can then integrate them into a variety of other positions, including supine, prone, quadruped, kneeling, half-kneeling, standing, etc.

Some of the foundational principles that are essential to a successful Feldenkrais experience include paying attention to the quality of the movement, doing the movements slowly and with minimal effort, resting frequently between movements to avoid physical and mental fatigue, and avoiding pain and discomfort.

To learn more about the Feldenkrais method, the reader is encouraged to contact the Feldenkrais Guild of North America or search for additional publications, course information, etc on the Internet.

5 Ls of Lifting

In the late 1980s, physical therapists at the Southside Health Institute in Bay Shore, NY, developed a useful education tool for the instruction of proper lumbar spine lifting mechanics. What came to be known as the 5 Ls of Lifting technique (Figure 20-24) was ultimately published in the *Physical Therapy Forum*.[28] However, because this publication was discontinued a few years later, the information was no longer available. Consequently, it is now being made available a second time with a few minor revisions. In addition to lifting, this technique can be adapted for bending, pushing/pulling loads, etc.

To serve as a memory jogger, each of the five instructions begins with the letter L, representing the 5 lumbar vertebrae as follows:

➡ L1: Load
➡ L2: Lever
➡ L3: Legs
➡ L4: Lordosis
➡ L5: Lungs

A brief explanation of the 5 Ls will serve to educate the patient in the theory behind the technique.

Patients should always check the load prior to lifting in the event that additional help and/or the use of a mechanical device is indicated. He or she may also decide not to attempt such a lift depending on the load involved.

The lever arm should always be kept as short as possible. Because Torque = Force x Lever Arm, the one aspect of the equation that is controllable is the distance from the object being lifted to the patient's center of rotation (ie, the torque or lever arm). Consequently, the patient should always get as close as possible to the item being lifted. It is also important to realize that a patient's torso has its own weight. Consequently, the mere act of bending can be potentially stressful to the lower back.

Regarding the lumbar lordosis, there is much controversy. Some advocate lumbar flexion, while others recommend functional neutral or hyperextension for lifting. Although the concept of a neutral spine makes the most sense, the author's experience is that patients mitigate their risk of injury by accentuating their lumbar lordosis. This position, if tolerated, loads the lumbar facets and "locks" the lumbar spine in its "close-packed" position. Consequently, unless unable to do so, which is rarely the case, patients are instructed to "hollow" their lower back and to maintain this position throughout the lift.

The next instruction relates to the use of the legs rather than the use of the back muscles. This is perhaps the most crucial component of a correct lift. Good lifting technique is contingent upon flexible and stable ankles, strong knee extensors, flexible hips, strong gluteal muscles, and good balance. Consequently, the patient is instructed to bend at the hips and knees and not at the waist. A lesson in "hip-hinging" with a stable trunk is often necessary for patients who are accustomed to bending at the waist. Patients should feel the load of the lift in their legs, not in their backs!

The final instruction is a safeguard especially related to heavy loads or lifts to which the patient is unable to get close and thereby minimize the lever arm (eg, working over a car, lifting a patient out of bed). As observed with weight lifters, a deep inhalation followed by pursed lip exhalation increases intra-abdominal pressure, which in turn stabilizes the trunk. Consequently, the final but very useful instruction in the 5 Ls of lifting technique involves the use of the lungs as a means of adding additional protection to the lumbar spine.

Though not one of the original 5 Ls, added protection to the low back can certainly be obtained by activating the core stabilizers for the duration of the lift. There is one final recommendation to consider regarding lifting. Patients should avoid twisting "like the plague." There's only one thing worse than lifting with the back forward bent at the waist, and that is to lift with the back forward bent and twisted at the waist!

References and Bibliography

References

1. Panjabi M. The stabilizing system of the spine. Part I. Function, dysfunction, adaptation and enhancement. *J Spinal Disord*. 1989;5:383-389.

2. Panjabi M. The stabilizing system of the spine. Part II. Neutral zone and stability hypothesis. *J Spinal Disord*. 1992;5:393-397.

3. Paris SV. Physical signs of instability. *Spine*. 1985;10(3):277-279.

4. Macnab I. *Backache*. Baltimore, Md: Williams & Wilkins; 1977.

5. McKenzie RA. *The Lumbar Spine: Mechanical Diagnosis and Therapy*. New Zealand: Spinal Publications; 1981.

6. Paris SV. Anatomy as related to function and pain. *Orthop Clin North Am*. 1983;14(3):475-489.

7. Adams MA, May S, Freeman BJC, et al. Effects of backward bending on lumbar discs. Relevance to physical therapy treatments for low back pain. *Spine*. 2000;25(4):431-437.

8. Kuslich SD, Ulstrom CL, Michael CJ. The tissue origin of low back pain and sciatica. *Orthop Clin North Am*. 1991;22(2):181-187.

9. Kramer J. *Intervertebral Disk Diseases, Causes, Diagnosis, Treatment, and Prophylaxis*. 2nd ed. New York, NY: Thieme Medical Publishers; 1990.

10. Beattie PF, Brooks WM, Rothstein JM, et al. Effect of lordosis on the position of the nucleus pulposus in supine subjects. *Spine*. 1994;19:2096-2102.

11. Fennell AJ, Jones AP, Hukins DWL. Migration of the nucleus pulposus within the intervertebral disc during flexion and extension of the spine. *Spine*. 1996;21:2753-2757.

12. Vleeming A, Mooney V, Dorman T, Snijders C, Stoeckart R. *Movement, Stability & Low Back Pain: The Essential Role of the Pelvis*. New York, NY: Churchill Livingstone; 1997.

13. Adams M, Bogduk N, Burton K, Dolan P. *The Biomechanics of Back Pain*. Edinburgh: Churchill Livingstone; 2002.

14. Gonnella C, Paris SV, Kutner M. Reliability in evaluating passive intervertebral motion. *Phys Ther*. 1982;62(4):436-444.

15. Ward RC. *The Myofascial Release Concept*. East Lansing, Mich: Michigan State University, College of Osteopathic Medicine; 1986.

16. Travell JG, Simons DG. *Myofascial Pain and Dysfunction: The Trigger Point Manual. Vol 2. The Lower Extremities*. Baltimore, Md: Williams & Wilkins; 1992.

17. Butler DS. *Mobilization of the Nervous System*. Melbourne: Churchill Livingstone; 1991.

18. Butler DS. *The Sensitive Nervous System*. Adelaide: Noigroup Publications; 2000.

19. Cyriax J. *Textbook of Orthopaedic Medicine, Vol. One: Diagnosis of Soft Tissue Lesions*. London: Bailliere Tindall; 1978.

20. Hertling D, Kessler RM. *Management of Common Musculoskeletal Disorders: Physical Therapy Principles and Methods*. Philadelphia, Pa: Lippincott-Raven; 1996.

21. Richardson C, Jull G, Hodges P, Hides J. *Therapeutic Exercise for Spinal Segmental Stabilization in Low Back Pain*. Edinburgh: Churchill Livingstone; 1999.

22. Kelly E. *Emily Kelly's Common Sense Pilates*. London: Lorenz Books; 2000.

23. Nachemson A. The lumbar spine. An orthopaedic challenge. *Spine*. 1976;1:50-71.

24. Kaltenborn FM. *Basic Evaluation and Mobilization Techniques*. 2nd ed. Minneapolis, Minn: OPTP; 1993.

25. Janda V. Central nervous motor regulation and back problems. In: Korr I, ed. *The Neurobiologic Mechanisms in Manipulative Therapy*. New York, NY: Plenum Press; 1978.

26. Posner-Mayer J. *Swiss Ball Applications for Orthopedic and Sports Medicine. A Guide for Home Exercise Programs Utilizing the Swiss Ball*. Denver, Colo: Ball Dynamics International Inc; 1995.

27. Jackson-Wyatt O. Feldenkrais method and rehabilitation. In: Davis CM, ed. *Complementary Therapies in Rehabilitation*. Thorofare, NJ: SLACK Incorporated; 1997.

28. O'Sullivan JJ, Ellis JJ, Makofsky HW. The 5 Ls of lifting. *Physical Therapy Forum*. 1991;3-6.

Bibliography

Beighton PH, Grahame R, Bird H. *Hypermobility of Joints*. 3rd ed. London: Springer-Verlag; 1999.

Biondi B, Drinkwater-Kolk M. *Functional Stabilization Training*. Course Manual, Back in Action Seminars; 1991.

Caplan D. *Back Trouble: A New Approach to Prevention and Recovery*. Gainesville, Fla: Triad Publishing Company; 1987.

Corning-Creager C. *Therapeutic Exercises Using Foam Rollers*. Berthoud, Colo: Executive Physical Therapy; 1998.

Donelson R, Grant W, Kamps C, Medcalf R. Pain response to sagittal end-range spinal motion: a prospective, randomized, multicentered trial. *Spine*. 1991;16(6):S206-S212.

Donelson R, Aprill C, Medcalf R, Grant W. A prospective study of centralization of lumbar and referred pain: a predictor of symptomatic discs and anular competence. *Spine*. 1997;22(10):1115-1122.

Donatelli RA, Wooden MJ. *Orthopaedic Physical Therapy*. 3rd ed. New York, NY: Churchill Livingstone; 2001.

Dutton M. *Manual Therapy of the Spine: An Integrated Approach*. New York, NY: McGraw-Hill; 2002.

Ellis JJ. *LPI: Lumbo-Pelvic Integration, A Course Workbook*. Patchogue, NY: 1990.

Evans C, Oldrieve W. A study to investigate whether golfers with a history of low back pain show a reduced endurance of transversus abdominis. *Journal of Manual & Manipulative Therapy*. 2000;8(4):162-174.

Fairbank J, Pynsent P. *The Oswestry Disability Index*. Spine. 2000;25(22):2940-2953.

Gracovetsky S, Farfan H, Helleur C. The abdominal mechanism. *Spine*. 1985;10:317-324.

Greenman PE. *Principles of Manual Medicine*. 2nd ed. Philadelphia, Pa: Lippincott Williams & Wilkins; 1996.

Grodin AJ, Cantu RI. *MF-1, Myofascial Manipulation*. Course Notes, Marietta, Ga: Institute of Graduate Physical Therapy Inc; 1991.

Gross J, Fetto J, Rosen E. *Musculoskeletal Examination*. 2nd ed. Cambridge, Mass: Blackwell Science; 2002.

Irion JM. Use of the gym ball in rehabilitation of spinal dysfunction. *Orthop Ther Clin North Am*. 1992;1(2):375-398.

Johnson GS, Saliba-Johnson V. The application of the principles of PNF for the care of lumbar spinal instabilities. *Journal of Manual & Manipulative Therapy*. 2002;10(2):83-105.

Kay AG. An extensive review of the lumbar multifidus: anatomy. *Journal of Manual & Manipulative Therapy*. 2000;8(3):102-114.

Konin JG, Wiksten DL, Isear JA, Brader H. *Special Tests for Orthopedic Examination*. 2nd ed. Thorofare, NJ: SLACK Incorporated; 2002.

Lawlis GF, Cuencas R, Selby D, McCoy CE. The development of the Dallas Pain Questionnaire, an assessment of the impact of spinal pain on behavior. *Spine*. 1989;14(5):511-515.

Long AL. The centralization phenomenon, its usefulness as a predictor of outcome in conservative treatment of chronic low back pain (a pilot study). *Spine*. 1995;20(23);2513-2521.

Magee DJ. *Orthopedic Physical Assessment*. 4th ed. Philadelphia, Pa: WB Saunders; 2002.

Maitland G, Hengeveld E, Banks K, English K, eds. *Maitland's Vertebral Manipulation*. Oxford: Butterworth Heinemann; 2001.

Manheim C. *The Myofascial Release Manual*. 3rd ed. Thorofare, NJ: SLACK Incorporated; 2001.

McGill SM, Cholewicki J. Biomechanical basis for stability: an explanation to enhance clinical utility. *J Orthop Sports Phys Ther*. 2001;31(2):96-100.

Morgan D. Concepts in functional training and postural stabilization for the low-back-injured. *Topics in Acute Care and Trauma Rehabilitation*. 1988;8-17.

Morrill Ramsey S. Feldenkrais movement principles in physical therapy. *Advance for Physical Therapists and PT Assistants*. 1999;7.

Olson KA, Joder D. Diagnosis and treatment of cervical spine clinical instability. *J Orthop Sports Phys Ther*. 2001;31(4):194-206.

Prentice WE, Voight ML eds. *Techniques in Musculoskeletal Rehabilitation*. New York, NY: McGraw Hill; 2001.

Robertson S. Integrating the fascial system into contemporary concepts on movement dysfunction. *Journal of Manual & Manipulative Therapy*. 2001;9(1):40-47.

Sahrmann SA. *Diagnosis and Treatment of Movement Impairment Syndromes*. St. Louis, Mo: Mosby-Year Book; 2002.

Saidoff DC, McDonough AL. *Critical Pathways in Therapeutic Intervention, Extremities and Spine*. St. Louis, Mo: Mosby-Year Book; 2002.

Saunders R, Piela C. *Functional Capacity Evaluation: The Saunders Method*. Chaska, Minn: The Saunders Group; 1998.

Saunders HD, Saunders R. *Evaluation, Treatment, and Prevention of Musculoskeletal Disorders*. 3rd ed. Chaska, Minn: The Saunders Group; 1993.

Taylor SJ, Taylor AE, Foy MA, Fogg AJB. Responsiveness of common outcome measures for patients with low back pain. *Spine*. 1999;24(17):1805-1812.

Waddell G. Nonorganic physical signs in low back pain. *Spine*. 1980; 5(2):117-125.

Westlake L. *Get on the Ball: Develop a Strong Core and Lean, Toned Body*. New York, NY: Marlowe and Co; 2002.

Winkle D, Aufdemkampe G, Matthijs O, Meijer OG, Phelps V. *Diagnosis and Treatment of the Spine, Nonoperative Orthopaedic Medicine and Manual Therapy*. Gaithersburg, Md: Aspen Publishers; 1996.

Zemach-Bersin D, Reese M. *Sensory Motor Learning Systems, Audio Tape Program User's Guide*. Berkeley, Calif: Sensory-Motor Learning Systems; 1983.

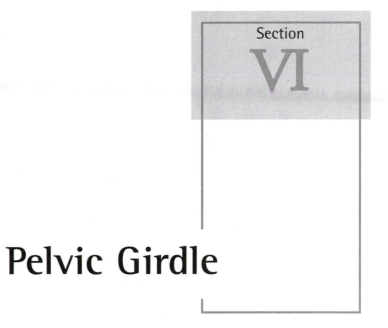

Section

VI

Pelvic Girdle

Examination and Evaluation of the Pelvic Girdle

It is now recognized that the sacroiliac (SI) joint retains mobility throughout life.[1] It is also well established that the sacroiliac joints can be a source of painful symptoms, especially when affected by inflammatory diseases such as ankylosing spondylitis, but also in conditions of mechanical impairment as occurs at the other synovial joints of the body.[2] According to Greenman,[3] the challenge confronting manual therapists is the ability of the clinician to identify a significant sacroiliac dysfunction when present. This, he says, is where more basic science and clinical research are needed. Regarding its contribution to patient care, Greenman says the following of the pelvic girdle, "The osseous pelvis has a significant contribution to the functional capacity of the musculoskeletal system and warrants appropriate investigation and management in all patients."[3] This author isn't convinced of its role in the management of "all patients," but clearly as a component of the lumbar-pelvic-hip complex, its role in low back and pelvic pain needs to be appreciated.

Because the ilium is capable of motion on the sacrum that is distinct from motion of the sacrum between the paired ilia, the sacroiliac joint can be functionally separated into the iliosacral and sacroiliac joints. It is believed that iliac motion is related to function of the lower extremity, whereas sacral motion is more related to the lumbar spine. The author believes that the complex mechanics of sacral motion (ie, sacroiliac), with its four "imaginary" axes, dictate that the subject of sacral examination/evaluation and intervention are best covered in an advanced course.

Consequently, this textbook will deal exclusively with the examination/evaluation and intervention of iliosacral impairment, which will enable the novice practitioner to manage a significant majority of patients with mechanical disorders of the pelvis. If a disorder of the sacroiliac complex is suspected and has not responded to manual correction of the lumbosacral junction nor iliosacral complex, then referral to a practitioner with advanced knowledge and skill in this area is warranted.

In the pelvic girdle, there are two systems that contribute to mechanical stability—the osteoarticularligamentous and the myofascial. Vleeming et al[4,5] and Lee[6] refer to these two systems as "form" and "force closure," respectively. Instability is defined by Lee as, "A loss of the functional integrity of a system which provides stability."[6] The manual examination of the pelvis in this chapter focuses on signs of instability, which include the presence of subluxations (ie, positional faults or misalignments) that often develop as a result of the underlying hypermobility. Through the process of inspecting pelvic asymmetry (A), range of motion (R), and tissue texture abnormality (T), the most common iliosacral (ie, anterior iliac rotation, posterior iliac rotation, and superior iliac shear or upslip) and pubic symphysis subluxations (ie, superior and inferior shears) can be identified, so that the proper manual intervention is rendered. In this way form closure is addressed and stability improved. Force closure, as in other regions of the body, is restored through normalization of myofascial function. This will be accomplished by stretching and "releasing" what is tight and strengthening and "retraining" what is weak.

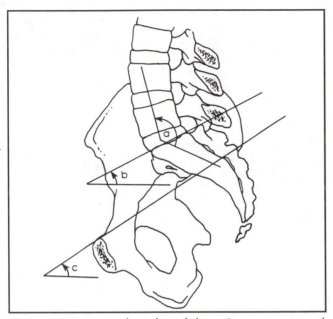

Figure 21-1. Normal angles of the spine, sacrum, and pelvis. a = lumbosacral angle (140 degrees), b = sacral angle (30 degrees), and c = pelvic angle (30 degrees) (reprinted with permission from Magee DJ. *Orthopedic Physical Assessment*. 3rd ed. Philadelphia, Pa: WB Saunders; 1997).

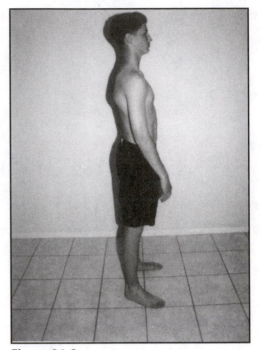

Figure 21-2a.

Structural Exam (Asymmetry of Bony Landmarks)

As with the other examination procedures covered thus far, the patient's pelvic girdle will be observed laterally, posteriorly, and anteriorly. In addition to observing alignment, key pelvic landmarks will also be palpated for positional asymmetry.

From a lateral perspective, there are three angles in the pelvis worth noting. They are the lumbosacral angle (140 degrees), the sacral angle (30 degrees), and the pelvic angle (30 degrees) as illustrated in Figure 21-1. Without necessarily measuring these angles, the therapist observes for deviations from normal. An acceptable clinical description may include normal, increased, or decreased angulation. For example, as the sacral base moves anterior and inferior, the sacral angle is described as having decreased. In geometric terms, this represents an increased acuity of the sacral angle. On the contrary, as the base moves posterior and superior, the sacral angle is described as having increased, which represents decreased acuity of the sacral angle. Movement of the sacral base anterior and inferior is referred to as sacral flexion, nutation, or anterior nutation, whereas movement of the sacral base in a posterior and superior direction is referred to as sacral extension, counternutation, or posterior nutation. There is a tendency to avoid the use of flexion and extension in this regard

because of the way in which sacral motion is described in the craniosacral literature. In craniosacral terms, sacral flexion is equivalent to counternutation, whereas sacral extension is equivalent to nutation. Consequently, the terms nutation and counternutation serve us better.

Regarding the normal pelvic angle (ie, inclination) in stance, the posterior superior iliac spine (PSIS) should always be slightly superior to the anterior superior iliac spine (ASIS) consistent with a 30-degree angle to the floor. In addition to a lateral inspection of the bony pelvis, the therapist is encouraged to begin the process of integrating the entire lower half of the body into the examination process (ie, from T6 to the feet). This includes a description of the mid/lower thoracic region, lumbar lordosis, pelvic tilt, hips, knees, ankles, and feet (Figure 21-2a).

Because of the interdependence of the lumbopelvic region and the lower limb, special attention should be given throughout the postural examination to such biomechanical and structural relationships as true versus functional leg length disparity; hip joint alignment; genu valgum, varum, and recurvatum; the quadriceps or Q-angle; tibial varum; tibial torsion; rearfoot/forefoot varus and valgus; compensatory rearfoot pronation; Feiss line; first ray position; hallux rigidus; functional hallux limitus; hallux abductovalgus; etc.

From a posterior perspective, the therapist should assess for a lateral shift of the trunk, signs of pelvic obliquity in the frontal plane, unilateral pelvic rotation in the sagittal plane, contour of the buttock region, and lower limb position as mentioned above (Figure 21-2b).

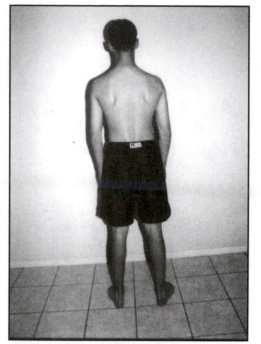

Figure 21-2b.

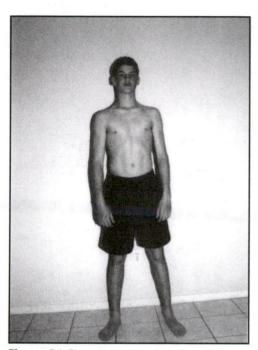

Figure 21-2c.

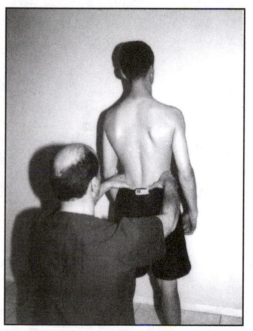

Figure 21-3a. Iliac crest assessment in standing.

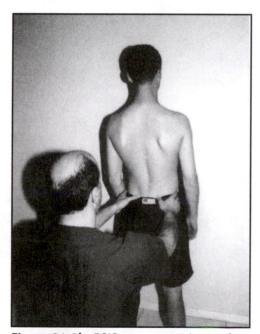

Figure 21-3b. PSIS assessment in standing.

In addition to assessing for these asymmetries, the anterior perspective offers the optimal view of hip joint position as well (Figure 21-2c).

The second aspect of the examination for pelvic girdle asymmetry includes the palpation of key bony landmarks. The pelvic/hip landmarks used for this purpose include the iliac crest, PSIS, ischial tuberosity, greater trochanter, ASIS, and the pubic tubercle.

The patient is first examined in the standing position. Posteriorly, the therapist palpates the iliac crests (Figure 21-3a), the PSISs at their inferior aspect (Figure 21-3b), and the greater trochanters at their superior aspect (Figure 21-3c). Whereas the iliac crests and greater trochanters are compared for asymmetry in height, the PSISs are assessed for differences in height and posterior prominence. When comparing for structural differences in height, osteopathic physicians suggest placing one's dominant eye in the midline of the patient's body.

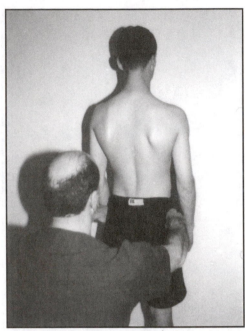

Figure 21-3c. Greater trochanter assessment in standing.

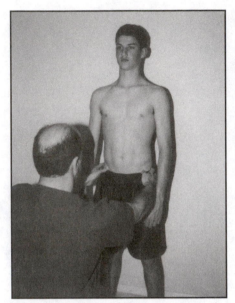

Figure 21-4. ASIS assessment in standing.

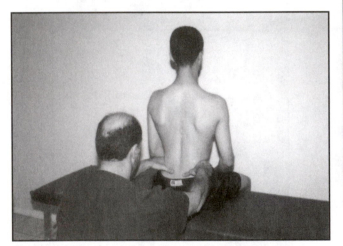

Figure 21-5a. Iliac crest assessment in sitting.

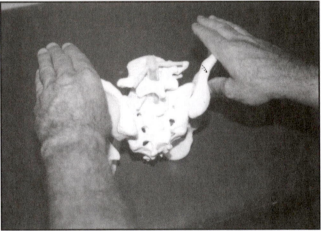

Figure 21-5b. Iliac crests.

Anteriorly, the standing patient's ASIS are palpated at their inferior aspects and assessed for asymmetry in height and anterior prominence (Figure 21-4). In sitting, the following landmarks are assessed: the iliac crests, PSIS, and ASIS (Figures 21-5a to 21-5f). In supine, the following landmarks are evaluated: the iliac crests (Figure 21-6a), ASIS (Figure 21-6b), and the pubic tubercles (Figures 21-6c and 21-6d). Because of the sensitive nature of the pubic region, it is suggested that the examiner ask the patient for permission to assess these bony landmarks. A picture of the bony anatomy is sometimes helpful in allaying the patient's apprehension. It is also recommended that the patient assist the therapist by finding his or her own pubic symphysis first and then from a superior direction, the therapist palpates

the patient's pubic tubercles (approximately 2 cm lateral to the pubic symphysis) for asymmetry in height and anterior prominence.

The final position for the comparison of bony landmarks in the osseous pelvis is prone lying. With the patient in a prone position, the therapist palpates the iliac crests (Figure 21-7a), PSIS (Figure 21-7b), and the ischial tuberosities (Figures 21-7c and 21-7d). Because we are dealing with iliosacral impairments only, there is no need at this point to palpate sacral landmarks (ie, the sacral sulcus and inferior lateral angle) for asymmetry. This, however, would be a component of the advanced examination involving sacroiliac impairment. Because the ilium rotates and translates in the same direction, the PSIS may become more prominent with posterior rotation and less prominent with anterior rotation. Conversely, the ASIS may become more prominent with anterior iliac rotation; less prominent with posterior rotation.

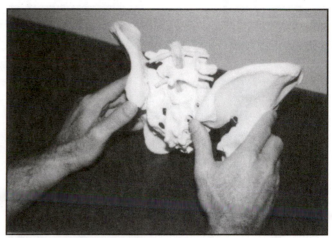

Figure 21-5c. PSIS assessment in sitting.

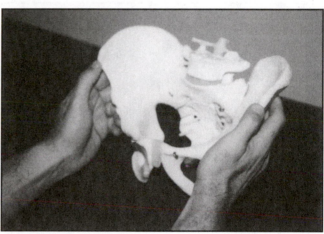

Figure 21-5d. PSIS location.

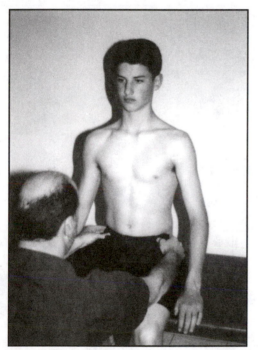

Figure 21-5e. ASIS assessment in sitting.

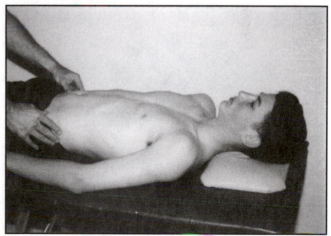

Figure 21-5f. ASIS location.

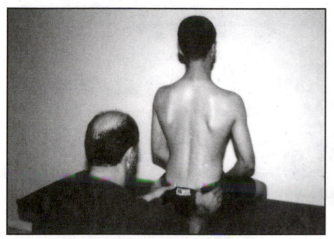

Figure 21-6b. ASIS assessment in supine.

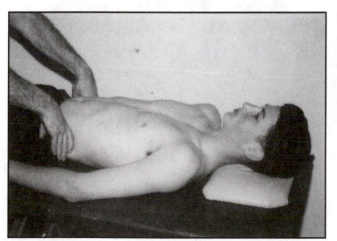

Figure 21-6a. Iliac crest assessment in supine.

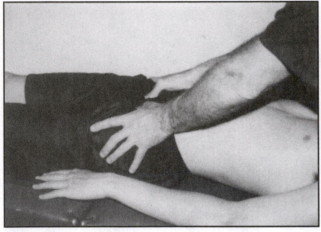

Figure 21-6c. Pubic tubercle assessment in supine.

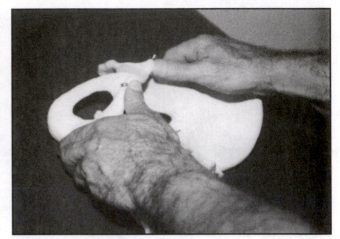

Figure 21-6d. Pubic tubercle location.

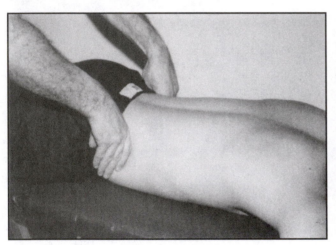

Figure 21-7a. Iliac crest assessment in prone.

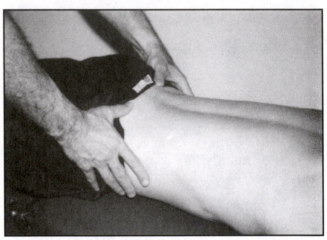

Figure 21-7b. PSIS assessment in prone.

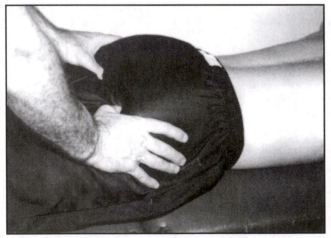

Figure 21-7c. Ischial tuberosity assessment in prone.

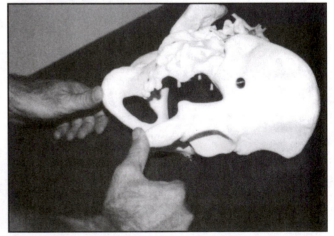

Figure 21-7d. Ischial tuberosities.

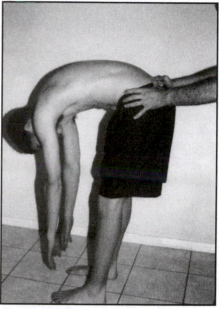

Figure 21-8.

The expected asymmetry in pelvic landmarks associated with iliosacral and pubic symphysis subluxation is as follows in all five of the following impairments:

1. Anterior iliac rotation on the right
   a. Superior right PSIS versus the left
   b. Inferior right ASIS versus the left
2. Posterior iliac rotation on the left
   a. Inferior left PSIS versus the right
   b. Superior left ASIS versus the right
3. Upslip of the right ilium (superior shear)
   a. Superior right iliac crest versus the left
   b. Superior right PSIS versus the left
   c. Superior right ASIS versus the left
   d. Superior right ischial tuberosity versus the left (6 mm or more)
   e. Level greater trochanters in standing (this finding distinguishes an iliac upslip from a leg length discrepancy)
4. Inferior pubic shear on the right ("down pube")
   a. Inferior right pubic tubercle versus the left
5. Superior pubic shear on the left ("up pube")
   a. Superior left pubic tubercle versus the right

Although it is useful for the therapist to begin considering the cause of these asymmetries early in the examination process, the therapist must avoid the temptation to make a diagnosis of iliosacral impairment prior to the completion of the remaining aspects of the exam, namely iliosacral mobility, soft tissue findings, and special tests, including provocation maneuvers.

Iliosacral Mobility Tests (Range of Motion)

The author has found the three iliosacral mobility tests described in this section to be extremely useful in the diagnosis of iliosacral impairment. They are as follows:

1. The standing flexion test
2. The one-legged stork or Gillet test
3. The long sitting test

The Standing Flexion Test

The standing patient is asked to forward bend as the therapist's thumbs monitor motion at the inferior aspect of the PSIS, bilaterally. The test (Figure 21-8) is considered positive for iliosacral impairment on the side in which the PSIS moves first and/or more superior. This represents a fixation, whereby the ilium becomes "bound" to the sacrum, resulting in premature movement and/or greater excursion on the affected side. A positive test is not specific as to the nature of the impairment but simply reveals that there is one. The therapist must integrate the other findings of the examination, including the history, to determine the specific impairment present.

There are at least four reasons for a false positive (ie, poor specificity) result with the standing flexion test. They are as follows:

1. A tight hamstring on the contralateral side
2. Iliac posterior rotation hypermobility on the contralateral side
3. A short leg on the contralateral side
4. Osseous (structural) asymmetry of the PSISs

If a leg length discrepancy is suspected, a lift should be used under the short leg prior to the test. If this is not done to balance pelvic alignment, the test is invalid.

The One-Legged Stork or Gillet Test

The stork or Gillet test can be used in a variety of ways to test both iliosacral as well as sacroiliac impairment. When used as a test for iliosacral impairment, it can detect restrictions in both posterior as well as anterior iliac rotation. It can also be applied separately to the superior aspect (upper pole) of the iliosacral joint, which consists of the shorter "arm" of the L-shaped surface and to the inferior aspect (lower pole) that consists of the longer "arm." L. Faye[7] likens the iliosacral joint surface to a "boot," whereby the superior articular surface (S1 segment) is above the "ankle" and the inferior surface (S2 and S3 segments) makes up the "foot" of the "boot."

Consequently, in the diagnosis of iliosacral impairment, the one-legged stork or Gillet test will be used to test motion loss in four different ways. They are as follows:

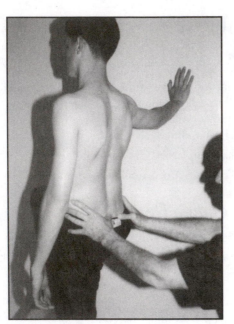

Figure 21-9a.

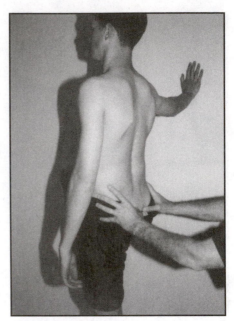

Figure 21-9b.

1. Superior iliosacral joint, posterior iliac rotation, right and left
2. Inferior iliosacral joint, posterior iliac rotation, right and left
3. Superior iliosacral joint, anterior iliac rotation, right and left
4. Inferior iliosacral joint, anterior iliac rotation, right and left

Superior Iliosacral Joint, Posterior Iliac Rotation

The patient is asked to raise his or her right knee to chest while holding for support. The therapist examines motion of the right ilium by palpating the inferior aspect of the right PSIS with the right thumb, while simultaneously palpating the S2 segment of the sacrum at the median sacral crest with the left thumb (Figure 21-9a). With normal iliosacral posterior rotation, the PSIS moves slightly inferior and lateral relative to the S2 segment. Restricted posterior rotation at the superior iliosacral joint (ie, the upper pole) is consistent with an anterior iliac rotation subluxation (misalignment) or an iliac shear lesion. In some patients, the PSIS actually moves superiorly, which suggests marked restriction. The left side is then tested accordingly.

Inferior Iliosacral Joint, Posterior Iliac Rotation

The patient performs the same knee-to-chest motion maneuver as in the previous exercise. However, in order to test right inferior or lower pole motion, the therapist places

his or her left thumb over the sacral apex at the hiatus, while the right thumb is placed at the same level on the posterior/inferior aspect of the right ilium (Figure 21-9b). With normal motion, the right iliac contact will move slightly anterior, inferior, and lateral in relation to the left thumb. Restricted motion is consistent with a right-sided, anterior iliac rotation or iliac shear misalignment (inferior shear or downslip is extremely rare). The left side is then tested accordingly.

Superior Iliosacral Joint, Anterior Iliac Rotation

As mentioned above, the one-legged stork or Gillet test can also be used to test for restricted anterior iliac rotation (ie, "reverse stork"). For those who use the term *marcher's test* instead of stork or Gillet, the following exam procedure is referred to as the "reverse marcher's test."

To assess upper pole anterior iliac rotation on the right side, the standing patient is instructed to bring his or her left knee to chest, while the therapist maintains contact at the S2 segment (in the midline) with the left thumb and the right PSIS with the right thumb (Figure 21-9c). As the left ilium rotates posteriorly and forces the sacrum into counternutation, a relative "anterior rotation" of the right ilium is induced. This is appreciated by the right PSIS "moving" superior and lateral relative to the sacrum. This is an example of "relative motion," whereby the change in iliac position, relative to the moving sacrum, is what the therapist is assessing. For example, a moving car passing a stationary car in the opposite direction can be said to cause relative "motion" of the stationary car when in fact it has not moved.

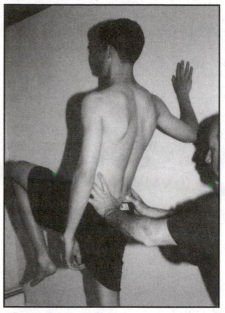

Figure 21-9c.

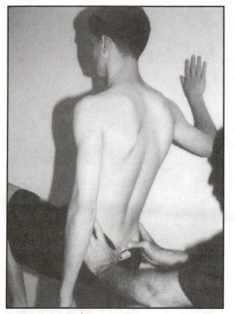

Figure 21-9d.

Consequently, the patient must bring the left knee high enough to his or her chest in order for the left ilium to recruit the sacrum and counternutate it. Should the right PSIS fail to "move" in a superior and lateral direction, it is said to be restricted. Restricted anterior iliosacral rotation implies that the ilium is "stuck" in either posterior rotation or a sheared position at the upper pole. The left side is then tested, accordingly, by having the patient raise his or her right knee high to the chest.

Inferior Iliosacral Joint, Anterior Iliac Rotation (Figure 21-9d)

The final of the four variations of the stork test involves an examination of anterior iliac rotation at the inferior aspect of the iliosacral joint ("reverse stork," lower pole). This, again, applies the principle of "relative motion" as described above. However, unlike the procedure demonstrated in Figure 21-9c, the examiner's thumb contacts now monitor motion at the lower pole by placing his or her left thumb over the sacral apex at the hiatus, while the right thumb makes contact with the posterior/inferior aspect of the right ilium at the same level (Figure 21-9d). To test the right side, the patient raises the left knee high to the chest in order to force the sacrum into counternutation. A normal response is observed when the therapist's right thumb moves superior and lateral relative to the left thumb. Motion restriction in conjunction with the expected asymmetry in iliac landmarks points to either a posteriorly rotated right iliac bone with impairment of motion at the inferior aspect or lower pole of the right iliosacral joint or to a right iliac shear (superior much more likely than inferior). The definitive diagnosis, however, cannot be made until the examination of tissue texture abnormality and special

tests are completed. The left side is tested, similarly, by reversing the thumb contacts and having the patient raise his or her right knee to the chest.

With all four variations of the stork test, an assessment of end-feel provides additional diagnostic information about impaired joint function.[8]

The Long Sitting Test

The long sitting test is also commonly used as an indicator of iliosacral impairment. The patient performs a bridging maneuver in order to obtain neutral alignment of the pelvis. The therapist then compares the length of the medial malleoli with the legs flat on the table (Figure 21-10a). This is followed by a similar comparison with the patient in the long sitting position (Figure 21-10b). A posterior iliac rotation misalignment is suspected when a short ipsilateral medial malleolus in supine becomes longer than the contralateral side in the long sitting position. An anterior iliac rotation is suspected when the ipsilateral medial malleolus changes from long in supine to short in long sitting versus the contralateral leg (Figure 21-11).

Soft Tissue Palpation (Tissue Texture Abnormality)

The inspection for signs of tissue texture abnormality in the pelvis is crucial in the diagnosis of somatic impairment. As with the other regions of the musculoskeletal system, the therapist is looking for the presence of the following associated indicators of a mechanical disorder: tenderness,

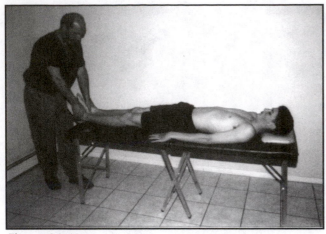

Figure 21-10a.

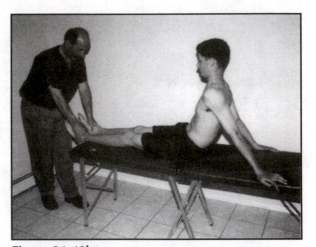

Figure 21-10b.

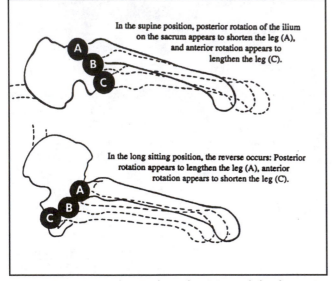

In the supine position, posterior rotation of the ilium on the sacrum appears to shorten the leg (A), and anterior rotation appears to lengthen the leg (C).

In the long sitting position, the reverse occurs: Posterior rotation appears to lengthen the leg (A), anterior rotation appears to shorten the leg (C).

Figure 21-11. Mechanical explanation of the long sitting test (reprinted from Saunders HD, Saunders R. *Evaluation, Treatment, and Prevention of Musculoskeletal Disorders*. 3rd ed. Chaska, Minn: The Saunders Group; 1993. Used with permission from the Saunders Group, Inc. © 1993).

tightness, hypertonia, fibrosis, swelling, and alterations in tissue texture, including a ropy, stringy, or boggy feel to the tissues. In addition to these aspects of the soft tissue examination, the therapist must also include the assessment of myofascial extensibility and muscle length.

The soft tissue structures amenable to examination in the pelvic region include the following:

1. Baer's SI point: 2 inches from the umbilicus on a line from the umbilicus to the ASIS (tenderness is often associated with a sacroiliac impairment).

2. Iliopsoas muscle: Medial to the sartorius muscle, medial and deep to the ASIS.

3. Pubic symphysis, inguinal ligament at its medial attachment, and the rectus abdominis at its distal attachment.

4. Quadratus lumborum muscle.

5. Iliolumbar ligament: Running from the transverse processes of L4 and L5 to the anterior surface of the iliac crest.

6. Posterior sacroiliac ligaments: Consisting of a deep layer of short interosseous ligaments running from the intermediate and lateral sacral crest to the rough sacropelvic surface of the ilium; the long interosseous ligaments extending from the median and lateral sacral crest, diagonally in a superior direction across the sacral sulcus, and attaching to the PSIS of the ilium. Particularly prominent is the long dorsal SI ligament,[9] which is a thickened band extending from the PSIS to the lateral sacral crest (it resists sacral counternutation and is thought to cause the all-to-common tenderness at the PSIS, when it comes under tension). The posterior, together with the anterior sacroiliac ligaments, are referred to as the intrinsic ligaments of the sacroiliac joint.

7. Gluteus maximus, medius, and minimus muscles.

8. Piriformis muscle: Palpable in the posterior buttock, deep to the gluteus maximus muscle, at the intersection of two lines. One line extends from the ASIS to the ischial tuberosity, while the other line runs from the PSIS to the greater trochanter.

9. Short lateral rotators of the hip (superior/inferior gemellus, obturator internus and externus, and the quadratus femoris): Deep to the gluteus maximus, anterior to the sciatic nerve, coming off the upper end of the greater trochanter. The obturator internus, lying between the two gemelli, is partly an intrapelvic muscle and partly a hip muscle.

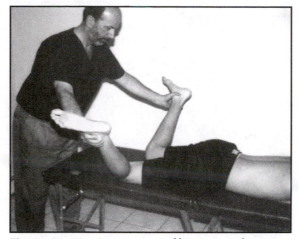

Figure 21-12a. Assessment of hip internal rotation prone.

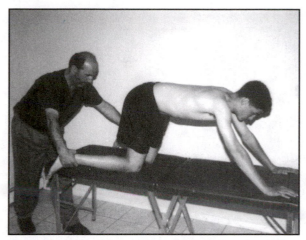

Figure 21-12b. Assessment of hip internal rotation quadruped.

10. Tensor fascia latae: The therapist performs myofascial inspection from its proximal attachment at the anterior iliac crest and ASIS to its distal insertion into the lateral patellar retinaculum, anterolaterally, and into Gerdy's tubercle at the lateral proximal tibia via the iliotibial tract, posterolaterally.

11. Pelvic floor muscles: Although optimal access to these intrapelvic muscles requires either a rectal or vaginal approach, the ischiococcygeus, iliococcygeus, and pubococcygeus muscles can be partly accessed just medial, posterior, and anterior to the ischial tuberosity with the patient in the hooklying position.

12. Adductor longus, brevis, magnus, gracilis, and pectineus muscles at the lower borders of the pelvis, pubic ramus, ischial ramus, and ischial tuberosity.

13. Hamstring muscles at their attachment into the ischial tuberosity.

14. Sacrotuberous ligament is a triangular-shaped structure connecting the PSIS, SI joint capsule, coccyx, and the ischial tuberosity with connecting fibers from the biceps femoris muscle a common finding. The tendons of the deepest laminae of the multifidus often extend into the sacrotuberous ligament. Its role is to resist sacral nutation and posterior iliac rotation. Consequently, the sacrotuberous ligament becomes palpably tender and taut in the presence of a posterior iliac misalignment.

15. Sacrospinous ligament is a triangular-shaped structure that lies under the sacrotuberous ligament, extending from the inferior lateral angle of the sacrum to the ischial spine. The sacrospinous ligament separates the greater from the lesser sciatic foramen. Like the sacrotuberous ligament, it resists sacral nutation and posterior iliac rotation. The iliolumbar, sacrotuberous, and sacrospinous ligaments are collectively referred to as the extrinsic sacroiliac ligaments.

Following the direct palpatory examination of the aforementioned tissues, the therapist should evaluate the length of all the postural muscles of the pelvis and hip that are prone to tightness (eg, rectus abdominis, sacrospinalis, quadratus lumborum, piriformis, hamstrings, adductors, tensor fascia latae, iliopsoas, etc). Hip flexor length can be tested with the Thomas, Ely, and/or the TRI muscle test (covered in the following chapter); the tensor fascia latae is tested with Ober's test. A tight piriformis is distinguished from a tight hip capsule by the range of hip internal rotation in prone versus quadruped (Figures 21-12a and 21-12b). Because the piriformis is an external rotator of the hip in neutral and an internal rotator above 60 degrees of hip flexion,[10] a restriction of internal rotation in neutral prone lying that normalizes in quadruped points to muscle tightness. However, restricted hip joint internal rotation in both positions points to stiffness of the hip joint capsule.

Manual muscle testing of the weak phasic muscles of the pelvis and hip (ie, the oblique abdominals, gluteus maximus, medius, and minimus, etc) can be performed at this point or in the special test section to follow.

Special Tests

Tests that mechanically stress the SI joint structures in order to reproduce the patient's symptoms are called *provocation tests*. These tests do not assess for asymmetries, range of motion deficits, nor tissue texture abnormality, but rather help to determine whether the SI joint is the anatomic source of the pain regardless of whether the underlying problem is due to disease or mechanical impairment. The provocation tests described in this section have substantial intertherapist reliability.[11,12] They have not, however, been tested for sensitivity nor specificity, and they do not discriminate between iliac misalignment on the sacrum (ie, iliosacral impairment) and sacral misalignment within the

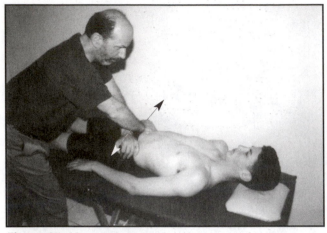

Figure 21-13.

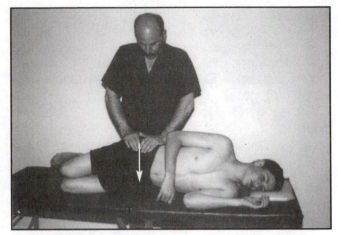

Figure 21-14.

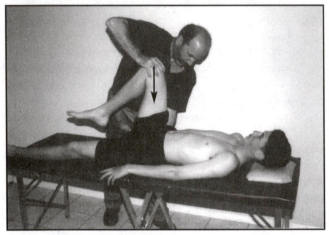

Figure 21-15.

paired ilia (ie, sacroiliac impairment). They include the following:

1. Distraction or "gapping" test
2. Compression test
3. Posterior shear or "thigh thrust" test
4. Pelvic torsion test

The Distraction or "Gapping" Test

In this test (Figure 21-13), the therapist applies a posterior and lateral force to both ASISs in order to distract or gap the anterior aspect of the SI joints and stretch the anterior SI ligaments. Reproduction or exacerbation of the patient's pelvic pain constitutes a positive response.

The Compression Test

In this test (Figure 21-14), the therapist applies downward pressure to the uppermost iliac crest directed toward the opposite iliac crest with the patient in side lying. This test purports to stretch the posterior SI joint ligaments and compress the anterior aspect of the SI joint. The test is positive if the patient's symptoms are either reproduced or worsened.

The Posterior Shear or "Thigh Thrust" Test

In this test (Figure 21-15), the therapist imparts a posterior shearing stress on the SI joint through downward pressure on the supine patient's flexed femur. For optimal application, the therapist blocks motion of the sacrum with one hand while applying the downward force through the femur with the other. Excessive hip adduction should be avoided lest the test becomes overly stressful to the joint and produces false positive results. The hip quadrant test does, however, involve compression with adduction, but this is a provocation test for the hip joint and will be mentioned subsequently. Again, provocation of the patient's pelvic pain is considered a positive test response.

The Pelvic Torsion Test

With the patient in supine and the left knee pulled to the patient's chest, the therapist applies overpressure to the left leg (Figure 21-16), causing end-range left posterior iliac rotation. In the meantime, the right hip is held in extension with the leg off the end of the table. It is expected that a left posterior iliac rotation subluxation will react to this end-range stress. However, the test is not specific for this given misalignment, but introduces sufficient stress to the left SI joint to provoke symptoms in a variety of positional faults, including, but not limited to, posterior iliac rotation. The torsion test is then repeated on the right side by simply reversing all manual contacts and having the patient pull the right knee to his or her chest instead. This maneuver is also referred to as Gaenslen's sign[13] and can be performed in the side lying position as well.[14]

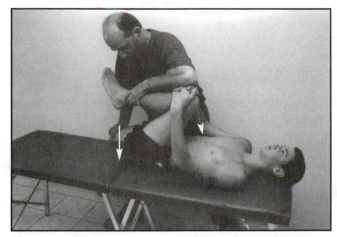

Figure 21-16.

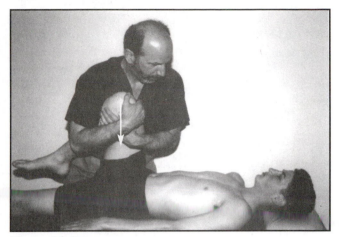

Figure 21-17.

When attempting to determine whether the patient's symptoms are pelvic in origin, it is necessary to perform a clarifying exam of the hip joints. There are many orthopaedic provocation tests of the hip (eg, Patrick's test, anterior and posterior labral tear test, torque test), but the one that the author has found the most useful is Maitland's hip quadrant or "scour" test (Figure 21-17). It assesses degenerative changes in the articular surfaces of the hip, including labral irregularities. The posterior and lateral aspects of the joint capsule are stretched, and the articular cartilage and labrum are compressed. The supine patient's hip is passively moved through an arc of flexion in adduction from 90 and 140 degrees where the knee is pointing toward the patient's opposite shoulder. Compression of the hip is maintained through the femur at all times as demonstrated. Throughout the arc, the femur should lie midway between medial and lateral rotation. A positive response for a hip disorder includes pain, guarding, apprehension, crepitus, etc. A small abnormality is often felt as a "bump" along the smooth arc of this circle. In addition to the hip quadrant test,[15] this section would not be complete without mentioning the goniometric assessment of hip joint range of motion, including an inspection of flexion, extension, abduction/adduction, medial, and lateral rotation. As noted in the soft tissue section of the examination, hip muscle length and strength must also be included in every examination of the pelvic girdle. Because of the significant influence of the hip postural (eg, hamstrings, iliopsoas, adductors, tensor fascia latae) and phasic (eg, gluteus maximus, gluteus medius) muscles on the alignment and function of the iliosacral joints, an approach that seeks to balance these influences by stretching what's tight and strengthening what's weak will certainly help many individuals. It is the author's philosophy, however, that combining stretching and strengthening procedures together with myofascial and articular manipulation yields the best outcomes possible. To that end, let us proceed to the chapters on manual therapy intervention!

22

Connective Tissue Techniques and Stretching Procedures for the Pelvic Girdle

Pelvic/Urogenital Diaphragm Release

Myofascial pain and dysfunction of the muscles of the pelvic floor causes pain to be felt in the perineum, urogenital structures, the posterior pelvic floor, the sacrococcygeal region, the vagina, the anococcygeal region, and the posterior thigh. The levator ani muscle is the most widely recognized source of referred pain in the perineal region. Referred pain from the levator ani may be felt in the sacrum, coccyx, rectum, perirectal area, vagina, or low back and be aggravated by lying on the back and by defecation. Terms used to describe pelvic pain of levator ani muscle origin include levator spasm syndrome, levator ani spasm syndrome, levator syndrome, and pelvic floor syndrome. Though not a likely occurrence, there is the potential for entrapment of the pudendal nerve and the internal pudendal vessels by the obturator internus muscle in the lesser sciatic foramen. Should this occur, perineal pain or dysesthesia can result.[16]

The pelvic/urogenital diaphragm release (Figure 22-1) is a "three-dimensional"/transverse fascial plane technique not unlike the thoracic inlet and respiratory diaphragm releases described in Chapter 5. As with any "three-dimensional"/transverse fascial plane release, the "4 Ms" procedure (also described in Chapter 5) is an excellent way of performing either a direct or indirect myofascial release technique of the pelvic floor. Manheim[17] reports that the reflex relaxation of the pelvic/urogenital diaphragm

achieved through myofascial release therapy has proven useful in easing the pain of endometriosis and premenstrual cramps and may help relieve chronic low back pain and deep hip joint pain.

Using the "4 Ms" procedure, the therapist molds, melds, monitors, and moves the tissues between the bottom hand placed under the sacrum and the top hand placed lightly over the pubic symphysis. The hands should be perpendicular to the patient's body and parallel to each other. The choice of whether to proceed with a direct fascial stretch or an indirect method, whereby tissue ease is sought, is dependent upon the patient's symptoms and level of tissue reactivity as discussed in Chapter 3. Because of the sensitivity of this region, the author recommends beginning with a gentle indirect approach in which myofascial relaxation or "unwinding" is achieved. The use of direct myofascial stretching is performed when the tissues require it. A slight degree of tissue compression, prior to either indirect or direct technique, is often useful in enhancing the release of tissue tension. As always, the purpose of this "three-dimensional"/transverse plane myofascial intervention is to relax, soften, and restore normal elasticity/pliability to the tissues between the therapist's two hands. Before proceeding, an explanation, along with the appropriate anatomy pictures, serves to allay the patient's apprehension. If the therapist is of the opposite gender of the patient, it is wise to have another person of the same gender as the patient in the treatment room during the application of the technique.

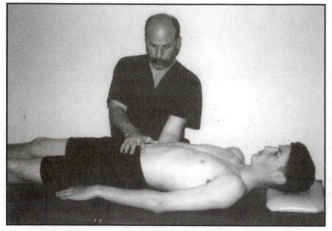

Figure 22-1.

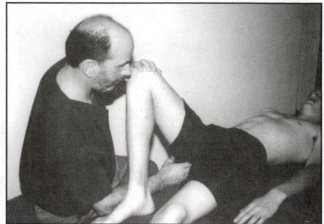

Figure 22-2.

Pelvic Floor Fascial Technique

The remainder of the manual connective tissue techniques in this section fall into the category of direct fascial techniques, otherwise known as myofascial manipulation, soft tissue mobilization, deep tissue massage, etc. As with the examination of this area in the previous chapter, the patient is placed in the hooklying position on the treatment table as demonstrated (Figure 22-2). Because of the proximity of the external genitalia and anus to the myofascial point of entry, this manual intervention requires the utmost respect for the patient's dignity and self-respect. It is strongly recommended that a third person be present in the treatment room and that this person be of the same gender as the patient. When children are involved, it is necessary for a parent or guardian to be present. An appropriate anatomic illustration of the pelvic floor musculature should be shown to the patient, parent, etc, prior to the application of the technique, including an explanation of the clinical purpose for the use of this procedure (in many clinics, a written, informed consent is required for this and perhaps all therapeutic procedures as an added measure of legal protection for the therapist and the facility). The patient must understand his or her right to refuse such treatment at any time. In addition to the above considerations, proper draping technique of the patient's perineal area should be a priority.

With fingernails that are appropriately trimmed, the therapist applies light digital pressure with two or three fingers to the area medial and anterior to the ischial tuberosity, while abducting the ipsilateral thigh for optimal access. It is the musculature of the pelvic diaphragm located between the ischial tuberosity, laterally, the coccyx posteriorly, the anus, medially, and the transversus perinei superficialis, superiorly, that are amenable to gentle direct fascial technique. Though direct skin contact is preferable, this procedure can be performed over a pair of shorts, sweatpants, or a towel. The objective is to release tension and tightness in this region of the pelvis through the application of gentle, direct manual pressure. The attachment sites of the muscles of the pelvic diaphragm into the entire ischial region of the innominate bone are likely areas of soft tissue impairment. For those patients who suffer with chronic pelvic floor pain syndromes related to myofascial involvement, there is nothing that is more useful than the direct manual "release" of this area.

Piriformis Fascial Technique

The piriformis muscle is thick and bulky in most individuals, but occasionally it is thin and sometimes absent. The Belgian anatomist Adrian Spigelius coined its name, which in Latin means "pear shaped." Travell and Simons[16] report that in approximately 85% of cadavers, the sciatic nerve passes anterior to the piriformis and between its fibers and the rim of the greater sciatic foramen. In approximately 10% of cadavers, the peroneal portion of the nerve passes through the piriformis and the tibial portion travels anterior to it. In 2% to 3%, the peroneal portion loops above and then posterior to the muscle, while the tibial portion passes anterior to it; both portions lie between the muscle and the rim of the greater sciatic foramen. In less than 1% of cadavers, an undivided sciatic nerve pierces through the piriformis muscle. When the piriformis is sufficiently enlarged to fill the foramen, entrapment of the superior and inferior gluteal nerves and blood vessels, the sciatic nerve, the pudendal nerve and vessels, the posterior femoral cutaneous nerve, and the nerves supplying the gemelli, obturator internus, and quadratus femoris muscles is a possibility. When sciatic nerve entrapment is present, there are usually signs of L5 and S1 nerve root involvement.

In the presence of sacroiliac or iliosacral misalignment, contraction of the piriformis loads the joint and thus can mimic sciatic pain. Piriformis tightness may also subject the sacrum to abnormal rotary stress and produce or exacerbate

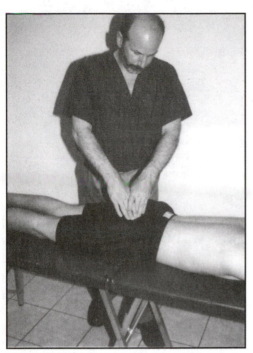

Figure 22-3a.

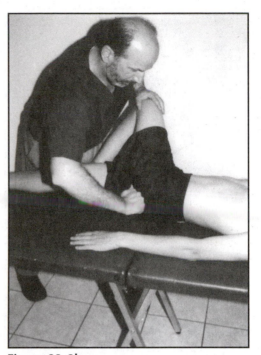

Figure 22-3b.

a pelvic dysfunction. Myofascial pain of the piriformis may cause symptoms to develop proximal to the gluteal cleft and at the posterior, superior, and medial border of the hip joint with possible referral down the buttock and into the posterior thigh. Symptoms tend to be aggravated by sitting; by a prolonged combination of hip flexion, adduction, and medial rotation; or by activity. However, before the painful symptoms can truly be considered to be of piriformis origin, the clinician must first clear the lumbar spine, sacroiliac region, and hip joint as discussed in previous sections. Compensatory hypertonicity (ie, muscle substitution) of the piriformis is often seen in the presence of gluteus maximus weakness.

To access the piriformis muscle in the prone-lying patient, the point of intersection of two imaginary lines, as described during the examination, is used as a guide. One line runs from the ASIS to the ischial tuberosity; the other from the PSIS to the greater trochanter. As illustrated in Figure 22-3a, the direct fascial technique known as "strumming" is an excellent way of "freeing" the piriformis muscle and its fascial attachments. Other methods include muscle play, circular friction with the thumb or elbow (used when more force is required), "steamrolling," etc. After applying soft tissue mobilization in the neutral range, the technique can progress to treatment under stretch, as illustrated in Figure 22-3b. As with all connective tissue techniques, the goal is to relax, soften, lengthen, and mobilize tense, restricted, and painful myofascial tissues. A small amount of soft tissue massage cream (ie, Deep Prep II [Smith & Nephew, Germantown, Wisc]) is recommended.

Tensor Fascia Latae Fascial Technique

The term *pseudotrochanteric bursitis* refers to the pain and tenderness caused by myofascial impairment of the tensor fascia latae (TFL). Patients with this disorder describe painful symptoms in the lateral hip extending down the anterolateral aspect of the thigh; they are often misdiagnosed as having trochanteric bursitis. These patients usually have difficulty lying on the involved side because of pressure on the tender region, and they often cannot lie on the contralateral side without a pillow between their knees because of the tight iliotibial band (ITB).

The TFL assists with flexion, abduction, and medial rotation of the hip. The tendinous fibers of the posterolateral half of the TFL join the longitudinal middle layer to form the ITB, which has two components at the knee: the iliopatellar band and the iliotibial tract. The iliotibial tract courses distally to its insertion at Gerdy's tubercle at the lateral proximal tibia; the iliopatellar band reinforces the lateral retinaculum, which adds stability to the lateral aspect of the knee. The iliopatellar band is connected to the iliotibial tract through the patellotibial ligament. There are several other iliotibial tract attachments, including the lateral intermuscular septum, the lateral femoral condyle, Gerdy's tubercle at the lateral proximal tibia, the lateral capsular ligament, the biceps femoris tendon, and the fibula. The ITB is influenced by both the gluteus maximus and the TFL from which it arises. At the knee, the ITB is an extensor from 0 to 30 degrees and a flexor when the knee is

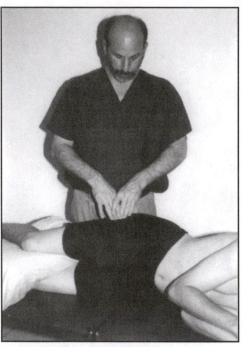

Figure 22-4a.

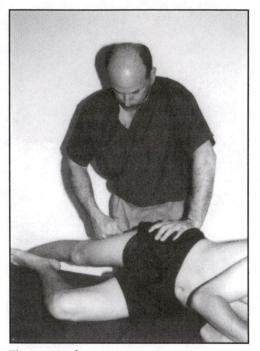

Figure 22-4b.

flexed 30 degrees or more.[18] This information is helpful when performing stretches of the TFL/ITB, incorporating both hip and knee motions. Compensatory hypertonicity of the TFL is often seen in the presence of gluteus medius weakness.

Direct fascial technique of the TFL is performed in side lying with the affected side up. A pillow is placed between the patient's knees to maintain a neutral position of the hip (Figure 22-4a). All previous manual methods, including "strumming," "steamrolling," "sculpting," etc, are applied to the bony attachments, fibers of the TFL and ITB, junction of the TFL and ITB and gluteus maximus/ITB, anterior and posterior edges of the ITB, and distally at the lateral femoral condyle, lateral retinaculum, patella, Gerdy's tubercle, and the fibula. The same soft tissue techniques can then be applied with the TFL in a stretched position (Figure 22-4b). This is the classic Ober's test position, in which the therapist stabilizes the iliac bone with one hand and performs the direct fascial technique with the other. The ITB tends to be most taut in knee extension, with the hip placed in slight extension, external rotation, and adduction. Again, a small amount of soft tissue massage cream is recommended.

Piriformis Stretch

The piriformis muscle, as discussed, is often tight and therefore in need of effective stretching. Because it assists with external rotation of the hip before 60 degrees of flexion and internal rotation after 60 degrees,[10] the manner in which it is stretched must differ based upon hip position. Consequently, two different stretching procedures will be shown to ensure full flexibility of the muscle throughout the hip joint's range of motion.

To stretch the left piriformis muscle below 60 degrees of hip flexion, the supine patient's left foot is placed to the right of the right lower leg with the foot flat on the table. Standing on the patient's right side, the therapist directs the patient's left distal femur toward the right into adduction and internal rotation (Figure 22-5a). At the barrier of motion, the postisometric relaxation (PIR) technique can be applied to enhance the stretch by having the patient perform a submaximal, isometric contraction of the abductors/external rotators for 6 seconds, followed by a stretch into the new range. After three cycles of the PIR/stretch technique, the patient's limb is returned slowly to the rest position (the left ASIS can be held down during the stretch to enhance control).

To stretch the left piriformis with the hip in more than 60 degrees of hip flexion (Figure 22-5b), the supine patient's left hip is passively moved into a combination of flexion, adduction, and external rotation (ie, left knee to the right shoulder). The therapist again stands on the side opposite the stretch and controls the PIR/stretch procedure by placing his or her hands on the patient's left knee (again, the patient's left ASIS can be stabilized with the left hand to enhance control during the stretch). For those patients who feel pain in the anterior hip area, the amount of hip adduction should be decreased and the external rotation increased. To perform these two stretches to the right piriformis muscle, all directions and contacts are simply reversed.

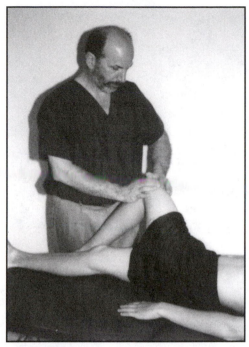

Figure 22-5a.

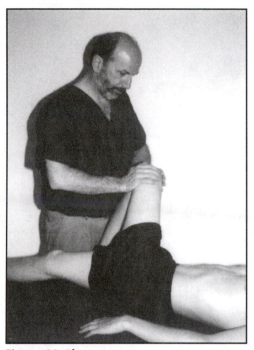

Figure 22-5b.

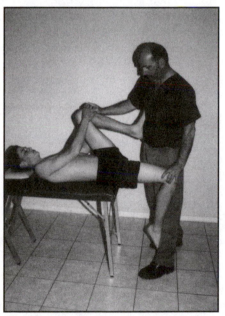

Figure 22-6.

Tensor, Rectus, Iliopsoas Muscle Stretch

A modification of the Thomas test position is to have the patient lying at the end of the table with one knee pulled tightly to the chest and the other leg dangling off the end with the knee relaxed in flexion (Figure 22-6). This modified Thomas position was first referred to as the TRI

muscle position by Ellis[19] since it assesses and treats three related muscles simultaneously (ie, the tensor fascia latae, rectus femoris, and iliopsoas). The utility of this position involves its ability to evaluate and treat tightness in these three postural muscles quickly and easily. For evaluation purposes, the patient's lumbar spine ideally should remain flat on the table at all times, while the suspended limb should be in the midline with the posterior thigh flat on the table surface and the knee flexed to 90 degrees. By contrast, tightness of the TRI muscles will cause deviation of limb position (ie, hip abduction, internal rotation, and flexion with TFL tightness; knee extension and/or hip flexion with tightness of the rectus femoris; and hip flexion/external rotation with tightness of the iliopsoas). In addition to observing for the effect of muscle tightness on the position of the femur, end-feel is noted and passive overpressure is applied to hip extension and knee flexion. By stabilizing the ASIS inferiorly, iliacus tightness[20] can be distinguished from psoas tightness (ie, the "iliacus test"). Tightness of the iliacus can also induce anterior rotation of the ipsilateral iliac bone, when the femur is fixed (ie, iliacus contraction in reverse action).

As an intervention, the same position is used while the therapist performs postisometric stretching of the TRI muscles. In addition, the therapist can add direct fascial technique in the stretched position of the muscle, especially of the TFL, while maintaining hip extension, adduction, and external rotation. In the presence of iliosacral hypermobility, the patient's pelvis should be stabilized with a strap or SI belt while the TRI muscles are being stretched.

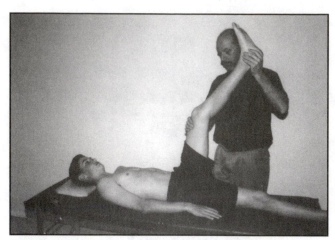

Figure 22-7.

Hamstring Stretch

The importance of stretching tight hamstrings (Figure 22-7) cannot be over emphasized. It is a muscle that directly affects the lumbopelvic region, hip joint, and knee and indirectly affects the entire kinetic system, including the cervicothoracic area, by virtue of its tendency to displace the center of gravity posteriorly. When bilaterally tight, compensatory forward head carriage may ensue. In the presence of unilateral tightness, there is the tendency for posterior iliosacral rotation to occur on the ipsilateral side. In addition, the biceps femoris is believed to be a myofascial "link" between the foot, ankle, and pelvic girdle through its connection to the fibular head. For example, rearfoot pronation displaces the fibular head anteriorly, which places the lateral hamstring under tension. This in turn introduces tension into the sacrotuberous ligament, which has the potential to affect the alignment and function of both the sacrum and ilium.

Hamstring tightness predisposes athletes and dancers to recurrent injuries. This is especially true when it is substituting for weakness of the ipsilateral gluteus maximus muscle. The astute clinician must also be mindful that adverse sciatic nerve tension, secondary to a lumbar disc derangement, will facilitate hamstring hypertonicity and predispose the hamstring to recurrent muscle strains. Consequently, the lumbar spine must always be examined before a definitive diagnosis of a hamstring "pull" is made. Conversely, in patients with a documented herniated lower lumbar disc, the hamstring must at some point be treated with connective tissue techniques and stretching because of its tendency to tighten in response to L5 and S1 nerve root compression.

Direct fascial technique to the hamstrings will not be described here. However, the therapist should consider using the same soft tissue techniques to "free-up" the hamstrings as used elsewhere. The manual stretch is performed on the supine patient in the 90 degrees/90 degrees position. As with all stretches, the postisometric relaxation component is an extremely useful addition. If iliosacral hypermobility is a concern, the patient's pelvis should be stabilized with a strap or SI belt for the duration of the stretch. Otherwise, the hamstring stretch may displace the ilium in posterior rotation.

Hip Adductor Stretch

The adductor longus, brevis, magnus, gracilis, and pectineus muscles are postural muscles that tend to become facilitated, hypertonic, and tight. According to Sahrmann,[21] the combination of hip adduction, medial rotation, and anterior pelvic tilt in standing lengthens the piriformis muscle, subjecting it to stress and strain, possibly leading to sciatic nerve entrapment. In the presence of hip adductor tightness, the TFL may also come under strain, causing pseudotrochanteric bursitis. In addition, tightness of the hip adductors may cause weakness of the gluteus medius muscle, which would undermine its important role in pelvic stability during ambulation.

In the presence of tight hip adductors, the standing patient may appear to have a longer leg on that side by virtue of a higher iliac crest.[21] This is in contrast to tightness of the hip abductors, which will lower the iliac crest on the affected side. To confirm this finding, the patient's pelvis will become level when the side with the tight adductors is adducted slightly. Conversely, the patient with tight abductors need only abduct slightly to level the pelvis. Regarding an additional effect of unilateral adductor tightness, the pubic ramus may be sheared inferiorly on the affected side in response to a strong isometric adductor contraction. Such would be the case if a soccer player missed the ball and struck the nonyielding ground instead.

"Rider's strain"[22] is characterized by the combination of painful isometric adduction and tenderness at either the musculotendinous or tenoperiosteal junction (a note should be made that painful isometric adduction is also present with fracture or neoblastic invasion of the os pubis).

Referred pain from myofascial injury and impairment of the hip adductors includes discomfort just below the inguinal ligament, deep groin pain, and referred symptoms into the hip, anteromedial thigh, and as far downward as the knee and shin.

To stretch the hip adductors, the therapist stands on the affected side, facing the supine patient's feet. In order to provide pelvic stability for a more effective stretch, the contralateral hip is slightly abducted with the leg placed over the edge of the table. The adductor stretch is then performed as follows (Figure 22-8):

1. The therapist abducts the patient's tight side via heel contact.

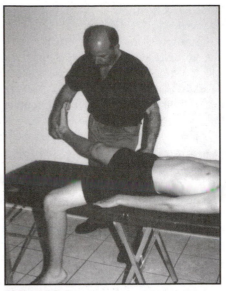

Figure 22-8.

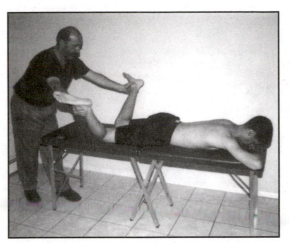

Figure 22-9a.

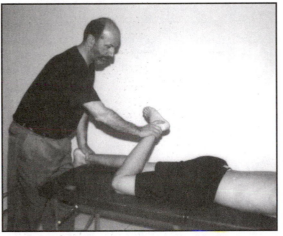

Figure 22-9b.

2. The other hand contacts the superior aspect of the patient's greater trochanter.

3. At the barrier of abduction, the therapist performs three repetitions of postisometric relaxation (ie, 6 second submaximal isometric contractions followed by relocalization to the new barrier of abduction).

4. If, in addition to the adductor tightness, the therapist detects inferior femoral glide restriction, a graded mobilization can be added with the hip in the abducted position. Through the arthrokinetic reflex mechanism,[23] the improved capsular mobility will theoretically inhibit adductor tone while facilitating tone and strength of the gluteus medius muscle.

Hip Rotator Stretch

The prone position is used to both assess and treat myofascial tightness of the external and internal rotators of the hip. As illustrated (Figure 22-9a), the external rotators of the hip (ie, the obturator externus/internus, quadratus femoris, piriformis, gemellus superior/inferior, gluteus maximus, posterior fibers of the gluteus medius, sartorius, and biceps femoris muscles) can be stretched bilaterally using postisometric relaxation technique (PIR). The hip internal rotators (ie, the gluteus minimus, anterior fibers of the gluteus medius, tensor fascia latae, semitendinosus, and semimembranosus muscles) can also be stretched using PIR in prone lying, but performed one limb at a time (Figure 22-9b).

Myofascial Leg Pull

The myofascial leg pull (Figure 22-10) is performed with the patient in supine. There are two variations of this technique that the author finds extremely useful. One is the indirect approach and the other is the direct approach. The indirect approach requires an appreciation of inherent tissue motion and seeks to relax myofascial tissues by passively moving them in the direction of tissue ease. Consequently, the myofascial tissues of the lower extremity are "unwound" the way a tangled telephone cord would be if allowed to follow its "path of least resistance." The indirect technique is useful when dealing with increased muscle tone of peripheral origin (ie, nociceptively mediated hypertonicity).

The direct myofascial leg pull is a "shotgun" type of approach that enables the therapist to stretch and mobilize several myofascial structures simultaneously. It imparts a vigorous stretch to the tissues and should, therefore, only be used in the presence of low reactive myofascial tightness.

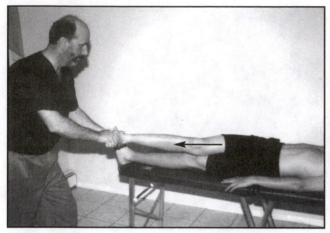

Figure 22-10.

The myofascial leg pull applies longitudinal traction to the leg with the patient supine. The ankle is passively dorsiflexed and the leg is moved successively into abduction and external rotation, followed by adduction and internal rotation. The patient is then rolled onto his or her other side as hip adduction/internal rotation is progressed, while also maintaining strong ankle dorsiflexion. The knee remains in the extended position throughout all phases of the leg pull. Unlike the indirect approach, which involves moving into tissue "ease," the direct technique intentionally moves into tissue "bind," where restrictive barriers are challenged and mobilized. It is an efficient treatment method that enables the therapist to stretch several areas of tightness in a short period of time. It can also be used, diagnostically, to determine the exact locus of myofascial tightness using multiaxial or combined motions. When areas of restriction are identified in this manner, the multiaxial stretch is maintained until a release of tension is perceived. This usually occurs within 30 seconds, but may take more or less time depending upon the severity of the tightness. As a general rule, the patient should not be stretched into the painful range. At the first indication of adverse neural tension, the technique should be aborted.

Pelvic Girdle Manual Therapy

According to Greenman,[3] muscle energy technique is an osteopathic manual medicine intervention that "involves the voluntary contraction of a patient's muscle(s) in a precisely controlled direction, at varying levels of intensity, against a distinctly executed counterforce applied by the operator." Though Dr. TJ Ruddy's "resistive duction" was probably the earliest form of what became known as muscle energy technique (MET), Dr. Fred L. Mitchell is generally acknowledged as the "father" of the system.

Purposes of MET include lengthening a shortened, contractured, or spastic muscle; strengthening a physiologically weakened muscle or group of muscles; reducing localized edema and congestion; and mobilizing an articulation with restricted mobility.

In the pelvic girdle, some have suggested that MET works by contracting a muscle in "reverse action," thus providing a "neuromuscular mobilization" for the purpose of realigning a subluxation or positional fault. Regardless of the theoretical mechanism of action, these treatment techniques have become the mainstay of manipulative intervention of the pelvis for years and will be applied to four of the five most common impairments affecting the iliosacral joint and pubic symphysis (ie, anterior and posterior iliac rotation and superior and inferior pubic shears). Because the iliac upslip requires additional force to correct, a manual thrust rather than MET will be described subsequently.

Because of the potential for confusion regarding the sequencing of the various lumbopelvic interventions covered thus far, guidelines will be provided at the end of this section to address this issue. In addition, more information will be provided on the subject of the effect of lower limb alignment on the pelvis and vice versa.

Anterior Iliac Rotation: Muscle Energy/Manipulation

➡ Lesion: Right anterior iliac rotation

➡ Motion Restriction: Right posterior iliac rotation

➡ C (Chief Complaint):

1. Diffuse right posterior lumbosacral and sacroiliac pain reported, with referral into the right buttock and posterior thigh.

2. Sitting usually more comfortable than standing or ambulating.

➡ H (History):

1. Missed golf or baseball swing.

2. Bowling.

3. Direct blow to the posterior sacroiliac joint, creating hyperextension of the hip.

➡ A (Asymmetry of Bony Landmarks):

1. Right PSIS is higher than the left in all positions (possibly anterior also).

2. Right ASIS is lower than the left in all positions (possibly anterior also).

3. Right medial malleolus is longer than the left in supine.

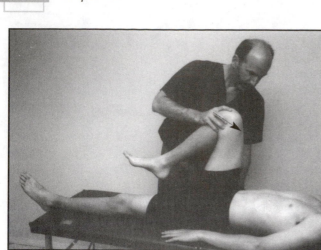

Figure 23-1.

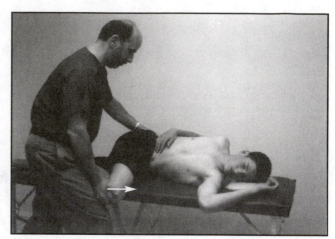

Figure 23-2.

➡ R (Range of Motion):

1. Standing flexion test is (+) on the right.

2. Stork test is (+) on the right at the upper and/or lower pole.

3. Long sitting test is (+) with the right medial malleolus changing from long to short as the patient moves from supine to long sitting.

4. Restricted right hip external rotation.

➡ T (Tissue Texture Abnormality):

1. Right sacrotuberous ligament is lax.

2. Right hip flexors may be hypertonic, tight, and tender (TRI muscles).

3. Baer's SI point is tender and tight on the right.

➡ S (Special Tests):

1. Some, if not all, sacroiliac provocation tests will reproduce or exacerbate the patient's chief complaint (ie, compression, distraction, posterior shear, and pelvic torsion tests).

2. Normal neurological exam.

3. Shortened swing phase on the right side.

4. Pain with extremes of right hip extension.

Two muscle energy techniques and one joint manipulation will be described and illustrated for correction of a right-sided anterior iliac rotation misalignment. The right side has been chosen because of the higher incidence of anterior iliac rotations on the right. To correct an anterior iliac rotation on the left side, all contacts and directions would be reversed.

Supine MET for Anterior Iliac Rotation on the Right

The therapist stands on the patient's right side with his or her fingers of the left hand medial to the patient's PSIS in the sacral sulcus (Figure 23-1). Meanwhile, the patient's right hip is flexed to the first motion barrier at the iliosacral joint in posterior iliac rotation (ie, the "feather edge" of the restrictive barrier). The patient is asked to resist further right hip flexion to a count of 6 seconds. Following a 3-second relaxation phase, the right ilium is repositioned against the new motion barrier in further posterior iliac rotation. The process is repeated two additional times for a total of three repetitions. Following the MET, the patient is reassessed for signs of improvement.

There are at least two mechanisms to explain the realignment of the bony pelvis following the application of muscle energy. The first is related to the neurophysiologic effect of hip extensor contraction (ie, the gluteus maximus and hamstrings). Through reciprocal inhibition, contraction of the hip extensors reduces tone in the hip flexors. This reduction in tone of the TRI muscles allows the iliac bone to "derotate" in a posterior direction and resume its normal anatomic relationship with the sacrum. The second mechanism involves the kinesiologic effect of working muscles in "reverse action." In this case, an isometric contraction of the hip extensors with fixation of the distal insertion will cause movement at the proximal origin. This therapeutic movement will theoretically realign the iliac bone from an anteriorly rotated position into its normal relationship with the sacrum.

Side Lying MET for Anterior Iliac Rotation on the Right

The patient lies on the unaffected left side. The therapist localizes right posterior iliac rotation through the right lower limb to the restrictive barrier by placing the fingers of his or her left hand in the sacral sulcus just medial to the left PSIS (Figure 23-2). When the "feather edge" of the restrictive barrier in the direction of posterior iliac rotation is reached, the patient's right foot is placed over his or her left knee and kept there (slight adduction of the right thigh

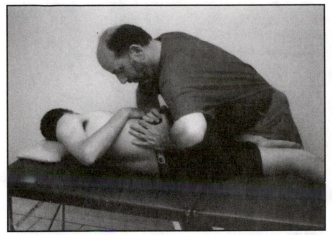

Figure 23-3a.

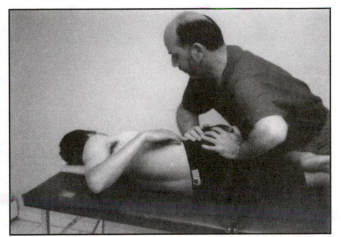

Figure 23-3b.

is helpful in decompressing the right iliosacral joint posteriorly). The lumbar spine is then "locked" by rotating it right via the left arm from above down, including the lumbosacral junction.

The MET is performed by having the patient perform a submaximal isometric contraction of the right hip extensors against the therapist's right hand. The appropriate instruction is, "Don't let me move your right knee up." Following a 6-second contraction, the ilium is relocalized through further hip flexion against the new barrier as determined through palpation at the sacral sulcus. This process is repeated a total of three times, and the patient is immediately reassessed.

Side Lying Manipulation for Right Anterior Iliac Rotation

If additional force is required to reduce the anterior iliac subluxation, the patient is then manipulated in the side lying position as follows:

1. The patient remains in the same side lying position as illustrated in Figure 23-2. However, the amount of right hip flexion will vary slightly, depending on which pole is being mobilized.

2. For an upper pole impairment of posterior iliac rotation, the right PSIS is engaged with the therapist's left pisiform contact (Figure 23-3a); for a lower pole impairment of posterior iliac rotation, the patient's right ischial tuberosity is engaged with the therapist's left pisiform contact (Figure 23-3b). The right hand makes contact with the ASIS regardless of which pole is being mobilized.

3. The manipulation involves a simultaneous "push" with both hands, causing posterior iliac rotation to occur, as if "turning a wheel," at the restrictive barrier. The posterior rotation can be graded 1 through 4, as indicated, for up to 1 minute with one or two brief pauses along the way.

Posterior Iliac Rotation: Muscle Energy/Manipulation

⇒ Lesion: Left posterior iliac rotation

⇒ Motion Restriction: Left anterior iliac rotation

⇒ C (Chief Complaint):

1. Pain usually localized to the left sacroiliac joint and ipsilateral buttock.

2. Pain described as deep, achy, sore, tight, etc.

3. Pain may be referred into the posterior thigh but not below the knee as with neurologic or radicular pain.

⇒ H (History):

1. Repeated unilateral standing on the left side.

2. Fall on the left buttock in trunk flexion.

3. Vertical thrust through the extended left leg.

4. Lifting in the forward bent position with the knees locked.

5. Female intercourse strain with the hips flexed.

⇒ A (Asymmetry of Bony Landmarks):

1. Left PSIS is lower than the right in all positions (possibly posterior also).

2. Left ASIS is higher than the right in all positions (possibly posterior also).

3. Left medial malleolus is shorter than the right in supine.

⇒ R (Range of Motion):

1. Standing flexion test is (+) on the left.

2. "Reverse stork" is (+) on the left at the upper and/or lower pole.

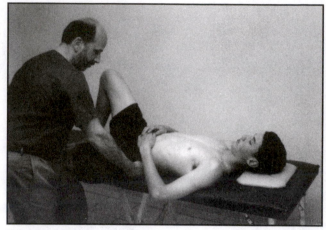

Figure 23-4.

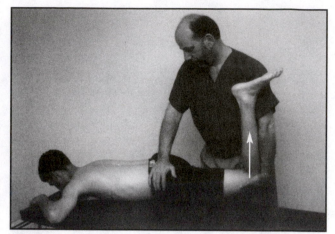

Figure 23-5.

3. Long sitting test is (+) with the left medial malleolus changing from short to long as the patient moves from supine to long sitting.

4. Restricted left hip internal rotation.

➡ T (Tissue Texture Abnormality):

1. Left sacrotuberous ligament is taut and tender.

2. Left hamstrings may be hypertonic, tight, and tender.

3. Baer's SI point is tender and tight on the left.

➡ S (Special Tests):

1. SI joint provocation tests are (+) on the left.

2. Normal neurological exam.

3. Shortened stride length on the left.

Two muscle energy techniques and one joint manipulation will be described and illustrated for a left-sided posterior iliac rotation misalignment. The left side has been chosen because of the higher incidence of posterior iliac rotations on the left. To correct this impairment on the right side, all manual contacts and directions are simply reversed.

Supine MET for Posterior Iliac Rotation on the Left

The therapist stands on the patient's left side. The patient's right foot is placed flat on the treatment table with the right knee comfortably flexed (Figure 23-4). While monitoring left iliosacral motion at the sacral sulcus with the fingers of the right hand, the therapist lowers the left thigh from a flexed position until the "feather edge" of the restrictive barrier in anterior iliac rotation is reached. Three seconds after a 6-second isometric contraction of the iliopsoas, the iliac bone is relocated to the new motion barrier by lowering the thigh in the direction of hip extension. Following three repetitions of MET, the pelvis is reassessed. To lessen the therapist's effort, his or her left thigh can assist with the support of the patient's left lower limb. This is especially helpful when the patient is larger than the therapist. To provide further assistance, a stool can be placed under the therapist's left foot.

The correction of posterior iliac rotation with MET can be explained both neurologically as well as mechanically. Neurologically, an isometric contraction of the iliopsoas muscle will decrease tone in the hamstrings through reciprocal inhibition, allowing the ilium to reposition itself more ideally on the sacrum. Mechanically, an isometric contraction of the iliopsoas with distal fixation will anteriorly rotate the ilium against its restrictive barrier, thus normalizing iliosacral alignment.

Prone MET for Posterior Iliac Rotation on the Left

The therapist stands on the patient's right side with the patient positioned in prone lying. To stabilize the right ilium, the patient's right foot is placed on the floor or on a stool with the right hip flexed between 75 to 90 degrees. The therapist monitors left iliosacral motion with the fingers of his or her right hand, while the patient's left thigh (flexed at the knee) is extended and slightly adducted in order to reach the restrictive barrier of left anterior iliac rotation (Figure 23-5). At the beginning of the restrictive barrier, three repetitions of MET are applied using the hip flexors isometrically. The following are crucial factors in performing an effective iliosacral MET:

1. Precise localization to the first barrier sensed (ie, the "feather edge"). A forceful engagement of the restrictive barrier may result in muscle hypertonicity.

2. Counterstability of the contralateral ilium.

3. Controlled submaximal isometric contraction for 6 seconds, which ramps up and down slowly.

4. Postcontraction relaxation for up to 3 seconds.

5. Precise relocalization to the new motion barrier.

6. Sensitivity to patient comfort at all times.

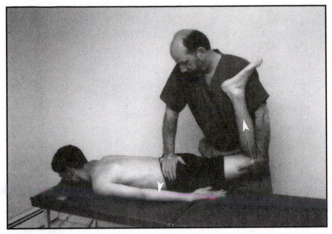

Figure 23-6.

Prone Manipulation for Left Posterior Iliac Rotation

When additional force is required to reduce a "stubborn" subluxation, the patient is then manipulated as follows:

1. The patient remains in the same position as in Figure 23-5 (ie, prone with the right foot on the floor). However, left hip position will differ depending on which pole is being mobilized.

2. For restriction at the upper pole of the left iliosacral joint, the therapist's right pisiform contact performs a mobilization over the left iliac crest in an anterior, superior, and lateral direction as the left extended/adducted thigh maintains the position of the left iliac bone at the restrictive barrier (Figure 23-6). For a lower pole impairment, the manual contact is over the left PSIS and mobilized in the same three directions (ie, anterior, superior, and lateral).

3. A graded mobilization is performed for up to 1 minute with one or two brief pauses along the way.

Iliac Upslip (Superior Shear): Manipulation

➡ Lesion: Right iliac upslip (superior shear)

➡ Motion Restriction: Inferior iliac shear

➡ C (Chief Complaint):
  1. Traumatically induced right sacroiliac pain localized to the SI joint or referred distally into the right buttock and thigh.

➡ H (History):
  1. Vertical fall on the right ischium.
  2. Unexpected step off a curb or "missed" step on stairs onto the right leg.

➡ A (Asymmetry of Bony Landmarks):
  1. Right PSIS is higher than the left in all positions.
  2. Right ASIS is higher than the left in all positions.
  3. Right iliac crest is higher than the left in all positions.
  4. Right ischial tuberosity is 6 mm higher (thumb width) than the left in prone lying.
  5. The greater trochanters are level in standing.

➡ R (Range of Motion):
  1. Standing flexion test is (+) on the right.
  2. Stork test is (+) on the right at the upper and/or lower pole.
  3. "Reverse stork" is (+) on the right at the upper and/or lower pole.

➡ T (Tissue Texture Abnormality):
  1. Right sacrotuberous ligament is lax.
  2. Right quadratus lumborum may be hypertonic, tight, and tender.
  3. Right gluteus medius may become lengthened and tender.

➡ S (Special Tests):
  1. Baer's SI point is tender and tight on the right.
  2. SI joint provocation tests are (+) on the right.
  3. Normal neurological exam.
  4. Antalgic gait with weight bearing on the right.

Unlike the rotatory impairments of the iliosacral joint, muscle energy is ineffective. This is because the underlying fixation is more articular in nature than myofascial. In fact, grade 1 to 4 mobilization is also inadequate because the ilium often becomes "locked" onto the sacrum, requiring a strong manipulative force to "unlock" it. Although manipulative thrust should generally not be taught on the introductory level, there is no other option for the iliac upslip but a thrust procedure (ie, grade 5). In terms of potential injury, the risk-to-benefit ratio overwhelmingly supports the use of the long axis thrust; if taught properly, there is only minimal risk to the patient. Regarding the side selected, there is no indication that iliac upslips are more prevalent on one side than the other. The choice, therefore, to examine and treat the right side was a random one. The examination findings and intervention are simply reversed for an iliac upslip on the left.

Supine Manipulation of an Iliac Upslip on the Right

The efficacy of this manipulative thrust is markedly increased when an assistant is used to stabilize the contralateral ilium. The technique can be broken down as follows:

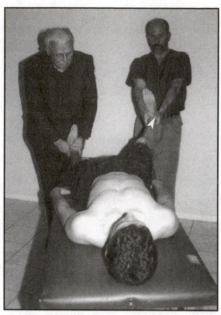

Figure 23-7.

1. The therapist grasps the patient's right ankle just proximal to the malleoli (Figure 23-7).

2. The iliosacral joint is placed in its loose-packed position by abducting the right hip 10 to 15 degrees.

3. To ensure that the long axis thrust affects the iliosacral joint and not the hip, the therapist close-packs the abducted hip by internally rotating it to end-range.

4. The assistant positions his or her thigh against the patient's left foot to prevent inferior movement of the left lower limb.

5. The therapist performs a grade 3 long axis traction maneuver through the right lower extremity by leaning back with extended arms.

6. Without giving up the strong long axis traction, the therapist leans forward by flexing the elbows. On the count of "three," the patient is told to cough (a cough theoretically distracts the SI joints momentarily), at which time the therapist imparts a quick thrust through the leg. If done correctly, the iliac upslip is reduced, often but not always, with an associated "thud" or "clunk." When practicing this maneuver on normal subjects, the amount of force should be kept to a minimum lest an inferior iliac shear (ie, downslip) results.

If an upslip has occurred, there is often associated laxity of the SI ligaments. Consequently, SI belt fixation is recommended postmanipulation to allow for proper healing and restabilization. If the SI joint remains unstable despite prolonged belt fixation, a course of prolotherapy is indicated. This physician-based intervention involves the injection of proliferant solutions into the ligaments for the pur-

pose of stimulating the proliferation of collagen, thereby enhancing joint stability. For further information, the reader is referred to the text *Diagnosis and Injection Techniques in Orthopaedic Medicine* by Dorman and Ravin.

Prior to performing the manipulative thrust described above, the therapist should review the contraindications to spinal manual therapy listed in Chapter 3. Regarding the pregnant patient with mechanical impairment of the pelvic girdle, the author recommends that novice practitioners not perform the thrust maneuver described above. However, gentle MET can be safely and effectively applied to rotatory impairments throughout a woman's pregnancy.

Though presented as separate and distinct impairments, it is important to appreciate that anterior and posterior iliac rotations are sometimes superimposed on an iliac upslip. When this is the case, the upslip should always be managed first.

Superior/Inferior Pubic Shears: "Shotgun" Technique

➡ Lesion 1: Right inferior pubic shear ("Down pube")

➡ Motion Restriction: Superior pubic shear on the right

➡ C (Chief Complaint):

  1. Pain and tenderness over the medial attachment of the right inguinal ligament.

  2. Diffuse and variable pain reference over the right SI joint, anterior groin, and thigh.

➡ H (History):

  1. During a soccer kick, the foot hits the ground rather than the ball, shearing the pubic symphysis inferior on the ipsilateral side.

  2. Common in postpartum females.

➡ A (Asymmetry of Bony Landmarks):

  1. Right pubic tubercle is inferior versus the left.

➡ R (Range of Motion):

  1. Standing flexion test is (+) on the right.

➡ T (Tissue Texture Abnormality):

  1. Tenderness at the medial attachment of the right inguinal ligament.

  2. Right hip adductors may be hypertonic, tight, and tender.

➡ S (Special Tests):

  1. Normal neurological examination.

  2. Antalgic gait with weight bearing on the right.

➡ Lesion 2: Left superior pubic shear ("Up pube")

➡ Motion Restriction: Inferior pubic shear on the left

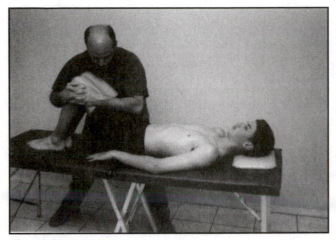

Figure 23-8a.

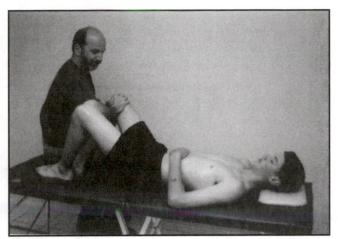

Figure 23-8b.

➡ C (Chief Complaint):

  1. Pain and tenderness over the medial attachment of the left inguinal ligament.

  2. Lower abdominal discomfort on the left.

  3. Possible secondary symptoms at the left SI joint.

➡ H (History):

  1. Rectus abdominis asymmetry (ie, tight left, weak right).

  2. Vertical fall on the left ischium.

➡ A (Asymmetry of Bony Landmarks):

  1. Left pubic tubercle is superior versus the right.

➡ T (Tissue Texture Abnormality):

  1. Tenderness at the medial attachment of the left inguinal ligament.

  2. Left distal insertion of the rectus abdominis may be hypertonic, tight, and tender.

➡ S (Special Tests):

  1. Normal neurological examination.

  2. Antalgic gait with weight bearing on the left.

  3. Resisted trunk flexion provokes local pain at the left symphysis pubis.

The sides selected for examination and treatment purposes represent the common patterns of impairment seen in the pubic region (ie, inferior pubic shear on the right and superior pubic shear on the left). Why we see these patterns in the pelvis and elsewhere in the body is unclear at this time.

Though specific techniques for each of the pubic shear dysfunctions are available, there is one technique that has the ability to correct the alignment of the pubic symphysis in either case. This procedure is referred to as the "shotgun" or "blunderbuss" technique.[24]

"Shotgun" Technique for Superior/Inferior Pubic Shears

There are two phases to this muscle energy technique. The first phase involves a contraction of the hip abductor muscles, while the second uses an isometric contraction of the adductors. Although it is the adductor contraction that realigns the pubic symphysis (sometimes with an associated "click" or "pop"), the abductor contraction beforehand markedly enhances the efficacy of this technique. Theoretically, through reciprocal inhibition, an isometric contraction of the abductors relaxes and resets the tone in the adductors for a more optimal contraction. By applying distal resistance at the knees, the therapist forces the adductor muscles to pull the inferior pubic rami laterally, causing a momentary distraction of the pubic symphysis. It is during this distraction that superior and inferior pubic shears often correct. An audible "pop" is not necessary for a correction to occur, but patients often see this as a confirmation that the problem has been "fixed."

To perform the "shotgun" technique, the supine patient's hips and knees are flexed with both feet on the table. The therapist then grasps both knees in the adducted position and resists hip abduction three times for a count of 6 seconds each (Figure 23-8a). The therapist then places his or her forearm between the patient's knees and asks for a strong bilateral adductor contraction for 3 to 6 seconds (Figure 23-8b). One contraction is often sufficient, but a second one can be attempted if the therapist chooses. The patient is immediately reassessed for signs of improvement.

Before proceeding to the final chapter on the pelvic girdle (ie, therapeutic and home exercises), two essential concepts need to be addressed. The first is related to the issue of treatment sequencing in the patient with somatic impairment of the lumbar-pelvic-hip complex, while the second deals briefly with the interrelationship between the lumbopelvic region and the lower extremity.

The recommended treatment sequence for a lumbar-pelvic-hip impairment is as follows:

1. Direct fascial technique and stretching of the tight postural muscles of the hip joints.

2. Mobilization/manipulation of the hips, which is not covered in this text.

3. Myofascial release/direct fascial technique of the lower thoracic/lumbar spine.

4. Mobilization/manipulation of the lower thoracic/lumbar spine (type 2, non-neutral impairment not covered in this text).

5. Myofascial release/direct fascial technique of the pelvic floor/diaphragm.

6. Correction of superior/inferior pubic shears.

7. Correction of superior/inferior iliac shears (inferior is rare).

8. Correction of sacroiliac impairment (not covered in this text: torsions, unilateral and bilateral nutation/counternutation).

9. Correction of anterior and posterior iliac rotations.

10. Recovery of core stability/lower abdominal and gluteal muscle strength.

Priority is always given to a McKenzie derangement, as it can be the most disabling and the most serious of the mechanical afflictions of the lumbopelvic region.

Regarding the inter-relationship between the lumbopelvic region and the lower extremity, it must be appreciated that the pelvis is the mechanical link between the lower limb and the trunk. Whether analyzing function or impairment of the hip, knee, foot, and ankle, one must always consider the role of the lumbopelvic region. When analyzing function or impairment of the lumbopelvic region, one must always consider the role of the muscles and joints of the lower extremity. To examine and treat each part independent of the whole is to deprive the patient of proper care. In fact, the author would say that it is irresponsible! Specializing in the foot and ankle or in the spine and pelvis is not the problem. The problem is when one fails to recognize the "unity of the body" and its total interdependence. The author has seen many low back patients helped when attention was paid to their lower extremity impairment and vice versa. It all comes back to the philosophy that finding and managing the source of the problem (ie, the area of greatest restriction) will yield great dividends in the end!

Therapeutic and Home Exercises for the Pelvic Girdle

In order to maintain proper alignment of the pelvic joints following manual therapy, the patient is expected to be diligent with his or her home program. As with the other areas covered thus far, successful outcomes are dependent upon the patient's willingness to commit to the home program. The home exercises described and illustrated below are simple to instruct and perform. However, not unlike taking medicine, the patient must strictly adhere to the regimen.

Pubic Shear Dysfunction: Self-Correction

To maintain proper alignment of the pubic symphysis, the patient performs a modification of the "shotgun" technique in the sitting position (Figure 24-1a). Following three 6-second isometric abductor contractions, the patient contracts the hip adductors against the unyielding resistance of his or her arm for 3 to 6 seconds (Figure 24-1b). This cycle can be repeated two to three times and performed every few hours as needed to maintain normal alignment until stability has returned to the region.

Anterior Iliac Rotation: Self-Correction

To self-correct the right side (Figure 24-2), the supine patient is instructed to make use of two muscle groups. By performing simultaneous isometric contractions of the right hip extensors and the left hip adductors, the corrective force is imparted to the right iliosacral joint. The patient is instructed to bring the right knee to chest and interlock his or her fingers behind the posterior thigh while the left foot engages the left side of the table. As the patient pushes his or her right thigh into the interlocked fingers, the left foot is pushed into the side of the table for a count of 6 seconds and repeated two to three times every few hours until stability returns to the region. The purpose of the left-sided hip adductor contraction is to provide counterstability as the right ilium is being mobilized.

Posterior Iliac Rotation: Self-Correction

To self-correct impairment on the left side (Figure 24-3), the exact same maneuver employed in the self-correction of an anterior iliac rotation on the right is used. This time, the hip adductors are used to mobilize the left ilium into anterior rotation, while the hip extensors are used to provide counterstability on the right. Again, the contraction is performed for 6 seconds and repeated two to three times every few hours.

Piriformis Self-Stretch

In keeping with the changing mechanics of the piriformis muscle below and above 60 degrees of hip flexion,[10]

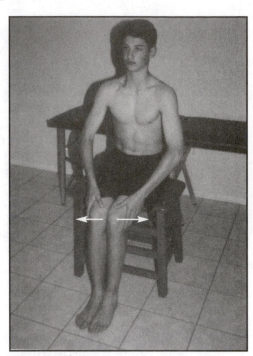

Figure 24-1a.

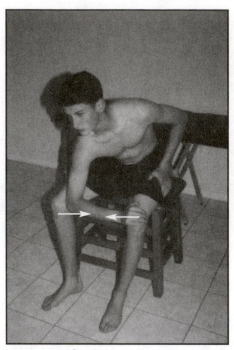

Figure 24-1b.

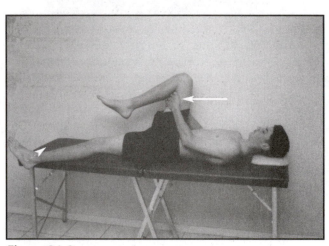

Figure 24-2.

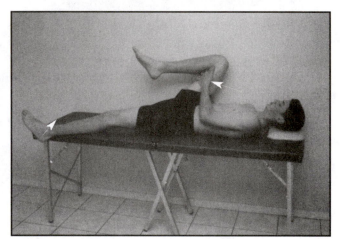

Figure 24-3.

the patient is instructed to stretch the muscle in two positions as illustrated. Below 60 degrees of flexion, the supine patient stretches the right side by placing his or her right foot immediately on the outside of the left knee with the foot flat. The right knee is then pulled across the body so that the right hip is flexed, adducted, and internally rotated (Figure 24-4a). The patient holds this position for a count of 30 seconds and repeats the stretch three times, several times per day.

To stretch the right piriformis muscle above 60 degrees of flexion, the hooklying patient places his or her right foot over the left knee. The right knee is then pulled toward the left elbow so that the right hip is flexed, adducted, and externally rotated (Figure 24-4b). The stretch is held for 30

seconds and repeated three times, several times per day. The patient can switch sides and repeat on the left.

The patient must not feel discomfort in the groin and must be careful to stop the stretch should radicular symptoms be perceived in the lower extremity. If the stretch is performed too vigorously, compression of the sciatic nerve can occur.

Iliopsoas Self-Stretch

The patient is positioned in the half-kneeling position with the right knee flexed and the right foot flat (Figure 24-5). To stretch the left iliopsoas muscle, the patient preposi-

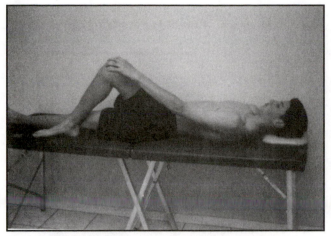

Figure 24-4a.

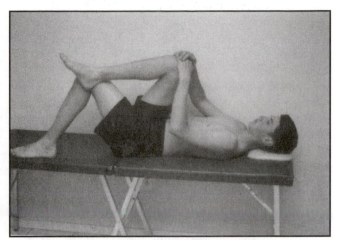

Figure 24-4b.

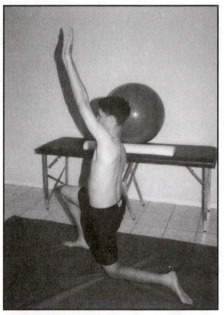

Figure 24-5.

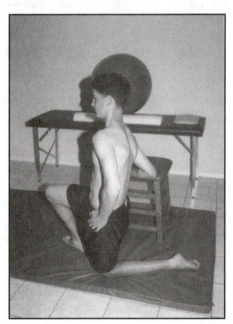

Figure 24-6.

tions the lumbar spine in posterior pelvic tilt and the left hip in internal rotation and extension. The stretch is achieved by having the patient "lean into" the left anterior hip and thigh without arching the low back. For those patients who desire a more aggressive stretch, trunk side bending to the right can be added with the left arm overhead. The stretch is held for up to 30 seconds and repeated three times, several times per day. The patient can switch sides and repeat on the right. For patients who have difficulty with kneeling because of knee pain, a pillow can be placed under the affected knee. If this is still problematic, the patient can perform the TRI muscle stretch over the end of a bed.

Tensor Fascia Latae Self-Stretch

The half-kneeling position is again utilized, but the prepositioning of the hip is different than for the iliopsoas. To stretch the left tensor fascia latae muscle, the left hip is positioned in external rotation and extension while the lower abdominals and gluteus maximus maintain a posterior pelvic tilt (Figure 24-6). The stretch is felt in the anterolateral aspect of the left hip as the patient translates his or her hips from right to left. Bookhout[24] suggests that the patient place his or her right hand on a chair for support. The stretch is brought to the point of perceived tightness but not to the point of pain, and held for 30 seconds. Each stretch is repeated three times and performed several times per day. The same stretch is performed on the right side as necessary.

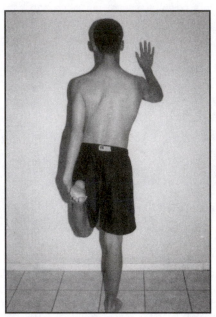

Figure 24-7.

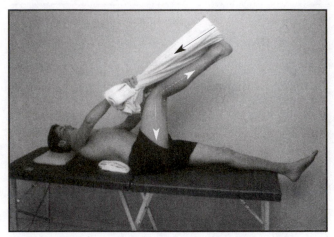

Figure 24-8.

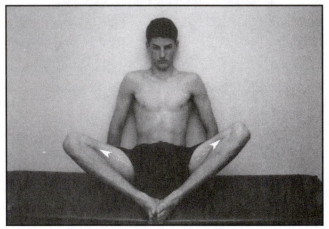

Figure 24-9.

Rectus Femoris Self-Stretch

The left rectus femoris is easily and effectively stretched by having the patient grasp the left ankle with his or her left hand and use the wall for standing support with the right hand (Figure 24-7). The stretch is achieved by performing a posterior pelvic tilt while simultaneously flexing the left knee. The stretch is held for 30 seconds and repeated three times. The right rectus femoris is then stretched similarly.

Hamstring Self-Stretch

A towel roll is placed under the lumbar curve to maintain a neutral lordosis. To easily and effectively stretch the hamstrings, the patient is instructed to use a sheet or beach towel. One hand controls the degree of knee extension, while the other hand controls the leg raise via the sheet placed over the distal aspect of the foot (Figure 24-8). The patient maintains the stretch for 30 seconds and repeats it three times, several times a day. Care must be taken to ensure that the stretch is of a muscular nature and at no time should radicular symptoms (eg, numbness, tingling) be experienced.

Hip Adductor Self-Stretch

This stretch (Figure 24-9) appears in the text, *Bourdillon's Spinal Manipulation*.[24] The patient sits with his or her back to the wall, maintaining a neutral lordosis. The soles of the feet are brought together as the hips are abducted and externally rotated. The patient's hands are placed on the floor behind his or her hips to assist in lifting and anteriorly rotating the pelvis. The patient slowly and carefully performs an anterior pelvic tilt and immediately feels the stretch in the groin area, bilaterally. The stretch is held for 30 seconds and repeated three times, several times a day.

Strengthening the Gluteus Maximus—Bridging Regimen

The final therapeutic exercise involves a strengthening regimen of the gluteus maximus muscles. These primary extensors of the hip play an important role in ambulation, running, and jumping. Patients with chronic low back pain often demonstrate weakness of these important phasic muscles. Patients who have problems with recurring hamstring strains often have tight hamstrings as a consequence of substituting for weak gluteal muscles. Once the hamstrings have been manually "released" and stretched, it is important to retrain the gluteus maximus.

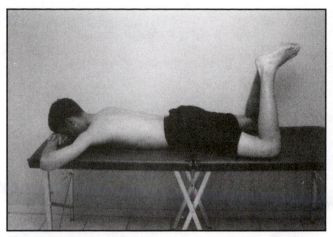

Figure 24-10.

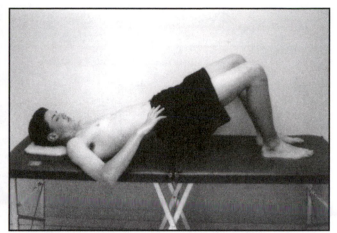

Figure 24-11a.

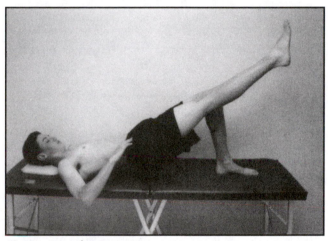

Figure 24-11b.

Recently, Yerys et al[23] have demonstrated the connection between anterior hip joint mobility and gluteus maximus strength. In keeping with the arthrokinetic reflex discussed previously in this text, the gluteus maximus muscle should not be retrained until the requisite degree of hip extension is present. Consequently, it once again behooves the therapist to mobilize impaired joint structures before strengthening inhibited and weak muscles.

Prior to commencing the bridging exercises, the patient may require a remedial session in gluteus maximus recruitment. One simple way of isolating these muscles is to have the prone patient resist bilateral isometric hip external rotation by pushing both feet together as illustrated (Figure 24-10). Once the sensorimotor "connection" has been made, the patient is ready to move on.

The hooklying patient is instructed to perform a posterior pelvic tilt followed by a bridge maneuver involving hip and not lumbar extension. The patient is also instructed to place both hands over the ASISs so that the pelvis remains level at all times (Figure 24-11a). The bridge is held for a count of 5 to 10 seconds and repeated 10 times, three times per day.

The more demanding phase of the bridging regimen involves straightening one leg at a time for 5 to 10 seconds, while maintaining a level pelvis as per ASIS palpation (Figure 24-11b). With time and improved strength/endurance, the extended leg can be held for up to 30 seconds. This can be incorporated into motion as the patient makes the letters of the alphabet (A through M) with one foot; N through Z with the other, while maintaining a level pelvis. If the patient cannot maintain a bridge without excessive lumbar extensor tone, or low back pain develops, the exercise should be terminated.

References and Bibliography

References

1. Vleeming A, Wingerden JP, van Dijkstra PF, Stoeckart R, Snijders CJ, Stijnen T. Mobility in the SI-joints in old people: a kinematic and radiologic study. *J Clin Biomech.* 1992;7:170-176.

2. Vleeming A, Mooney V, Dorman TA, Snijders CJ, Stoeckart R. *Movement, Stability and Low Back Pain: The Essential Role of the Pelvis.* New York, NY: Churchill Livingstone; 1997.

3. Greenman PE. *Principles of Manual Medicine.* Philadelphia, Pa: Lippincott, Williams & Wilkins; 1996.

4. Vleeming A, Stoeckart R, Volkers ACW, Snijders CJ. Relation between form and function in the sacroiliac joint. Part 1: clinical anatomical aspects. *Spine.* 1990;15(2):130-132.

5. Vleeming A, Volkers ACW, Snijders CJ, Stoeckart R. Relation between form and function in the sacroiliac joint. Part 2: biomechanical aspects. *Spine.* 1990;15(2):133-136.

6. Lee D. Instability of the sacroiliac joint and the consequences to gait. *Journal of Manual & Manipulative Therapy.* 1996; 4(1):22-29.

7. Schafer RC, Faye LJ. *Motion Palpation and Chiropractic Technique: Principles of Dynamic Chiropractic.* Huntington Beach, Calif: The Motion Palpation Institute; 1989.

8. Petersen CM, Hayes KW. Construct validity of Cyriax's selective tension examination: association of end-feels with pain at the knee and shoulder. *J Orthop Sports Phys Ther.* 2000;30(9):512-527.

9. Vleeming A, Pool-Goudzwaard AL, Hammudoghlu D, Stoeckart R, Snijders CJ, Mens JMA. The function of the long dorsal sacroiliac ligament, its implication for understanding low back pain. *Spine.* 1996;21(5):556-562.

10. Hertling D, Kessler RM. *Management of Common Musculoskeletal Disorders: Physical Therapy Principles and Methods.* Philadelphia, Pa: Lippincott-Raven; 1996.

11. Laslett M, Williams M. The reliability of selected pain provocation tests for sacroiliac joint pathology. *Spine.* 1994;19(11): 1243-1249.

12. Laslett M. Pain provocation sacroiliac joint tests: reliability and prevalence. In: Vleeming A, Mooney V, Dorman T, Snijders C, Stoeckart R, eds. *Movement, Stability & Low Back Pain: The Essential Role of the Pelvis.* New York, NY: Churchill Livingstone; 1997.

13. Gross J, Fetto J, Rosen E. *Musculoskeletal Examination.* 2nd ed. Cambridge, Mass: Blackwell Science; 2002.

14. Konin JG, Wiksten DL, Isear JA, Brader H. *Special Tests for Orthopedic Examination.* 2nd ed. Thorofare, NJ: SLACK Incorporated; 2002.

15. Maitland GD. *Peripheral Manipulation.* 2nd ed. London: Butterworth; 1977.

16. Travell JG, Simons DG. *Myofascial Pain and Dysfunction: The Trigger Point Manual, Vol. 2 The Lower Extremities.* Baltimore, Md: Williams & Wilkins; 1992.

17. Manheim C. *The Myofascial Release Manual.* 3rd ed. Thorofare, NJ: SLACK Incorporated; 2001.

18. Tomberlin JP, Saunders HD. *Evaluation, Treatment, and Prevention of Musculoskeletal Disorders.* Vol 2. 3rd ed. Chaska, Minn: The Saunders Group; 1994.

19. Ellis JJ. *LPI, Lumbo-Pelvic Integration, A Course Workbook.* Patchogue, NY: Author; 1990.

20. Eland DC, Singleton TN, Conaster RR, et al. The "iliacus test": new information for the evaluation of hip extension dysfunction. *J Am Osteopath Assoc.* 2002;102(3):130-142.

21. Sahrmann SA. *Diagnosis and Treatment of Movement Impairment Syndromes.* St. Louis, Mo: Mosby-Year Book; 2002.

22. Cyriax J. *Textbook of Orthopaedic Medicine.* London: Bailliere Tindall; 1978.

23. Yerys S, Makofsky H, Byrd C, Pennachio J, Cinkay J. The effect of mobilization of the anterior hip capsule on gluteus maximus strength. *Journal of Manual & Manipulative Therapy.* 2002;10(4):218-224.

24. Isaacs ER, Bookhout MR. *Bourdillon's Spinal Manipulation.* 6th ed. Boston, Mass: Butterworth-Heinemann; 2002.

Bibliography

Alderink GJ. The sacroiliac joint: review of anatomy, mechanics, and function. *J Orthop Sports Phys Ther.* 1991;13(2):71-84.

Beal MC. The sacroiliac problem: review of anatomy, mechanics, and diagnosis. *J Am Osteopath Assoc.* 1982;81(10):667-679.

Bemis T, Monte D. Validation of the long sitting test on subjects with iliosacral dysfunction. *J Orthop Sports Phys Ther.* 1987;8(7):336-345.

Boyling JD, Palastanga N, eds. *Grieve's Modern Manual Therapy: The Vertebral Column.* 2nd ed. Edinburgh: Churchill Livingstone; 1994.

Cibulka MT, Delitto A, Koldehoff RM. Changes in innominate tilt after manipulation of the sacroiliac joint in patients with low back pain, an experimental study. *Phys Ther.* 1988;68(9):1359-1370.

DonTigny RL. Mechanics and treatment of the sacroiliac joint. *Journal of Manual & Manipulative Therapy.* 1993;1(1):3-12.

Dorman TA, Ravin TH. *Diagnosis and Injection Techniques in Orthopaedic Medicine.* Baltimore, MD: Williams & Williams; 1991.

Dutton M. *Manual Therapy of the Spine: An Integrated Approach.* New York, NY: McGraw-Hill; 2002.

Kostopoulos D, Rizopoulos K. *The Manual of Trigger Point and Myofascial Therapy.* Thorofare, NJ: SLACK Incorporated; 2001.

Magee DJ. *Orthopedic Physical Therapy.* 4th ed. Philadelphia, Pa: WB Saunders; 2002.

Riddle DL, Freburger JK. Evaluation of the presence of sacroiliac region dysfunction using a combination of tests: a multicenter intertester reliability study. *Phys Ther.* 2002;82(8):772-781.

Rocabado M. *Pelvic Girdle, Course Manual.* Boston, Mass: Rocabado Institute; 1984.

Schwarzer AC, Aprill CN, Bogduk N. The sacroiliac joint in chronic low back pain. *Spine.* 1995;20(1):31-37.

Spagnoli R. *Spinal Orthopedics, Evaluation and Treatment of Somatic Dysfunction in the Lumbar Spine and Pelvic Girdle, A Course Workbook.* Centereach, NY: Author; 1995.

Van der Wurff P, Hagmeijer RHM, Meyne W. Clinical tests of the sacroiliac joint: a systematic review. Part 1: reliability. *Man Ther.* 2000;5(1):30-36.

Walker JM. The sacroiliac joint: a critical review. *Phys Ther.* 1992;72(12):904-916.

From the Classroom to the Clinic

The Evidence for Spinal Manual Therapy and Therapeutic Exercise

Looking at the ubiquitous use of manual therapy and my own personal preferences for many manual techniques, it is with sorrow that I observe how the great edifice of manual therapy has been built upon the shakiest of foundations. I understand how the great American patriot John Adams felt when he was forced by his principles to reluctantly face reality and defend British soldiers accused in the Boston massacre. As Adams observed during that defense: 'Facts are stubborn things; and whatever may be our wishes, our inclinations, or the dictates of our passions, they cannot alter the state of facts and evidence.' So it must be with manual therapy.

We lack facts and evidence. Does this mean that manual therapy techniques do not work? No! It means that, whether we like it or not, our profession's endorsement of manual therapy is based on anecdotal observations and a shared faith, a belief that exists in the absence of evidence. I understand this because I too was a believer, one who accepted with enthusiasm and without critical thinking.

Jules M. Rothstein, PhD, PT
Editor's Note, *Physical Therapy,*
1992;72(12)

In 1996, Sacket et al[1] defined evidence based medicine (EBM) as the "conscientious, explicit, and judicious use of current best evidence in making decisions about the care of individual patients." Four years later, Sacket et al[2] described EBM as the "integration of best research evidence with clinical expertise and patient values." To determine "best evidence," Sacket et al rate[2] the type of study employed on a 1 through 5 scale with 1 being the ideal, whereas levels 4 and 5 fall into the category of "lower-level" research. In numerical order, they are as follows: randomized controlled trial (RCTs) = 1, cohort studies = 2, case-controlled studies = 3, case series without a control group = 4, and expert opinion = 5.

In this chapter, the author seeks to demonstrate that manual therapy is not built upon "the shakiest of foundations." Although many more RCTs are needed to demonstrate efficacy, there is more than "anecdotal observation" and a "shared faith" to support the use of manual therapy within the larger context of physical therapy. In essence, Dr. Rothstein has challenged the manual therapy community to either "put up or shut up." Such a challenge should provide the impetus for scholarly activity at a time when it is most needed. Manual therapists should, therefore, accept the challenge and move forward.

It's time for us to be held accountable for the claims that we make and ultimately for the living that we earn. According to the more recent description of EBM by Sacket et al,[2] we can surely claim "clinical expertise and patient values," but we can do better than that! As manual physical therapists who routinely incorporate therapeutic exercise into patient care, we should also be able to demonstrate the clinical effectiveness of these interventions with sound science as well.

To this end, the author has selected representative studies on various aspects of the practice of spinal manual therapy and therapeutic exercise (ie, diagnostic and interventional applications) with emphasis on patient outcomes.

Study #1: Jull G, Bogduk N, Marsland A. The accuracy of manual diagnosis for cervical zygapophyseal joint pain syndromes. Med J Aust. 1988;148(5):233-236.

Twenty consecutive patients from the Pain Clinic at the Princess Alexandra Hospital entered the study. There were 7 men and 13 women. Fourteen patients complained of neck pain and headache, 3 patients complained of neck and arm pain, and 3 patients complained of neck pain alone. All patients had chronic neck pain for at least 12 months.

In 11 patients, radiographically-controlled diagnostic nerve blocks were used to determine the presence or absence of a symptomatic zygapophyseal joint in the cervical spine. All 11 patients were then seen by a manipulative physiotherapist who had no knowledge of the results of the diagnostic nerve block. In the remaining 9 patients, the above sequence of events was reversed.

The manipulative physiotherapist, using a combination of PAIVMs and PPIVMs, correctly identified all 15 patients with proven symptomatic zygapophyseal joints. None of the five patients with asymptomatic joints were misdiagnosed. Furthermore, the therapist specified the correct segmental level of the symptomatic joint in each instance.

The researchers concluded the following, "Manual diagnosis by a trained manipulative therapist can be as accurate as radiologically-controlled diagnostic blocks in the diagnosis of cervical zygapophyseal syndromes." The authors do suggest, however, that further research into intertherapist reliability be performed before generalized claims about the reliability of manual diagnosis can be made.

Study #2: Donelson R, Aprill C, Medcalf R, Grant W. A prospective study of centralization of lumbar and referred pain. A predictor of symptomatic discs and annular competence. Spine. 1997;22(10):1115-1122.

Sixty-three patients (41 men, 22 women) with low back pain and varying degrees of lower extremity pain/altered sensation participated in this prospective, blinded study. Patients with a history of prior lumbar surgery, including chemonucleolysis, were excluded. The average age was 39.6 years, and all patient symptoms were present for greater than 3 months.

Upon entering the radiology clinic for the scheduled lumbar discography, each patient underwent a McKenzie assessment using repeated end-range lumbar test movements. Each examiner was a Diplomat in mechanical diagnosis and therapy, as well as a faculty member of the McKenzie Institute. One of three effects on pain was identified during each patient's mechanical assessment. They were rapid centralization or abolition of the referred pain ("centralizers"); no centralization, but peripheralization of pain in

one or more directions ("peripheralizers"); and no change in the distal-most pain location or intensity ("no change").

Immediately after the mechanical assessment, patients underwent lumbar discography by a single investigator "blinded" to the findings of the McKenzie exam. During disc injection, each patient was assessed for pain response by the discographer and a second observer. Provocation discography provides direct information about nuclear morphology and the status of the nuclear envelope; it is the "gold standard" for determining whether a disc is painful.

Results of the McKenzie assessment indicated that 31 patients (49.2%) were "centralizers," 16 patients (25.4%) were "peripheralizers," and the remaining 16 patients (25.4%) experienced "no change." Furthermore, of the 31 patients who were "centralizers," 23 (74%) had a positive discogram ($p < 0.0007$). Of those 23, the annular wall of the positive disc was competent in 21 patients or 91% ($p < 0.001$). Of the 16 patients (25.4%) who were "peripheralizers," 11 (69%) had a positive discogram ($p < 0.004$). Of those 11, the annular wall of the positive disc was competent in 6 (54%) patients ($p = 0.093$). Of the 16 patients (25.4%) whose pain showed "no change," only 2 (12.5%) had a positive discogram ($p < 0.001$); the annular walls of these two positive discs were both competent. Considering the high incidence of positive discograms in "centralizers" and "peripheralizers" and the low incidence in the "no change" group, the ability to distinguish between a positive and a negative discogram on the basis of pain responses alone was highly significant ($p < 0.001$). In patients with positive discograms, the "centralizers" demonstrated a significantly greater incidence of annular competence as compared to the "peripheralizers" ($p < 0.042$).

Based on these data, the researchers concluded that the McKenzie assessment process reliably distinguished discogenic from nondiscogenic pain ($p < 0.001$) as well as a competent from an incompetent annulus ($p < 0.042$) in symptomatic discs. In their discussion of spinal imaging procedures (eg, radiography, CT, MRI, and myelography), the authors point out that, unlike the McKenzie system, these procedures are unable to determine the source of the patient's painful symptoms. Although this is not the case with invasive discography, the authors are quick to suggest that the McKenzie assessment system, unlike discography, can easily and safely be implemented in the acute setting, allowing for the early identification of relevant response groups with minimal risk to the patient.

In summary, these researchers have demonstrated the clinical relationship between the centralization phenomenon, and a contained intervertebral disc herniation, the peripheralization phenomenon and the likelihood of a non-contained extruded disc, and the "no change" pattern of a nondiscogenic impairment. Consequently, these findings suggest an important role for the McKenzie method, not only in the mechanical diagnosis of discogenic symptoms, but also as a means of identifying those disc patients who are the most likely to benefit from nonsurgical, mechanical therapy. Although the findings of this study support the validity of the McKenzie internal disc model and the role of the annulus as a pain generator, the researchers still admit to not fully understanding "the precise neural mechanism by which pain centralizes."

Study #3: Schoensee SK, Jensen G, Nicholson G, Gossman M, Katholi C. The effect of mobilization on cervical headaches. J Orthop Sports Phys Ther. 1995;21(4):184-196.

Twelve subjects (between the ages of 20 to 50), satisfying the diagnostic criteria for cervical headache, were recruited, but 10 subjects (three males and seven females) went on to complete the study (one subject was hospitalized for appendicitis and the second subject was not included because of incomplete data). A single case A-B-A design was used for each of the 10 subjects in the study. The A phase consisted of data collection on headache frequency, duration, and intensity. The B phase, or treatment phase, consisted of two to three mobilization sessions per week, for 4 to 5 weeks, for a total of 9 to 11 treatment sessions. The subject then entered the second A, or withdrawal phase, duplicating the first phase and lasting approximately 1 month.

Treatment consisted of mobilization techniques to the limited or painful upper cervical segments (O-C1; C1,2; and C2,3) found on passive accessory and physiologic testing. The mobilizations included central and unilateral posteroanterior pressures described by Maitland and the following techniques described by Paris:

1. Inhibitory distraction.
2. Physiological rotation of C1,2 in sitting.
3. Occipital nod on the atlas.
4. Lateral pressures on the atlas.
5. Upslides and downslides on the upper cervical facets.

A one-way ANOVA for repeated measures on headache frequency, duration, and intensity was found to be statistically significant. Visual analysis of data plots also revealed a decrease in headache frequency, duration, and intensity from the baseline phase to the treatment phase. This improvement continued through the second A phase for frequency, but leveled off for both duration and intensity. Complete headache relief was obtained in 1 of the 10 subjects. The placebo effect was partially countered by the use of an additional baseline after treatment. The authors report finding the greatest impairment of motion at C2,3, which is in agreement with the findings of related studies on the topic.

In summary, this study revealed that mobilization of the upper cervical spine had a therapeutic effect in reducing the frequency, duration, and intensity of headaches in 10 patients suffering from cervical headache with 1 of the 10 experiencing complete headache relief.

Study #4: Schenk R, MacDiarmid A, Rousselle J. The effects of muscle energy technique on lumbar range of motion. Journal of Manual & Manipulative Therapy. 1997;5(4):179-183.

Considering that the goal of manipulation is to "restore maximal pain-free motion within postural balance," the Schenk et al study, with its focus on range of motion, is particularly relevant to our discussion of patient outcomes. When considering the connection between limited lumbar extension and the incidence of disc derangements in young adults, there is added significance.

The researchers included 26 subjects with limited lumbar spine extension. Subjects were randomly assigned to either the treatment group, which consisted of eight males and five females, or to the control, consisting of five males and eight females. The average age of the subjects was 25 years.

The study was a pretest-posttest design, comparing the effects of muscle energy technique (MET) on lumbar extension mobility in the treatment group versus an untreated control. The independent variable was the application of osteopathic MET; the dependent variable was the change in extension range of motion of the lumbar spine. Lumbar extension was measured with the bubble inclinometer (intrarater and interrater reliability for lumbar extension were r = 0.93 and r = 0.89, respectively).

The experimental group underwent eight sessions of MET (twice per week for 4 weeks), performed by a board certified orthopaedic clinical specialist who was also certified in orthopaedic manual physical therapy. At the conclusion of the intervention, all subjects were re-examined for changes in lumbar spine extension.

An independent group t-test revealed a statistically significant increase (p < 0.05) in lumbar extension range of motion in those who were treated with manual therapy versus those who weren't. The average range of lumbar extension for the treatment group was 13.8 degrees at pretest and 20.7 degrees at post-test. The average range of lumbar extension for the untreated control was 17.1 degrees at pretest and 16.7 degrees at post-test.

This study demonstrates the ability of a well-executed manual therapy intervention to significantly alter impaired lumbar extension for the better. Though the sample size was small and improvements in study design could be made (eg, improved examiner "blinding," enhanced placebo-control), the Schenk et al study does provide evidence in support of manipulative therapy. It is also written for clinicians by clinicians; unlike many outcome studies, the reader doesn't need a PhD to understand it!

Study #5: Mitchell UH, Wooden MJ, McKeough DM. The short-term effect of lumbar positional distraction. Journal of Manual & Manipulative Therapy. 2001;9(4):213-221.

A convenience sample of thirty patients presenting with low back pain and unilateral radiating symptoms, secondary to nerve-root irritation and associated with dermatomal sensory loss or weakness in a specific myotome, were included in this study. Patients with previous back surgeries, spinal stenosis, and unstable spondylolisthesis were excluded from the study. Patients were randomly assigned to the treatment or control group. The treatment group included 15 patients (9 females and 6 males) with an age range of 19 to 65 years. The control group also included 15 patients (8 females and 7 males) with an age range of 37 to 54 years. Each patient underwent a thorough examination, including a neuromuscular assessment to determine their eligibility for the study (13 patients in the treatment group exhibited specific sensory and two patients, specific motor impairment, while 15 patients in the control had specific sensory and three had weakness in a specific myotome). After signing the informed consent, the patients with even numbers were assigned to the treatment group consisting of 5 minutes of lumbar positional distraction; those with odd numbers were assigned to the control and were asked to "comfortably lie on the pain-free side," also for 5 minutes. A second examiner, blinded to the patient's group assignment, performed the post-intervention examination, which was identical to the initial examination and included an assessment of pain using a verbal digital scale (1 to 10), an assessment of the pain site with a body diagram, and a measurement of straight leg raise (SLR) height.

The Wilcoxon Signed-Ranks Test was employed to assess the difference between the pre/post pain-score in both groups. In the treatment group, there was a statistically significant improvement in symptoms ($p = 0.001$), whereas in the control there was no significant change noted ($p = 0.506$). Regarding pain location, 10 patients in the treatment group reported centralization, one reported peripheralization, and two reported "no change" in response to 5 minutes of positional distraction. In the control group, three patients reported "centralization," two reported peripheralization, and 10 reported "no change" in response to 5 minutes of comfortable side lying. Regarding SLR height, the treatment group demonstrated a statistically significant increase in height ($p = 0.005$), whereas the control group did not ($p = 0.884$). The authors indicate the "very high" reliability of the test and re-test SLR data in this study (ie, correlation coefficients of 0.99 and 0.989, respectively).

This study supports the clinical efficacy of lumbar positional distraction in three areas: diminished pain intensity, centralization of painful symptoms, and improvement in neurodynamic testing of the sciatic nerve with the classical SLR. The purpose of lumbar positional distraction is to decompress painful nerve roots by increasing space in the intervertebral foramina. Unlike the McKenzie approach, which claims to reduce the joint derangement and therefore cause centralization, positional distraction is a temporary measure that modulates, but does not, correct the underlying disorder. However, an intervention that readily decompresses "pinched nerves" with the simple use of a towel roll is welcome news to patients who suffer with these afflictions. In addition, where the McKenzie approach has limited effectiveness in achieving nerve root decompression (ie, extrusion of the disc with an incompetent annulus or stenosis of the lateral recess), positional distraction is an excellent alternative.

On the negative side, the researchers acknowledge that the sample size was small and that "only the very immediate effect of positional distraction was investigated and that the statistically significant difference should not be confused with a clinically important change." Be that as it may, manual physical therapists welcome the Mitchell et al study and look forward to seeing other clinical studies that confirm, with evidence, what clinicians have known experientially for years.

Study #6: Donelson R, Grant W, Kamps C, Medcalf R. Pain response to sagittal end-range spinal motion. A prospective, randomized, multicentered trial. Spine. 1991;16(6): S206-S212.

Patients with nonspecific low back pain (LBP) with or without referred leg pain presenting at 12 physical therapy clinics in five different countries (Australia, Canada, New Zealand, the United Kingdom, and the United States), were considered potential participants. Seventeen different examiners, 14 of whom had extensive experience with the McKenzie method, were involved in data collection. A total of 267 patients provided informed consent; however, after exclusions, 145 patients were included in the final study sample. Information on the location of a patient's pain at the time of the study was used to determine their Quebec Task Force (QTF) classification. Patients were then entered into one of two protocols based upon month-of-birth.

All patients were asked to record the location of symptoms on a pain drawing and the intensity of their central and most distal symptom on an analog scale. Thereafter, the protocols consisted of a sequence of single and repeated flexion and extension movements performed to the patient's available end-range, first standing and then while recumbent. The two protocols differed only in the order in which the flexion and extension movements were performed. Following each single movement and each repeated movement sequence, patients again recorded the intensity of their central pain and the location and intensity of their most distal symptom on a standardized form. Movements were repeated to a maximum of 4 sets of 10 repetitions with brief rest periods between each set of 10. Movements were terminated if the pain intensified or peripheralized.

Mantel-Haenszel chi-square analysis was used to explore group differences for categorical data and the Yates correction for continuity (z) to test distributions of proportions. The student t-test for unpaired samples was used to evaluate initial group differences in continuous variables; an analysis of covariance for repeated measures was employed to standardize patient's initial responses to a common starting point. Data analysis proceeded along two main lines of inquiry. The first involved whether changes in central pain intensity (CI), distal pain intensity (DI), and distal to most peripheral pain (DIST) could be attributed to the protocol used; the second was concerned with the relationship between symptom differences and the direction of movement. Based on the preliminary data analysis, an analysis model was constructed to assess differences recorded as patients were moved through the two protocols. Because CI, DI, and DIST changed after the performance of each movement sequence and consequently affected the patient's starting point for the subsequent movement sequence, analysis of covariance techniques statistically adjusted the results of one movement sequence to serve as a baseline for the next. Ultimately, a modified regression equation determined whether the groups known to be different from one another could be identified by the data and described by the model. Because the outcome variable (protocol) was categorical, logistic regression techniques were used to allow for the development of models of prediction for noncontinuous outcome variables. Specific design structures used to reduce potential bias included the multicentered, randomized, and prospective research design; standardization of the assessment process consisting of a set of written instructions; and the inclusion of examiners who had little or no experience in spinal care and who, therefore, were believed to have had no expectations of outcome.

Results demonstrated no significant differences between the two protocol groups for gender, age, QTF classification, work status, back and leg symptoms, or the number of past painful episodes. However, significant differences in responses to flexion and extension were found. Regardless of whether flexion preceded or followed extension, flexion increased intensity and peripheralized pain (ie, an increase in DIST) for the mean of both study groups, while extension decreased intensity and centralized pain (ie, a decrease in DIST). The statistical results from the testing of this model, were all significant at $p < 0.0001$. Only one of the 145 patients noted improvement in both flexion and extension during standing testing; no subject showed improvement in both directions while recumbent. This is an important finding when considering that spinal activity in general is considered beneficial for LBP patients. Forty percent improved with extension and worsened with flexion, whereas 7% improved with flexion and worsened with extension. This preference was highly significant ($p < 0.001$). Not only did one direction clearly centralize their symptoms, but the opposite direction typically intensified and/or peripheralized them. It was apparent that the performance of a single test movement frequently resulted in a different pain response than performing the same movement repetitively. The inclusion of single movements confounded the differences noted; when single movement

responses were deleted, results of analysis of repeated test movements were definitive.

In summary, regardless of the order of spinal movements, there were highly significant differences between the effects of flexion and extension test movements on pain intensity and distal location. Whereas end-range extension significantly decreased central and distal intensity and centralized referred pain, lumbar flexion significantly increased central and distal pain intensity and peripheralized the patient's symptoms. Furthermore, individual patients clearly had statistically significant directional preferences (ie, 40% of this study group improved with extension and 7% improved with flexion). In a previous study by Donelson et al,[3] a centralizing effect was identified in 87% of the patients compared to 47% in this study. The difference can be partially explained by the fact that, in the former study, the test movements were not limited to the sagittal plane. McKenzie has often stated that many patients whose pain does not centralize with repeated flexion or extension will experience centralization with lateral or rotational test movements. In the Donelson et al[3] study, the McKenzie method of achieving centralization, while concurrently discouraging positions and movements that cause peripheralization, yielded excellent patient outcomes in 92% of the cases and good outcomes in 6% of patients when these patients had symptoms for less than 4 weeks. In patients with symptoms lasting longer than 12 weeks, excellent or good outcomes were achieved in 81% of the cases.

Lastly and perhaps most importantly, this study demonstrates the ability of the McKenzie system to assist the clinician in determining the appropriate mechanical intervention for the patient. The notion that any form of exercise for LBP is therapeutic, regardless of its direction, must be reconsidered based upon these data.

Study #7: Farrell JP, Twomey LT. Acute low back pain, comparison of two conservative treatment approaches. Med J Aust. 1982;1:160-164.

Of 56 eligible patients, 48 completed the study. Patients of either gender were accepted into the study, if they met the following inclusion criteria:

1. Age range, 20 to 65 years
2. LBP experienced with lumbar movements or SLR
3. Intermittent or constant pain between T12 and the gluteal folds
4. LBP of 3 week's duration or less
5. A pain-free period of 6 months prior to the onset of the current episode

Patients were excluded if they had other treatment for the current episode, were pregnant, presented with frank neurological signs, had prior lumbar surgery, had a history of a lower thoracic/lumbar fracture, and showed evidence of systemic disease.

The patients were randomly assigned to one of two groups. The experimental group received passive mobilization and manipulation of the lumbar spine as described by Stoddart[4] and Maitland.[5] The control group received a regimen of microwave diathermy, isometric abdominal exercises, and ergonomic instructions. There were no significant differences between the treatment and control groups in terms of age, gender, low back pain history, and the duration of symptoms before treatment. All personnel involved in the examination/evaluation and intervention were physiotherapists who followed standardized measurement and treatment procedures. The assessment included an evaluation of functional limitations, pain severity, active lumbar movements with a lumbar spondylometer and rotameter, and straight leg raising with a standard goniometer. Patients were examined before the first treatment, immediately after the first treatment, after the third session, after the final session, and 3 weeks from the date of the initial treatment. Intraobserver tests showed no significant differences between measurements ($p < 0.01$); thus reinforcing the reliability of these devices. The patients as well as the examiner were "blinded."

Each patient was treated three times a week for up to 3 weeks. For a subject to be pronounced "symptom-free," it was necessary that he or she could perform all functional activities without difficulty, his/her subjective pain was either 0 or 1 on a 0 through 10 scale, and the objective measures of lumbar movements and SLR were pain-free with passive overpressure at the extreme of the patient's active range. If a patient met the criteria for discharge before 3 weeks, treatment was discontinued.

A Mann-Whitney U-test indicated a statistically significant difference between the two groups in the number of treatments needed to reach the symptom-free status ($p < 0.001$). The manipulative group required 3.5 ± 1.6 treatments, while the control required 5.8 ± 2.3 to reach the same result. An analysis of covariance indicated that the manipulative group had significantly greater lumbar extension following the last session ($p < 0.05$). However, this was not the case for the other active lumbar movements. Overall, the researchers were not impressed with significant differences in active lumbar range of motion between the two groups. At the end of the 3 weeks, there was no significant difference between the subjective pain ratings of the two groups, although the trend favored the manipulative group. Within 4 weeks of developing symptoms, 91% of all subjects recovered from their symptoms. This is consistent with other studies that report that the vast majority of patients with acute LBP are asymptomatic within 4 weeks of developing symptoms, regardless of the treatment received.

In summary, the findings of this study strongly suggest that patients with acute low back pain treated by passive mobilization/manipulation had a shorter mean duration of symptoms compared to those treated with microwave diathermy, isometric abdominal exercises, and ergonomic instructions. Though one can argue that the placebo effect was stronger in the manipulative group because of greater patient contact, it can also be argued that the control had the advantage of being instructed in proper body mechanics. The "bottom line" is that, despite an "advantaged" control group in several respects (ie, pain-relieving treatment, strengthening exercises, and ergonomic training), the manipulative group still demonstrated a superior clinical outcome!

Study #8: Hoehler FK, Tobis JS, Buerger AA. Spinal manipulation for low back pain. JAMA. 1981;245(18):1835-1838.

This was a randomized clinical trial (RCT) conducted on 95 patients with low back pain (LBP). Patients were selected from a group of 1880 patients referred to the University of California, Irvine, Medical Center Back Clinic between June 1973 and June 1979. Exclusion criteria consisted of prior manipulative treatment, disability income, pending litigation, prior back surgery, obesity, drug/alcohol abuse, and pain not amenable to manipulative therapy of the lumbosacral area.

After being admitted to the trial and signing the appropriate informed consent, patients were randomly assigned to either the experimental group or the control. Patients in the experimental group (56 subjects) received rotational manipulations of the lumbosacral spine consisting of a high velocity thrust maneuver with the intention of gapping the facet joints and stretching the paravertebral muscles of the lumbosacral area. Patients assigned to the control group (39 subjects) received soft tissue massage of the same area without the rotational thrust manipulation. The number of treatments received was at the discretion of the treating physicians. On discharge, each patient was re-examined by the same physician who performed the initial examination. The patient and physician performing the examinations were both "blinded" in this study. Subjective data came from questionnaires; the objective examination consisted of the SLR to the point of both pain and pelvic rotation, and the distance of the fingertips to the floor in standing forward flexion. Nonparametric statistics were used (ie, the Mann-Whitney U-test) because the data were only measurable on an ordinal scale and therefore not normally distributed. Correlations were measured by the nonparametric Spearman rank-order correlation coefficient; the criteria for statistical significance was $p < 0.05$ for a one-tailed test.

Although the pretreatment comparison of the two groups revealed a somewhat higher proportion of patients with "severe" or "very severe" pain complaints in the experimental group, there were no statistically significant differences regarding the origin of pain, rapidity of pain onset, the extent of pain on lateral bending, SLR to pain, SLR to pelvic rotation, and forward flexion. The experimental group also had a somewhat lower proportion of patients with "chronic" pain, but this too was not a statistically significant difference. Regarding the duration of treatment and number of treatments, the manipulative group exceeded the massage group in both categories. The authors acknowledge, "This effect is difficult to interpret and presents problems for any analysis of postdischarge data."

Moving on to outcome parameters, the data demonstrated the following immediate benefits of spinal manipulation over soft tissue massage:

1. The manipulation group showed more improvement than the control (p < 0.01) in four of six subjective measures of spinal flexibility, including walking, bending or twisting, sitting down in a chair, sitting up in bed, reaching, and dressing.

2. The manipulative group reported more pain relief than the control (p < 0.05).

3. The manipulative group demonstrated a statistically significant increase in SLR to pain after the first treatment (p < 0.01).

4. At discharge, the manipulative group demonstrated superior SLR to pelvic rotation, but this difference was not statistically significant (p > 0.05). One explanation for this lack of significance was the reduced number of patients represented in this particular comparison.

Regarding long-term improvement, apart from the perceived effectiveness of manipulation over massage at 3 weeks postdischarge (p < 0.05), manipulation did not appear to be significantly better than soft tissue massage. However, it must be noted that the two groups are similar in this regard because both showed substantial improvement. Furthermore, the long-term effectiveness of manipulation is difficult to assess because, given sufficient time, many patients with back pain will recover with or without intervention.

In summary, these data clearly show that spinal manipulation provides immediate subjective alleviation of LBP. The amount of relief produced by manipulation was significantly greater than the amount of relief produced by soft tissue massage of the affected areas. However, at discharge and following, there was no significant difference between the two groups because both showed substantial improvement. This raises another consideration in this study. The authors are pleased with their choice of soft tissue massage as the placebo-control intervention; however, one cannot help but see that soft tissue massage, in reality, is another form of manual therapy. To report that there was no significant difference between the two groups at discharge is another way of saying that both forms of intervention are equally effective. Consequently, the outcomes after the first session, at discharge, and at 3 weeks postdischarge indicate that these two manual therapy interventions were effective in the management of LBP.

Study #9: Sunshine W, Field T, Schanberg S, Quintino O, Kilmer T, Fierro K, Burman I, Hashimoto M, McBride C, Henteleff T. Massage therapy and transcutaneous electrical stimulation effects on fibromyalgia. J Clin Rheumatol. 1996;2:18-22.

Thirty female adult fibromyalgia syndrome (FMS) patients were recruited from local rheumatology practices. (Note: FMS was confirmed by a rheumatologist using criteria established by the American College of Rheumatology.) Patients averaged 49.8 years; were of middle income levels (on average); and were 32% Caucasian, 44% Hispanic, and 24% African American. The patients were randomly assigned (using a table of random numbers) to one of three groups: massage therapy, transcutaneous electrical nerve stimulation (TENS), and sham TENS. The three groups of women did not differ on the demographic variables of ethnicity, income, or age. The researchers responsible for pre- and post assessments were "blinded" to the group assignment of the patients. Assessments were made during the first and final sessions, sessions 1 and 10, respectively.

All pre- and post-tests were performed by the same rheumatologist. A global rating of pain was recorded by the rheumatologist on the first and last days of treatment. Patients were required to maintain their pharmacological regimen during the course of the study. The immediate effects of these interventions were measured by the State Trait Anxiety Inventory (STAI), the Profile of Mood States (POMS), and by stress hormone (cortisol) levels. The end-of-study effects (ie, the end versus the beginning of the study period) were assessed by the dolorimeter test; an interview on pain, sleep, and daily functioning; and by the CES-D (depression scale).

Massage therapy sessions consisted of moderate pressure stroking of the head, neck, shoulders, back, arms, hands, legs, and feet for 30 minutes. The TENS group received microamperage stimulation through the electroacuscope roller to the same areas as the massage group. The sham TENS group received the same tactile stimulation with the electroacuscope roller, however, with the machine turned off. Because the dials and knobs of the unit were hidden from view, the therapist and the patient were both "blinded" during this aspect of the study. Obviously, there was no way to double "blind" the massage group.

Analyses of the immediate treatment effects revealed the following:

1. The massage therapy group had lower state anxiety STAI (p = 0.001), lower depressed mood (POMS) scores (p = 0.05), and lower salivary cortisol levels (p = 0.05).

2. There were no statistically significant immediate treatment effects of either TENS or sham TENS.

Analyses of longer-term effects (first-session/last session measures) suggested the following:

1. The massage group had lower anxiety/depression scores and salivary cortisol (p = 0.05).

2. The TENS group demonstrated statistically significant improvement in all three measures (ie, anxiety, p = 0.01; depression, p = 0.01; cortisol level, p = 0.05).

3. No changes were noted in the sham TENS group.

4. The massage group improved on the rheumatologist's rating of clinical condition (p = 0.05) and dolorimeter value (p = 0.01); there were significantly fewer symptoms at the end of the study, including less pain, less pain over the last week, less stiffness, less fatigue, and fewer nights of difficult sleeping.

5. The TENS group only improved on the physician's assessment of clinical condition.

6. The sham TENS group also improved on the physician's assessment of clinical condition, but to a lesser degree than the other two groups.

In summary, this study of 30 adult female FMS patients demonstrated the following outcomes:

1. Soft tissue massage therapy was superior to TENS and sham TENS in reducing anxiety and depression.

2. Whereas both therapeutic massage and TENS significantly reduced anxiety, depression, and salivary cortisol levels on the last day of treatment, only massage showed these changes on both the first and last day of treatment.

3. Although the rheumatologist's assessment of the subject's clinical condition improved for all three groups, only the massage group improved on the dolorimeter and the subject's self-report of pain.

4. Only the massage group consistently reported significantly fewer symptoms by the end of the study, including less pain, stiffness, fatigue, and difficulty sleeping.

Whereas the emphasis in physical therapy education has historically been on the physiological effects of soft tissue mobilization/massage, this study clearly demonstrates the psychological benefits of this important manual therapy intervention as well.

Study #10: Saal JA, Saal JS. Nonoperative treatment of herniated lumbar intervertebral disc with radiculopathy: an outcome study. Spine. 1989;14(4):431-437.

The researchers used a retrospective cohort study design to analyze the results of a group of patients treated nonoperatively for lumbar intervertebral disc herniation. The available records of patients seen in the San Francisco Spine Institute and the SpineCare Medical Group in Daly City, California with a diagnosis of herniated lumbar intervertebral disc between January 1, 1985 and April 1, 1986 were reviewed. The inclusion criteria were as follows:

1. Diagnosed "herniated nucleus pulposus" (HNP) as per computerized tomography (CT) and/or magnetic resonance imaging (MRI).

2. Diagnosed lumbar radiculopathy based on a primary complaint of leg pain and a secondary complaint of back pain, a positive electromyogram (EMG) demonstrating the electrophysiologic presence of lumbar radiculopathy, and a positive SLR test reproducing leg pain at less than 60 degrees elevation.

3. Willingness to participate in an "aggressive" treatment program, including back school, exercise training to teach spinal stabilization (ie, dynamic maintenance of postural control, trunk, and general upper/lower body strengthening and flexibility exercises).

Epidural injections and/or selective nerve root blocks were to be used when indicated for pain control. All patients in the study had failed passive conservative management and were comparable clinically to the patients evaluated in surgical studies of herniated lumbar discs.

Exclusion criteria were as follows: previous lumbar spine surgery, and the presence of significant spinal stenosis or spondylolisthesis (ie, grade 3 on the Glenn scale).

A standardized questionnaire, including questions from the Oswestry Scale, pain self-rating, work status, and self-rating of outcome, were mailed to each patient who met the above criteria. Self-rating criteria were as follows:

1. Excellent: working full time, performing usual athletic activities.

2. Good: working full time but limited in performance of athletic activities.

3. Fair: working part time only, unable to participate in athletic activities.

4. Poor: unable to work and unimproved following treatment.

Out of a total of 347 consecutively identified patient records reviewed, 64 were included in the group to whom questionnaires were mailed. A total of 58 questionnaires were returned (91% response rate).

Data analysis included calculation of rates of return to work, average sick-leave time, subsequent surgery due to failure of "aggressive" conservative care, and a self-rating of outcome.

Of the 58 patients in the study, there were 36 men and 22 women with a median age of 35.5 ± 1.2 years. Thirteen (22%) were worker's compensation cases. Weakness of at least one grade on a 0 to 5 grading scale was noted in 37 patients (64%). Symptom duration averaged 4.6 ± 0.6 months. The mean postcare follow-up time was 31.1 ± 1.7 months. Six patients required surgery.

The "aggressive" treatment program utilized in this study consisted of two phases. The first was the pain control phase, and the second was the exercise training phase. Pain control consisted of physical therapy, pain-relieving modalities, back school, McKenzie exercises, non-narcotic analgesics, facet joint injections, corticosteroid epidural injections, acupuncture, etc. Exercise training included the use of techniques to improve soft tissue flexibility, joint mobility, joint stability, and aerobic capacity.

Results indicated a success rate, defined as excellent or good, of 83% in the entire study population; an impressive 96% success rate in the nonoperative cases. Forty-eight patients returned to work (83 ± 5.2% of the entire study population and 92 ± 3.5% of all non-operative patients), and 85 ± 5% of all patients returned to their previous jobs. The average sick-leave time was 3.8 ± 1 month; 26 patients (50 ± 6.9%) reported less than 1 week sick-leave. The self-rated reports for these patients were 15 excellent, 35 good, 2 fair, and 0 poor. The median Oswestry score for the excellent group was 16.6, the good group was 20, and the fair group was 32. Therefore, 20 patients who categorized themselves as good by self-report could fall into the excellent group. This would yield 31 excellent results and 14 good ones.

Eleven worker's compensation patients returned to work, with an average sick-leave time of 9 ± 3 months. Six patients required subsequent surgery after unsatisfactory improvement with the nonoperative program. Four of these patients had significant stenosis at the time of operation. One patient had progressive weakness and one, unable to complete the program, referred herself to surgery.

Eighteen patients (31%) were seen for a second opinion. All of these had been advised by a surgeon that they needed surgery as soon as possible to avoid long-term complications. Of these 18, 15 were nonoperative treatment successes, three scoring excellent on the self-rating reports and 12 scoring good. All 15 returned to work with an average sick-leave time of 13.6 weeks.

As per CT and/or MRI scans, extruded discs were seen in 15 patients. Of these, 11 had weakness. Eighty-seven percent (13 of 15) of these patients had good and excellent outcomes. The average sick-leave time for this group was 2 months and 92% of these patients returned to work. Three of the patients with extruded discs required subsequent surgery, one because of progressive weakness, and one who had significant lateral recess stenosis at the time of surgery. The third withdrew from the program and referred herself to surgery.

In summary, this study demonstrated that patients with HNP and radiculopathy can be successfully treated, nonsurgically. The sick-leave time and return to work rates were superior to rates reported for similar patients treated surgically. The presence of weakness did not adversely affect outcome in the treatment cohort. Disc extrusion was successfully managed 87% of the time. The premise that operative patients fare better in the first year, as noted by the average sick-leave time, is contrary to these outcome measures. Four of the six patients who failed "aggressive," nonsurgical treatment were found to have stenosis at subsequent lumbar spine surgery. Thus, failed aggressive nonoperative measures should probably warrant greater decompression than disc excision alone. From this study it appears that HNP combined with stenosis is associated with a different prognosis than HNP without. The results of this study also suggest that failed passive, nonoperative therapy is not a sufficient criterion for the decision to operate.

Study #11: Nicolakis P, Erdogmus B, Kopf A, Djaber-Ansari A, Piehslinger E, Fialka-Moser V. Exercise therapy for craniomandibular disorders. Arch Phys Med Rehabil. 2000;81:1137-114.

The objective of this "before-after" trial was to evaluate the use of exercise therapy for the treatment of craniomandibular disorders. Thirty patients (28 women and two men) with a mean age of 33.1 ± 11.0 years and diagnosed with anterior disc displacement (ADD) with reduction participated in this study. Patients were selected consecutively from patients consulting the Craniomandibular Disorders (CMD) Service at the Department of Dentistry, University of Vienna. At the 6-month follow-up, 26 patients remained in the study (two were not available and two were allocated to splint therapy because they were not satisfied with the treatment result).

Inclusion criteria included symptoms lasting at least 3 months, pain in the temporomandibular joint (TMJ) region, signs consistent with a diagnosis of TMJ ADD with reduction, joint clicking together with a straight or convex pathway finding on computerized axiography, and evidence of postural dysfunction.

Patients were examined by the same physiatrist in a standardized manner. After the examination, all patients were assigned to a waiting list for exercise therapy, serving as a no-treatment control period. The following outcome measures were used in this study:

1. Pain at rest was measured with a visual analogue scale (VAS).

2. Maximal pain during the "last 2 days" (pain at stress) was also measured with a VAS.

3. Patients were asked to rate their overall impairment in daily life activities with a VAS.

4. The maximal interincisal opening (MIO) was measured in millimeters (mm).

5. The change in self-perceived joint clicking from the outset to the end of treatment was measured on a four-point scale (ie, vanished, better, equal, and worse).

6. Perceived improvement of jaw pain was measured on a seven-point scale (ie, excellent, distinct improvement, moderate improvement, equal, moderate, distinct deterioration, severe deterioration).

7. Perceived improvement of jaw function was also measured on the same seven-point scale. The first four measures were recorded at baseline, immediately before, immediately after, and 6 months after exercise therapy, while the remaining measures (5 to 7) were recorded only at the second, third, and final examination.

Each patient was treated a minimum of five times, with each session lasting 30 minutes (usually two treatments per week were administered with the last two treatments given at intervals of 1 to 2 weeks to establish the home program). Exercise therapy included massage, stretching, gentle isometric exercises, guided opening and closing movements, manual TMJ distraction, disc/condyle mobilization, postural correction, and relaxation techniques. Patients were also instructed in a home program including some of the above-mentioned exercises for the TMJs, as well as postural and relaxation exercises. Exercise therapy was intended to improve coordination of the muscles of mastication, reduce muscle spasm, and alter the jaw-closing pattern.

According to a "before-after" trial, the time on the waiting list served as the control period. However, because time on the waiting list and treatment time were not equal, changes of all numerical parameters (ie, pain at rest, maximal pain, impairment of quality of life, and MIO) were normalized for daily changes for these two periods. Differences between this normalized data were analyzed with the t-test for paired samples. Descriptive data were analyzed by the chi-square test (ie, perceived jaw clicking, pain, and function). For statistical evaluation of perceived improvement of jaw pain and function, the seven-point scale was reduced to a three-point scale as follows: improvement (excellent, distinct improvement), no change (moderate or no improvement), and worse (distinct or severe deterioration). The Wilcoxon test was used to identify differences between baseline and pretreatment investigation, between pretreatment and post-treatment, and between pretreatment and the 6-month control.

Patients experienced symptoms of CMD for a mean of 2.6 years. Mean duration on the waiting list was 27 days and the mean duration of treatment was 39 days. Patients received a mean of 9.9 treatments. All patients completed treatment. Results revealed that the overall mean pain intensity was reduced significantly as a result of treatment. At the end of therapy, 87% of patients rated improvement in jaw pain as excellent or distinctly improved and 13% experienced a moderate pain reduction. Six months after treatment, 80% of the patients experienced improvement in jaw pain, with no patient reporting deterioration in contrast to his or her pretreatment condition. The effects of treatment on pain at rest, pain at stress, perceived improvement in jaw function, and maximal jaw opening (MIO) were all statistically significant ($p < 0.001$). TMJ clicking vanished in 13.3% and was reduced in another 13.3% after therapy. Six months later 11.5% reported that their clicking had not returned, while 15.4% indicated a reduction in joint clicking. However, a deterioration in clicking had occurred in one patient. At the 6-month follow-up, five of the remaining 26 patients were in need of treatment, four because of pain and one because of excessive clicking.

The authors point out that the results obtained in this study were superior to recent studies using occlusal appliances to treat patients with arthrogenous or myogenous temporomandibular pain and at least equal to studies using either physical therapy modalities or a multimodal approach utilizing a stabilization appliance, exercise therapy, muscle injections, and various forms of physical therapy.

The authors conclude this study with the following statement, "Exercise therapy seems to be useful in the treatment of anterior disc displacement with reduction and pain. The impairing symptoms, jaw pain, and restricted movement can be alleviated significantly."

Study #12: Bronfort G, Evans R, Nelson B, Aker PD, Goldsmith CH, Vernon H. A randomized clinical trial of exercise and spinal manipulation for patients with chronic neck pain. Spine. 2001;26(7): 788-799.

The objective of this prospective, parallel-group, randomized clinical trial was to compare the relative efficacy of rehabilitative neck exercise and spinal manipulation for the management of patients with chronic neck pain.

Patients 20 to 65 years who had a primary problem of mechanical neck pain persisting for 12 or more weeks were eligible for the study. Patients were excluded for referred neck pain, severe osteopenia, progressive neurologic deficits, vascular disease of the neck or upper extremity, previous cervical spine surgery, current or pending litigation, inability to work because of neck pain, spinal manipulative therapy (SMT) or exercise therapy within 3 months prior to study entry, or concurrent treatment for neck pain by other health care workers. Recruitment of patients was conducted over a 22-month period from October 1994 to July 1996. There were a total of 191 patients (113 females, 78 males).

Patients were randomized to one of three groups on the basis of a computer-generated list using a 1:1:1 allocation ratio. The three groups were as follows:

1. Spinal manipulation and low-technology exercise (38 females, 26 males, age 45 ± 10.5 years). At each visit, patients underwent treatment by one of nine chiropractors (15 minutes), followed by a supervised low-technology rehabilitative exercise session (45 minutes).

2. MedX exercise (38 females, 25 males, age 43.6 ± 10.5 years). These patients were seen by a physical therapist who, following stretching, upper body strengthening, and aerobic exercise using a dual-action stationary bike, performed dynamic, progressive resistive exercises on the MedX cervical extension and rotation machine (Med X Corp, Ocala, Fla).

3. Spinal manipulation (37 females, 27 males, age 44.3 ± 11.0 years). Patients in the SMT group received 15-minute sessions of chiropractic manipulation using short-lever, low-amplitude, high velocity thrust to the cervical spine. To balance for time and attention, all the patients attended 20 1-hour visits during the 11-week study period.

Outcome measures included patient self-report questionnaires administered twice at baseline; 5 and 11 weeks after the start of treatment; then 3, 6, and 12 months after treatment. Pain, the primary outcome measure, was rated with an 11-box scale (0 = no symptoms, 10 = highest severity of pain). The Neck Disability Index measured disability, while the Short Form (SF-36) was used to measure functional health status. The patients rated their improvement using a nine-point ordinal scale. Use of over-the-counter pain medication was assessed by a five-point scale, with choices from "none" to "every day." Finally, satisfaction with care was assessed by a seven-point scale with choices ranging from "completely satisfied" to "completely dissatisfied."

Cervical spine muscle strength, endurance, and range of motion were measured twice at baseline, then after 11 weeks of treatment by observers "blinded" to patient group assignment. Cervical isometric strength was measured by a computerized load-cell transducer dynamometer; the highest of three trials assessing maximal voluntary contraction for flexion, extension, and rotation were used for analyses. Static cervical endurance was measured by having the recumbent patient (supine for flexion, prone for extension) elevate his or her head, free of support with an attached weight, for up to 240 seconds. Dynamic endurance was recorded as the number of repetitions until failure. The attached weight for the static test corresponded to 60% of the maximal voluntary contraction; for the dynamic test, the attached weight was 25% of the maximal voluntary contraction. Active cervical rotation, flexion, extension, and lateral bending ranges of motion were measured with the CA6000 Spine Motion Analyzer (Orthopedic Systems Inc, Haywood, Calif).

The statistical analysis involved the use of a repeated measures analyses of covariance (ANCOVA) for each of the patient-rated outcomes. Repeated measures multivariate analyses of variance (MANCOVA) were used as overall tests of treatment differences incorporating the six patient-oriented outcomes for the short- and long-term. Change scores (week 11 minus baseline) in objective neck performance data were tested for group differences with an analysis of variance (ANOVA). Group differences were determined by the multiple comparison Newman-Keuls test. Effect sizes were calculated to standardize measurement units of the six outcomes and to help evaluate the importance of the magnitude of group differences under the curve. These summary measures were tested for group differences with ANOVA, and 95% confidence intervals were placed on group differences. To evaluate potential predictors of outcome, a multiple linear regression analysis was performed. A statistician independent of the study site performed the main analyses.

An analysis of short-term therapeutic outcomes revealed substantial improvement in all three study groups. However, except for satisfaction with care, which was significantly higher in the SMT with exercise group than SMT alone, there were no clinically important or statistically significant differences between groups.

Regarding neck performance outcomes, the SMT/exercise group demonstrated greater gains in strength, endurance, and range of motion than SMT alone ($p < 0.05$) after 11 weeks of treatment. The SMT/exercise group also demonstrated more improvement in flexion endurance and in flexion and rotation strength than the group treated with MedX ($p = 0.03$). Finally, the MedX group showed greater gains in extension strength and flexion-extension range of motion than the SMT group ($p < 0.05$).

An analysis of long-term therapeutic outcomes revealed that most of the improvement noted in all outcomes for the three groups at the end of the treatment phase was maintained during the post-treatment follow-up year. There was a group difference in patient-rated pain ($p = 0.02$) in favor of the two exercise groups. There was a group difference in satisfaction with care, with the SMT/exercise group superior to both MedX and SMT alone ($p = 0.002$). The remaining outcome measures showed no significant group differences for neck disability. There were no important differences for any of the patient-oriented outcomes between patients who regularly performed the recommended home exercises throughout the follow-up year (n = 46), those who did them occasionally (n = 51), or those who did not do them at all (n = 62). Overall, these analyses showed that, except for satisfaction with care, there were no important differences between SMT/exercise and MedX. The data did show that SMT/exercise was superior to SMT alone in terms of pain, satisfaction, and improvement and that MedX was superior to SMT in terms of pain.

Regression analyses showed that expectation was not a predictor for any of the outcomes. Although such side effects as temporary increases in neck pain or headache were reported in as many as 23 patients, the differential number of side effects across treatments was not statistically significant.

The following highlights of this study are worth repeating:

1. In the short term (ie, during the 11 weeks of intervention), all three treatments were associated with substantial improvement in patient-reported symptoms.

2. The SMT/exercise group was significantly more satisfied with care than the SMT alone group and the MedX group.

3. In terms of neck performance, at least twice as much improvement was observed in the SMT/exercise group over SMT alone.

4. The SMT/exercise group showed greater improvement in flexion endurance and flexion strength than the MedX group.

5. The tendency in the short term for the two exercise groups to perform better in the patient-oriented outcomes than the group treated with SMT alone continued throughout the follow-up year and cumulatively resulted in statistically significant group differences.

Based on these findings, the authors conclude their paper by stating, "Overall, the use of strengthening exercise, whether in combination with SMT or in the form of a high technology MedX program, appears to be more beneficial to patients with chronic neck pain than the use of spinal manipulative therapy alone."

In his commentary on this study, Rand S. Swenson, DC, MD, PhD, points out that the data give support to two important clinical concepts. The first is that exercises should be incorporated as a regular part of the treatment of patients with chronic neck pain and the second is that the significantly higher level of treatment satisfaction among the SMT/exercise group "could relate to the addition of a 'hands-on' component to the treatment protocol."

Some would say that the Bronfort et al study raises questions about the relative efficacy of spinal manual therapy. Though it is true that the manipulative group alone was inferior to the manipulative/exercise group in many respects, it must be pointed out that the merits of this combined approach to patient care (ie, spinal manual therapy plus therapeutic exercise) are underscored by this outcome study.

Study #13: Hoving JL, Koes BW, de Vet H, van der Windt D, Assendelft W, van Mameren H, Deville W, Pool J, Scholten R, Bouter LM. Manual therapy, physical therapy, or continued care by a general practitioner for patients with neck pain. A randomized controlled trial. Ann Intern Med. 2002;136(10): 713-722.

This randomized controlled trial (RCT) consisted of 183 patients between the ages of 18 to 70 years of age who had nonspecific neck pain for at least 2 weeks. Patients were referred to one of four research centers by 42 general practitioners. Patients with nonbenign causes of neck pain (ie, prior neck surgery, malignancy, neurologic disease, fracture, herniated disc, systemic rheumatic disease, etc) were excluded from the study (40 in all).

Patients were randomly assigned to one of three groups: manual therapy (n = 60), physical therapy (n = 59), and continued care from a general practitioner (n = 64). Manual therapy, consisting of specific nonthrust spinal mobilization, was performed once per week for 6 weeks by six experienced manual physical therapists acknowledged by the Netherlands Manual Therapy Association. Physical therapy, consisting of a combination of massage, heat application, interferential stimulation, stretching, manual traction, and active exercise therapy, was performed twice per week for 6 weeks. The treatment was performed by five experienced physical therapists with emphasis on therapeutic exercises (ie, postural correction, stretching, relaxation training, functional and active strengthening/range of motion exercises). These physical therapists, unlike the six manual physical therapists in the study, were not specialists in manual therapy. The third group received standardized care from his or her general practitioner, including advice on prognosis, psychosocial issues, self-care (eg, heat application, home exercises), ergonomics (eg, pillow size, work position), and encouragement to await further recovery. Patients were prescribed medication, including paracetamol or nonsteroidal anti-inflammatory drugs as needed. Ten-minute follow-up visits scheduled every 2 weeks were optional. Referral during the intervention period was discouraged. Two research assistants (experienced physical therapists), who were "blinded" to treatment allocation, performed physical examinations at baseline and follow-up.

Outcome data were collected after 3 and 7 weeks. Primary outcome measures focused on perceived recovery, pain, and functional disability, which was measured according to the Neck Disability Index. Secondary outcome measures included the severity of the most important functional limitation, rated by the patient on a numeric 11-point scale. Cervical range of motion was measured by using the Cybex Electronic Digital Inclinometer 320 (Lumex Inc, Ronkonkoma, NY). General health was measured according to the self-rated health index (scale 0 to 100) of the Euro Quality of Life scale. Patients recorded absences from work and analgesic use in a diary.

The differences in success rates for perceived recovery were analyzed by applying chi-square tests (univariate analysis). Likewise, differences in improvement rates for absence from work and use of analgesics were analyzed. For the continuous outcome measures, univariate analyzes of variance were applied to the differences between the baseline measurement and each of the follow-up measurements (mean improvement).

Multivariate analyses (multiple logistic regression and analyses of covariance) were performed to examine the influence of the following covariates: baseline value of an outcome measure, therapist, age, severity, research center, sex, duration of the current episode, prior episodes of neck pain, headache of cervical origin, radiating pain below the elbow, and patient preference for treatment. For all comparisons, a two-tailed P value of 0.05 was considered statistically significant.

In general, the outcome measures showed distinct differences, both within groups (compared with baseline) and among groups. These differences usually favored manual therapy more than physical therapy and physical therapy more than continued care. The success rate at 7 weeks was twice as high for the manual therapy group (68.3%) as for the continued care group (35.9%). Physical dysfunction, pain, and disability were less severe in the manual therapy group than in the physical therapy and continued care groups. Some differences in outcome measures were already statistically significant at 3 weeks. At 7 weeks, the success rate for physical therapy (50.8%) was higher than for continued care (35.9%), but this difference was not statistically significant. The success rates for manual therapy were statistically significantly higher than those for physical therapy. Manual therapy scored better than physical therapy on all outcome measures; however, not all differences were statistically significant. There were no statistically significant differences between groups on the Neck Disability Index; however, the Euro Quality of Life scale showed a statistically significant difference in favor of manual therapy compared with physical therapy and continued care. Regarding range of motion, both the manual therapy and physical therapy groups improved markedly when compared to the continued care group. Patients receiving manual therapy had fewer absences from work due to neck pain than the other groups, but the differences were not statistically significant. Regarding analgesic use, the manual and physical therapy groups demonstrated significantly less analgesic use compared with the continued care group.

In their discussion of the results, the authors make the following comments:

1. Manual therapy was more effective than continued care on almost all outcome measures.

2. Physical therapy scored slightly better than continued care, but most of the differences were, except for range of motion, not statistically significant.

3. Although manual therapy seemed to be more effective than physical therapy, differences were small for all outcome measures except for perceived recovery, which was statistically significant (the authors state that perceived recovery may be the most responsive outcome because it combines other outcomes, such as pain, disability, and patient satisfaction). Perceived recovery was also significantly greater when comparing manual therapy to continued care.

4. As expected, the manual therapy group demonstrated the largest increase in cervical spine range of motion.

5. The low disability scores on the Neck Disability Index at baseline may have left only a small margin for improvement. Other studies using the Neck Disability Index have found that function may not be severely limited in patients with nonspecific neck pain; therefore, it may lack sensitivity in this regard.

6. Mobilization, the passive component of the manual therapy strategy, formed the main contrast with physical therapy or continued care and was considered to be the most effective component.

Study #14: Sterling M, Jull G, Wright A. Cervical mobilization: concurrent effects on pain, sympathetic nervous system activity, and motor activity. Man Ther. 2001;6(2):72-81.

This study utilized a double blind, placebo-controlled, within-subjects design in which each subject experienced all three experimental conditions (ie, treatment, placebo, and control) in a randomized order. Thirty subjects (16 female and 14 male) with a mean age of 35.77 ± 14.92 years were recruited. Inclusion criteria consisted of mid to lower cervical spine pain of insidious onset, greater than 3 months duration with symptoms originating from the C5,6 segment, as determined by a manipulative physiotherapist. Exclusion criteria included a history of trauma or surgery to the cervical spine, evidence of radiculopathy, headache, dizziness or other cervical spine symptoms, diabetes, or peripheral vascular disease.

Three experimental conditions were applied: spinal manual therapy (SMT), placebo, and control. The SMT treatment consisted of a Maitland grade III PA technique to the articular pillar of C5,6 on the symptomatic side, while the placebo condition consisted of a manual contact at the C5,6 articular pillar on the symptomatic side, but with no movement of the vertebral segment. The control consisted of no physical contact between the subject and the researcher. The treatment and placebo conditions involved three 1-minute applications with a 1-minute interval between each. Two researchers were involved in the experiment. Researcher A recorded all pre- and post-experimental measures and was blind to the experimental condition applied. The experimental conditions were applied by researcher B who was an experienced manipulative physiotherapist. Researcher B was "blind" to data collection on each subject.

Three pain related measures were taken, including scores of the subject's neck pain with visual analogue scales (VAS), pressure pain thresholds (PPTs) over the symptomatic segment, and thermal pain thresholds (TPTs) also recorded at the C5,6 segment, bilaterally. In addition, two measures of sympathetic nervous activity were taken (skin conductance and skin temperature) as well as a measure of EMG activity in the sternocleidomastoid muscles during the "craniocervical flexion test" performed in supine. This test involved the use of an air-filled sensor to monitor flattening of the cervical lordosis during contraction of the longus colli. EMG recordings were taken at 22, 24, 26, 28, and 30 mmHg as the subject was asked to hold each position for 5 seconds. Prior to the main study, the reliability of the test measures utilized was established.

Based upon the postexperiment questionnaire, only three of the 30 subjects correctly identified the treatment session. Removal of their data did not significantly affect the results. A one-way ANOVA revealed decreased VAS scores at rest (p = 0.049). The Newman-Keuls test demonstrated a significant difference between treatment and control conditions, but no significant difference for treatment versus placebo condition. There was no significant main effect of condition for VAS scores at end of range cervical rotation (p = 0.381). Regarding the condition of PPTs on the symptomatic side, a two-way ANOVA revealed a significant main effect (p = 0.0042). The post-hoc analysis (Newman-Keuls test) demonstrated a significant difference between treatment and placebo and between treatment and control. There was no significant main effect of condition for TPTs.

A two-way ANOVA demonstrated a significant main effect of treatment condition for skin conductance (p < 0.002) and skin temperature (p < 0.002). Post-hoc analysis revealed a significant difference between treatment and placebo and between treatment and control for skin conductance and skin temperature.

A two-way ANOVA demonstrated a significant main effect of condition for EMG activity of the superficial neck muscles at pressure levels of 22, 24, and 26 mmHg (p < 0.0002). Post-hoc analysis demonstrated significant differences between treatment and placebo and between treatment and control at 22, 24, and 26 mmHg of pressure. The treatment condition induced decreases in EMG activity in the superficial neck flexor muscles by approximately 28% at 22 mmHg, 34% at 24 mmHg, and 21% at 26 mmHg. There was no significant reduction in EMG activity of the sternocleidomastoid muscles at 28 and 30 mmHg. The placebo condition induced increases in EMG activity of the superficial neck flexors by approximately 40% at 22 mmHg and 27% at 26 mmHg.

The findings of this study demonstrated that SMT had a hypoalgesic effect specific to mechanical nociception, but not thermal nociception; an excitatory effect on sympathetic nervous system activity; and an effect on motor activity in the cervical region, whereby there was significantly less activity of the superficial neck flexors (sternocleidomastoids, scalenes, and infrahyoids) in the staged craniocervical flexion test. This could imply facilitation of the deep neck flexor muscles with a decreased need for co-activation of the superficial neck flexors at the lower pressure levels of 22 to 26 mmHg. Although mechanical pain thresholds were increased in the order of 23% on the side of treatment, the authors acknowledge that the effect of SMT on VAS scores was less than expected, especially at the end of active movement. They suggest that the treatment technique utilized was not an adequate stimulus given that initial pain scores were low and of long duration. In these cases, more vigorous manual therapy techniques are probably indicated.

Given the combination of effects mentioned (ie, hypoalgesia, sympathoexcitation, and motor effects), the authors suggest that SMT may exert its initial effects by activating descending inhibitory pathways from the dorsal periaqueductal gray area of the midbrain (dPAG).

Study #15: Jull G, Trott P, Potter H, Zito G, Niere K, Shirley D, Emberson J, Marschner I, Richardson C. A randomized controlled trial of exercise and manipulative therapy for cervicogenic headache. Spine. 2002;27(17):1835-1843.

Two hundred patients, who met the diagnostic criteria for cervicogenic headache, participated in this prospective, multicenter, randomized controlled trial. Participants, ages 18 to 60 years, were recruited from general practitioners or through advertising in five centers located in capital cities in Australia. Inclusion criteria consisted of the following: unilateral or unilateral dominant side-consistent headache associated with neck pain and aggravated by neck postures or movement, joint tenderness in at least one of the upper three cervical joints as detected by manual palpation, and headache frequency of at least one per week over a period of 2 months to 10 years. Exclusion criteria specified bilateral headaches (typifying tension-type headache), features suggestive of migraine, any condition that might contraindicate manipulative therapy, involvement in litigation or worker's compensation, and physiotherapy or chiropractic treatment for headache in the previous 12 months. Those who fulfilled the symptomatic criteria underwent a physical examination of the cervical spine including manual palpation of the upper cervical joints relevant to the inclusion criteria. A preparatory intertherapist reliability study indicated excellent agreement between pairs of assessors in manual joint examination for subject eligibility.

The 200 subjects were then randomized into four groups: manipulative therapy group, exercise therapy group, combined therapy group, and a control group. Manipulative therapy consisted of both low as well as high velocity cervical mobilization techniques as taught by Maitland. The therapeutic exercise intervention consisted of low-load endurance exercises to train muscle control of the cervicoscapular region, especially the deep neck flexors, which have an important supporting function for the cervical region. The Stabilizer (Chattanooga Group Inc, Chattanooga, Tenn), an air-filled pressure sensor that monitors the slight flattening of the cervical curve that occurs with contraction of the longus colli, was used for feedback purposes. In addition, the serratus anterior and lower trapezius were trained using inner range holding exercises of scapular adduction and retraction; postural correction exercises were performed regularly throughout the day in the sitting position. The third intervention was a combination of manipulative therapy and exercise therapy applied on the same day. The control group received no physical therapy intervention. Usual medication was not withheld from any participant regardless of group allocation. Active treatment extended over a period of 6 weeks, including a minimum of 8 and a maximum of 12 treatments. Treatment was delivered by 25 experienced physiotherapists across trial centers. The nature of the interventions precluded any blinding of physiotherapists or participants to assigned treatments. However, blinded outcome assessment was conducted.

The primary outcome measure was a change in headache frequency from baseline to immediately after treatment and at month 12. Changes in headache intensity and duration and in neck pain were secondary outcome measures. Frequency was recorded as the number of headache days in the past week. Average intensity was rated on a VAS and duration was the average number of hours that headaches lasted in the past week. Neck pain and disability were measured using the Northwick Park Neck Pain Questionnaire. The participant-perceived effect of treatment and relief gained were rated on VASs. For analysis, pain medication was converted to a defined daily dose of analgesics using the Anatomic Therapeutic Chemical Code. The tertiary physical assessments included pain with neck movements (VAS). The three movements with the highest pain scores were evaluated at follow-up assessment. The pain provoked by manual palpation of the upper cervical joints (VAS) and the two joints exhibiting the highest tenderness scores at baseline were reassessed. Performance on the craniocervical muscle test as well as a photographic measure of the craniocervical angle, representing forward head posture, were also included in the assessment. In addition, several prognostic and evaluative assessments were made for baseline comparisons, including a full headache history, an MPQ, and a psychometric evaluation, the Headache-Specific Locus of Control Scale. Participants also rated the global perceived effect of treatment and the headache relief obtained.

Results demonstrated no differences in headache-related and demographic characteristics between the groups at baseline. The loss to follow-up evaluation was 3.5%. Wilcoxon analyses showed that manipulative therapy (MT), exercise therapy (ExT), and the combination thereof (MT + ExT) all significantly reduced headache frequency, intensity, and the neck pain index immediately after treatment; these differences were still evident at month 12 (p < 0.05 for all). The combined therapies were not significantly superior to either therapy alone, but 10% more patients gained relief with the combination. The exception was headache duration, for which combining MT + ExT was effective, but for which the effect of ExT was no greater than the control at the 7-week and 12-month end points. At the 12-month follow-up assessment, MT was not significantly different from the control group in terms of headache duration and neck pain. The results of the two-way ANOVA provided some evidence that MT + ExT was more beneficial initially in reducing pain produced on joint palpation than either therapy alone, but there was no indication that the additive effect was maintained at month 12.

The authors of this solid multicenter trial conclude that the conservative interventions of manipulative therapy and a specific exercise program were effective in the management of cervicogenic headache with statistically significant improvement in headache frequency and intensity and that the effects are maintained in the long term. Although there was no statistical evidence of an additive effect from combining interventions, 10% more participants receiving the combined therapy obtained good and excellent outcomes. This would support the use of combined MT and therapeutic and home exercises in the management of cervicogenic headache.

This concludes the author's attempt at providing evidence to suggest that the practice of manual therapy is not built upon the "shakiest of foundations." There is, in fact, an evolving science that demonstrates a fair degree of support for the types of interventions discussed in this text. Having said that, the author is well aware of the lack of acceptable science in the world of manipulative therapy. Many studies have an insufficient number of subjects; are not prospective, placebo-controlled, properly "blinded," nor statistically analyzed; and have often been published in journals that are not peer-reviewed. There is no doubt that we need to do better, and Dr. Rothstein and others, including the Philadelphia Panel Members,[6] are correct in challenging the status quo of manual therapy. The point of this literature review, however, is to ensure that the "baby is not thrown out with the bath water." The above studies demonstrate that a body of outcomes data is available to support the use of spinal manual therapy and therapeutic exercise. Are more RCTs needed? Absolutely and sooner rather than later!

Because of the clinical scope of this text, evidence from the basic science literature (ie, histology, anatomy, physiology, movement science, motor learning, articular neurology, pain science, etc) was not presented. Many good studies, especially in the area of connective tissue pathophysiology, have demonstrated the beneficial effects of mobilization. The reader is directed to the bibliography at the end of this section for further study.

In addition to individual studies on the efficacy of manual therapy and exercise, there are systematic reviews available that have been used to create meta-analyses of related literature. In many cases, these analyses have provided additional support for the use of manual therapy and exercise. For example, the Duke University Evidence-Based Practice Center published *Evidence Report: Behavioral and Physical Treatments for Tension-Type and Cervicogenic Headache*,[7] which concluded, "Manipulation is effective in patients with cervicogenic headache, but its efficacy in patients with tension-type headache is unproven." In his systemic review of the literature, DiFabio[8] concludes, "Overall, there was clear evidence to justify the use of manual therapy, particularly manipulation, in the treatment of patients who have back pain." In their large scale, multisite study on TMD diagnosis and treatment, Gaudet et al[9] found that, "Treated patients (TMD) report statistically and clin-

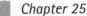

ically significant levels of improvement… but the weight of the evidence indicates that untreated TMD patients, as a group, do not improve spontaneously over time." Of significance to manual physical therapists is the fact that 43.7% of the 1212 treated TMD patients received "physical modalities," which upon further inquiry included the use of manual therapy, therapeutic, and home exercises.

In conclusion, an attempt has been made to present a defense of the practice of manual therapy and therapeutic exercise based upon the available evidence. As in a courtroom, where an attorney makes his or her best case in support of a given position, this chapter presents the case for the efficacy of manual therapy. The author would not be intellectually honest if he failed to acknowledge the fact that several studies have demonstrated poor interrater reliability using techniques of manual diagnosis. In fact, several of these studies are listed in the bibliography at the end of this chapter (eg, Potter and Rothstein, Binkley et al, Riddle and Freburger). Having said that, the author has selected 15 studies that are a representative cross-section of clinical approaches within the practice of modern manual therapy in hopes of making his case. The objective of this chapter was not only to respond to the critics, but also to balance the art of practice with a comparable degree of science so that at the end of the day, physical therapists will rise to the professional level to which we all aspire.

References and Bibliography

References

1. Sackett DL, Rosenberg WM, Gray JA, et al. Evidence based medicine: what it is and what it isn't. *BMJ*. 1996;312:71-72.

2. Sackett DL, Straus SE, Richardson WS, et al. *Evidence-Based Medicine: How to Practice and Teach EBM*. 2nd ed. New York, NY: Churchill Livingstone; 2000.

3. Donelson RG, Silva G, Murphy K. The centralization phenomenon: its usefulness in evaluating and treating sciatica. *Spine*. 1990;15:211-213.

4. Stoddard A. *Manual of Osteopathic Techniques*. London: The Anchor Press; 1977.

5. Maitland GD. *Vertebral Manipulation*. 5th ed. London: Butterworth-Heinemann; 1986.

6. Albright J, Allman R, Bonfiglio RP, et al. Evidence-based guidelines: application to clinical practice, Philadelphia Panel. *Phys Ther*. 2001;81(10):1629-1730.

7. McCrory DC, Penzien DB, Hasselblad V, Gray RN. *Evidence Report: Behavioral and Physical Treatments for Tension-Type and Cervicogenic Headache*. Durham, NC: Duke University Evidence-Based Practice Center; 2001.

8. DiFabio RP. Efficacy of manual therapy. *Phys Ther*. 1992;72(12):853-864.

9. Gaudet EL, Brown DT. Temporomandibular disorder treatment outcomes: first report of a large-scale prospective clinical study. *J Craniomandibular Pract*. 2000;18(1):9-20.

Bibliography

Akeson W. Collagen crosslinking alterations in joint contractures: changes in the reducible crosslinks in periarticular connective tissue collagen after nine weeks of immobilization. *Connect Tissue Res*. 1977;5:15-19.

Binkley J, Stratford PW, Gill C. Interrater reliability of lumbar accessory motion mobility testing. *Phys Ther*. 1995;75(9):786-792.

Bronfort G, Evans R, Nelson B, Aker PD, Goldsmith CH, Vernon H. A randomized clinical trial of exercise and spinal manipulation for patients with chronic neck pain. *Spine*. 2001;26(7):788-799.

Cibulka MT, Aslin K. How to use evidence-based practice to distinguish between three different patients with low back pain. *J Orthop Sports Phys Ther*. 2001;31(12):678-695.

Davidson CJ, Ganion LR, Gehlsen GM, Verhoestra B, Roepke JE, Sevier TL. Rat tendon morphologic and functional changes resulting from soft tissue mobilization. *Med Sci Sports Exerc*. 1997;29(3):313-319.

DiFabio RP. Myth of evidence-based practice. *J Orthop Sports Phys Ther*. 1999;29(11):632-634.

Donelson R, Grant W, Kamps C, Medcalf R. Pain response to sagittal end-range spinal motion. A prospective, randomized, multicentered trial. *Spine*. 1991;16(6)(Suppl):S206-S212.

Donelson R, Aprill C, Medcalf R, Grant W. A prospective study of centralization of lumbar and referred pain. A predictor of symptomatic discs and annular competence. *Spine*. 1997;22(10):1115-1122.

Farrell JP, Twomey LT. Acute low back pain: comparison of two conservative treatment approaches. *Med J Austr.* 1982;1:160-164.

Feine JS, Widmer CG, Lund JP. Physical therapy: a critique. *Oral Surg Oral Med Oral Pathol Oral Radiol Endod.* 1997;83:123-127.

Freburger JK, Riddle DL. Using published evidence to guide the examination of the sacroiliac joint region. *Phys Ther.* 2001;81(5):1135-1143.

Gehlsen GM, Ganion LR, Helfst R. Fibroblast responses to variation in soft tissue mobilization pressure. *Med Sci Sports Exerc.* 1999;31(4):531-535.

Gobel H, Heinze A, Heinze-Kuhn K, Jost WH. Evidence-based medicine: botulinum toxin A in migraine and tension-type headache. *J Neurol.* 2001;248(Suppl 1):34-38.

Gonnella C, Paris SV, Kutner M. Reliability in evaluating passive intervertebral motion. *Phys Ther.* 1982;62(4):436-444.

Haldeman S, Hooper PD. Mobilization, manipulation, massage and exercise for the relief of musculoskeletal pain. In: Wall PD, Melzack R, eds. *Textbook of Pain.* 4th ed. Edinburgh: Churchill Livingstone; 1999.

Hoehler FK, Tobis JS, Buerger AA. Spinal manipulation for low back pain. *JAMA.* 1981;245(18):1835-1838.

Hoving JL, Koes BW, de Vet HC, et al. Manual therapy, physical therapy, or continued care by a general practitioner for patients with neck pain. *Ann Intern Med.* 2002;136(10):713-722.

Hurwitz EL, Aker PD, Adams AH, Meeker WC, Shekelle PG, Barr JS Jr. Manipulation and mobilization of the cervical spine: a systematic review of the literature. *Spine.* 1996;21(15):1746-1760.

Jull G, Bokduk N, Marsland A. The accuracy of manual diagnosis for cervical zygapophyseal joint pain syndromes. *Med J Austr.* 1988;148(5):233-236.

Jull G, Trott P, Potter H, et al. A randomized controlled trial of exercise and manipulative therapy for cervicogenic headache. *Spine.* 2002;27(17):1835-1843.

Koes BW, Bouter LM, van Mameren H, et al. A randomized clinical trial of manual therapy and physiotherapy for persistent back and neck complaints: subgroup analysis and relationship between outcome measures. *J Manipulative Physiol Ther.* 1993;16:211-219.

Koes BW, Bouter LM, van Mameren H, et al. The effectiveness of manual therapy, physiotherapy, and treatment by the general practitioner for nonspecific back and neck complaints. A randomized clinical trial. *Spine.* 1992;17:28-35.

Korr IM, ed. *The Neurobiologic Mechanisms in Manipulative Therapy.* New York, NY: Plenum Press; 1978.

Lundy-Ekman L. *Neuroscience: Fundamentals for Rehabilitation.* 2nd ed. Philadelphia, Pa: WB Saunders; 2002.

Magee DJ, Oborn-Barrett E, Turner S, Fenning N. A systematic overview of the effectiveness of physical therapy intervention on soft tissue neck injury following trauma. *Physiotherapy Canada.* 2000;52(2):111-130.

McPartland J, Goodridge J. Counterstrain and traditional osteopathic examination of the cervical spine compared. *Journal of Bodywork and Movement Therapies.* 1997;1(3):173-178.

Mitchell UH, Wooden MJ, McKeough DM. The short-term effect of lumbar positional distraction. *Journal of Manual & Manipulative Therapy.* 2001;9(4):213-221.

Nicolakis P, Erdogmus B, Djaber-Ansari A, Piehslinger E, Fialka-Moser V. Exercise therapy for craniomandibular disorders. *Arch Phys Med Rehabil.* 2000;81:1137-1141.

Nicolakis P, Burak EC, Kollmitzer J, et al. An investigation of the effectiveness of exercise and manual therapy in treating symptoms of TMJ osteoarthritis. *J Craniomandibular Pract.* 2001;19(1):26-32.

Nilsson N, Christensen HW, Hartvigsen J. The effect of spinal manipulation in the treatment of cervicogenic headache. *J Manipulative Physiol Ther.* 1997;20(5):326-330.

O'Donoghue CE. Manipulation trials. In: Boyling JD, Palastanga N, eds. *Grieve's Modern Manual Therapy.* 2nd ed. Edinburgh: Churchill Livingstone; 1994.

Ottenbacher K, DiFabio RP. Efficacy of spinal manipulation/mobilization therapy. A meta-analysis. *Spine.* 1985;10(9):833-837.

Paydar D, Thiel H, Gemmell H. Intra and interexaminer reliability of certain pelvic palpatory procedures and the sitting flexion test for sacroiliac joint mobility and dysfunction. *Journal of the Neuromusculoskeletal System.* 1994;2(2):65-69.

Potter NA, Rothstein JM. Intertester reliability for selected clinical tests of the sacroiliac joint. *Phys Ther.* 1985;65:1671-1675.

Razmjou H, Kramer JF, Yamada R. Intertester reliability of the McKenzie evaluation in assessing patients with mechanical low-back pain. *J Orthop Sports Phys Ther.* 2000;30(7):368-389.

Riddle DL, Freburger JK. Evaluation of the presence of sacroiliac joint region dysfunction using a combination of tests: a multicenter intertester reliability study. *Phys Ther.* 2002;82(8):772-781.

Roddey TS, Olson SL, Grant SE. The effect of pectoralis muscle stretching on the resting position of the scapula in persons with varying degrees of forward head/rounded shoulder posture. *Journal of Manual & Manipulative Therapy.* 2002;10(3):124-128.

Rothstein JM. Manual therapy: a special issue and a special topic. *Phys Ther.* 1992;72(12):839-841.

Saal JA, Saal JS. Nonoperative treatment of herniated lumbar intervertebral disc with radiculopathy: an outcome study. *Spine.* 1989;14(4):431-437.

Sahrmann SA. *Diagnosis and Treatment of Movement Impairment Syndromes.* St. Louis, Mo: Mosby-Year Book; 2002.

Schenk R, Adelman K, Rousselle J. The effects of muscle energy technique on cervical range of motion. *Journal of Manual & Manipulative Therapy.* 1994;2(4):149-155.

Schenk R, MacDiarmid A, Rousselle J. The effects of muscle energy technique on lumbar range of motion. *Journal of Manual & Manipulative Therapy.* 1997;5(4):179-183.

Schoensee SK, Jensen G, Nicholson G, Gossman M, Katholi C. The effect of mobilization on cervical headaches. *J Orthop Sports Phys Ther.* 1995;21(4):184-196.

Seymour R, Walsh T, Blankenberg C, Pickens A, Rush H. Reliability of detecting a relevant lateral shift in patients with lumbar derangement: a pilot study. *Journal of Manual & Manipulative Therapy.* 2002;10(3):129-135.

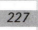

Shekelle PG, Adams AH, Chassin MR, et al. *The Appropriateness of Spinal Manipulation for Low-Back Pain: Indications and Ratings by a Multidisciplinary Expert Panel.* Santa Monica, Calif: Rand; 1991.

Shekelle PG, Adams AH, Chassin MR, Hurwitz EL, Brook RH. Spinal manipulation for low back pain. *Ann Inter Med.* 1992;117:590-598.

Smedmark V, Wallin M, Arvidsson I. Interexaminer reliability in assessing passive intervertebral motion of the cervical spine. *Man Ther.* 2000;5(2):97-101.

Sterling M, Jull G, Wright A. Cervical mobilization: concurrent effects on pain, sympathetic nervous system activity and motor activity. *Man Ther.* 2001;6(2):72-81.

Sunshine W, Field T, Schanberg S, et al. Massage therapy and transcutaneous electrical stimulation effects on fibromyalgia. *J Clin Rheumatol.* 1996;2:18-22.

Threlkeld AJ. The effects of manual therapy on connective tissue. *Phys Ther.* 1992;72(12):893-900.

Wall PD, Melzack R, eds. *Textbook of Pain.* 4th ed. Edinburgh: Churchill Livingstone; 1999.

Whittingham W, Nilsson N. Active range of motion in the cervical spine increases after spinal manipulation (toggle recoil). *J Manipulative Physiol Ther.* 2001;24(9):552-555.

Yuasa H, Kurita K. Randomized clinical trial of primary treatment for temporomandibular joint disk displacement without reduction and without osseous changes: a combination of NSAIDs and mouth-opening exercise versus no treatment. *Oral Surg Oral Med Oral Pathol Oral Radiol Endol.* 2001;91(6):671-675.

Case Studies

26

In order to apply the concepts and principles discussed in this text, this final chapter consists of a collection of case studies including questions and answers. These cases are representative of those patients typically seen in an outpatient physical therapy clinic and will hopefully facilitate the transition from the "classroom to the clinic." The answers can be found starting on p. 236.

Case #1

A 25-year-old female housewife presents with a chief complaint of painful clicking of the right temporomandibular joint. The patient reports that she is under stress with two small children at home and that in addition to her jaw symptoms, she also has recurring headaches, intermittent neck pain and stiffness, and occasional dizziness. The patient has no recollection of head, neck, or jaw trauma. The patient indicates that, according to her husband, she grinds her teeth at night. The patient's family physician is aware of her symptoms and has recommended psychological counseling.

1. Before physical therapy is initiated, to whom should this patient be directed?
   A. A rheumatologist to rule out osteoarthritis
   B. A neurologist to diagnose the cause of her headaches and dizziness
   C. A chronic pain center
   D. A physiatrist to determine which physical therapy modalities are indicated

2. Which of the following dental interventions may prove beneficial for this patient?
   A. Root canal
   B. Orthognathic surgery
   C. The Nociceptive Trigeminal Inhibition Tension Suppression System (NTI-tss) appliance
   D. Dental implantation

3. Facilitation of which cranial nerve is implicated in light of the patient's head, neck, and TMJ/facial complaints?
   A. Trigeminal
   B. Spinal accessory
   C. Facial
   D. Vestibulocochlear

4. The patient's TMJ clicking suggests which diagnosis?
   A. Capsular hypomobility
   B. Capsular hypermobility
   C. Internal derangement
   D. Myofascial pain and dysfunction

5. Which of the following is true of the upper cervical spine?

A. It can be the source of this patient's headaches

B. It can be the source of this patient's dizziness

C. It can contribute to this patient's TMJ impairment through trigeminal nerve facilitation

D. All of the above

Case 2

A 30-year-old male carpenter presents with a chief complaint of intractable left-sided low back and buttock pain secondary to a lifting injury on the job. The pain is acute (ie, less than 2 weeks) and the patient is unable to work. The Oswestry Disability Index, Version 2.0, revealed marked functional limitation in the following categories: lifting, sitting, sleeping, and social life. The patient was referred to your outpatient physical therapy clinic by his internist.

1. Your examination reveals normal neurologic function, but there is a right lateral shift with limited lumbar extension. What does your initial intervention involve?

A. Correction of the lateral shift

B. Flexion exercises

C. Extension exercises

D. Myofascial release/stretching of the right quadratus lumborum

2. If the patient's symptoms are not worsened by movement nor relieved by rest, what would be the correct course of action?

A. Use pain-relieving modalities to manage symptoms

B. Discuss proper body mechanics

C. Call the patient's physician regarding the possibility of viscerogenic pain referral

D. Instruct the patient in positional distraction

3. Providing that the patient responded well to the McKenzie approach (ie, lateral shift correction and extension exercises), which of the following is the least likely patient classification?

A. Derangement syndrome

B. Dysfunction syndrome

C. Postural syndrome

D. All of the above

4. What is the muscle most likely to be tender to palpation?

A. Right piriformis

B. Left hamstring

C. Left tensor fascia latae

D. Right iliopsoas

5. Assuming the presence of a lumbar derangement, what is the most likely category?

A. Derangement one

B. Derangement two

C. Derangement three

D. Derangement four

Case 3

A 60-year-old female physician presents with a long history of intermittent right-sided headaches. There is no family history of migraine. The patient reports sustaining a neck injury when falling off a horse at age 40. Stress is under control, but the patient spends several hours per week at her computer. The patient's headaches are always right-sided, of moderate to severe intensity, and nonthrobbing in nature. They are not associated with nausea, vomiting, or photophobia/phonophobia. Besides having a right hip replacement at age 55, the patient is otherwise healthy and physically fit.

1. Examination of postural alignment reveals marked forward head position. What is this acquired postural deformity associated with?

A. Occipital flexion/lower cervical extension

B. Occipital extension/lower cervical flexion

C. Occipital flexion/lower cervical flexion

D. Occipital extension/lower cervical extension

2. Examination also reveals moderate restriction of active cervical rotation to the right. What are the history and physical examination consistent with?

A. Migraine without aura

B. Headache secondary to a brain tumor

C. Cervicogenic headache

D. Subarachnoid hemorrhage

3. Where would the most symptomatic apophyseal joint in this patient's neck be expected to be found?

    A. C2,3 on the left

    B. C2,3 on the right

    C. C5,6 on the left

    D. C5,6 on the right

4. Entrapment of which of the following nerves gives rise to unilateral headache on the affected side?

    A. The long thoracic nerve

    B. The dorsal scapular nerve

    C. The suprascapular nerve

    D. The greater occipital nerve

5. Which column of gray matter in the CNS mediates headache of cervical origin?

    A. The trigeminocervical nucleus

    B. The locus ceruleus

    C. The nucleus dorsalis

    D. The caudate nucleus

Case 4

A 14-year-old female soccer player presents with chronic pain (ie, over 3 months duration) in the cervical and lumbar spine. She, like her parents, is round shouldered. She also reports an overall sense of restricted mobility, without pain, in the midback area. She was seen by an orthopaedic surgeon who diagnosed thoracic spine rotoscoliosis with an accentuated kyphosis. The deformity does not warrant surgery nor a spinal orthosis; therefore, physical therapy was recommended. The Present Pain Intensity (PPI) of the standard long-form McGill Pain Questionnaire revealed the pain to be distressing (ie, three out of a possible five).

1. Upon examination, a right thoracic convexity is observed from T5 through T11 with an associated rib hump located where?

    A. Right side

    B. Left side

    C. Right above T8, left below T8

    D. None of the above

2. Which muscle in the scapulothoracic region tends toward inhibition, hypotonicity, and weakness?

    A. The upper trapezius

    B. The levator scapulae

    C. The pectoralis minor

    D. The lower trapezius

3. The middle trapezius muscle is inhibited by restricted midthoracic:

    A. Flexion

    B. Extension

    C. Lateral flexion

    D. A and C

4. Tightness of which muscle restricts scapular upward rotation and consequently contributes to impingement of the glenohumeral joint?

    A. The levator scapulae

    B. The upper trapezius

    C. The latissimus dorsi

    D. A and C

5. This patient demonstrates the common pattern of:

    A. Thoracic hypomobility/cervical hypomobility

    B. Thoracic hypermobility/cervical hypermobility

    C. Thoracic hypomobility/cervical hypermobility

    D. Thoracic hypermobility/cervical hypomobility

Case 5

A 38-year-old male accountant sustained an injury to his right low back area while golfing 2 days prior to arriving in your outpatient clinic. The patient gives a history of "missing the golf ball" during an attempted drive on a par 5 with an immediate onset of pain in the right upper buttock region. The patient has had difficulty weight bearing on the right leg. The patient rated his pain as 7 out of 10 on a pain intensity numerical rating scale (PI-NRS).

1. Examination reveals a (+) standing flexion test on the right, (+) reverse stork at the upper pole of the right sacroiliac joint, and a (+) posterior shear test also on the right. From these findings and the patient's history, the following pelvic asymmetries are expected with the patient recumbent?

A. High ASIS/low PSIS on the right versus the left

B. High ASIS, PSIS, and iliac crest on the right versus the left

C. Low ASIS/high PSIS on the right versus the left

D. Low ASIS, PSIS, and iliac crest on the right versus the left

2. Regarding tissue texture abnormality, this muscle will have expected hypertonicity as a result of this injury?

A. The left hamstring

B. The right hamstring

C. The left iliopsoas

D. The right iliopsoas

3. Muscle energy technique to correct this iliosacral impairment utilizes the neurophysiologic principle of reciprocal inhibition via an isometric contraction of which of the following?

A. Right gluteus maximus

B. Right rectus femoris

C. Right hamstrings

D. A and C

4. Which of the following is involved in a grade 3 joint mobilization to the right iliac bone?

A. Large amplitude oscillations at the end of range

B. Small amplitude oscillations at the end of range

C. Large amplitude oscillations at the beginning of range

D. Small amplitude oscillations at the end of range

5. The proper sequence of intervention for this patient's condition includes addressing which of the following?

A. Reactivity, muscle strength, joint mobility, soft tissue extensibility, and alignment

B. Reactivity, soft tissue extensibility, joint mobility, alignment, and muscle strength

C. Alignment, muscle strength, joint mobility, soft tissue extensibility, and reactivity

D. Soft tissue extensibility, joint mobility, muscle strength, alignment, and reactivity

Case 6

A 45-year-old male English teacher presents with a 6-month history of progressive pain commencing in the right lumbosacral area and spreading into the right lower limb below the knee and into the right foot. The patient's lumbar spine x-rays and MRI were unremarkable. The patient has not responded to prior physical therapy and is interested in a second opinion. The patient has been seen by a family physician, orthopaedist, and neurologist and has been given a diagnosis of lumbar radiculopathy. A visual analogue scale revealed pain to be 6 out of 10 during the examination and 9 out of 10 at its worst.

1. Your evaluation includes a detailed history and a physical examination of:

A. Spinal and pelvic alignment

B. Active and passive lumbar range of motion

C. Sensation, muscle strength, DTRs, and neurodynamic tests (ie, femoral nerve, proximal sciatic nerve and its branches)

D. All of the above

2. The examination reveals the following findings: left lateral lumbar shift, centralization of symptoms with lumbar extension, peripheralization into the right leg with lumbar flexion, (+) straight leg raise on the right at 45 degrees, and enlargement of the right buttock. The above signs are all consistent with a McKenzie derangement six except for:

A. Right buttock enlargement

B. (+) Straight leg raise on the right

C. Left lateral lumbar shift

D. "Centralization" of symptoms with lumbar extension

3. Given the finding of an enlarged right buttock, what should be the next course of action?

A. Contact the patient's family physician regarding your concern

B. Proceed with McKenzie management of a lumbar derangement

C. Apply ice and electrical stimulation to the right buttock

D. Perform connective tissue techniques and stretching to the right piriformis muscle

4. Therapy is begun on the patient, but at patient rounds your colleagues express concern over the large right buttock. They suggest that you examine the right hip for limitation of hip flexion and to your surprise this motion is considerably limited and causes intense pain. You proceed with a further examination of hip range of motion and find that rotations are limited by pain with an "empty end-feel." Now that the Cyriax "sign of the buttock" has emerged, you immediately contact the patient's physician. What will an MRI of the pelvis confirm?

A. Piriformis spasm on the right

B. A torn long dorsal sacroiliac ligament on the right

C. A malignant neoplasm of the right iliac bone

D. Inflammation of the right sacroiliac joint

5. In retrospect you are trying to understand how a neoplasm could present like a McKenzie derangement six. What was the tumor compressing?

A. Right sural nerve

B. Right sciatic nerve

C. Right lateral femoral cutaneous nerve

D. Right obturator nerve

Case 7

A 50-year-old male truck driver presents with intermittent left-sided neck pain and muscle spasm. Pain-free periods could last several weeks, but the exacerbations are becoming more frequent and intense and are beginning to interfere with the patient's work. During one of his recent episodes, the patient experienced "tingling" in the middle finger of his left hand for several days. Neurologic examination is normal, but there is considerable impairment of neck mobility and the head-neck region appears laterally shifted to the right. The Neck Disability Index revealed that during an exacerbation there is moderate disability that interferes with his ability to drive long distances.

1. The patient's complaint of "tingling" in the middle finger of the left hand coupled with his other symptoms points to possible disc derangement at which segment?

A. C5,6 on the left

B. C5,6 on the right

C. C6,7 on the left

D. C6,7 on the right

2. Restricted segmental extension, rotation, and side-bending left is consistent with an apophyseal joint that is "stuck" in which position?

A. Closed position on the left

B. Open position on the left

C. Closed position on the right

D. Closed position on the left

3. If this patient's symptoms progress to the point of causing neurologic involvement, what would the most likely sign(s) consist of?

A. Triceps weakness on the left

B. Biceps weakness on the left

C. Hypoactive left biceps jerk

D. A and C

4. A type 2 impairment (FRS right) in the lower cervical spine is treated with postisometric relaxation (PIR) of which muscles?

A. Flexors, left rotators, and left side benders

B. Flexors, right rotators, and left side benders

C. Flexors, left rotators, and right side benders

D. None of the above

5. In the McKenzie system, at the time of the initial visit, this patient presents to you with which derangement?

A. One

B. Two

C. Three

D. Four

Case 8

The patient is a 17-year-old female basketball player who presents with recurrent aggravating backache. An MRI exam revealed degenerative disc disease at L4,5 with a mild retrolisthesis of L4. The patient wears a lumbar support during games, which provides temporary relief of painful symptoms. The Dallas Pain Questionnaire revealed that both daily activities interference and work/leisure activities were greater than 50%, indicating significant functional limitation. However, the anxiety/depression and social interest interference were not significantly elevated. The patient's orthopaedic surgeon referred the patient for spinal stabilization therapy.

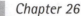

1. What most likely caused the patient's pain?

   A. Capsular hypomobility of the L4,5 facet joints

   B. Clinical "instability" at L4,5

   C. Myofascial pain

   D. Malingering

2. Strengthening of which muscle should prove beneficial to the patient?

   A. Sacrospinalis

   B. Multifidus

   C. Quadratus lumborum

   D. Rectus abdominis

3. Evidence suggests that this muscle plays a key role in providing core stability?

   A. Transversus abdominis

   B. Pubococcygeus

   C. Multifidus

   D. All of the above

4. How is an isolated contraction of the transversus abdominis achieved?

   A. Drawing the navel in toward the spine upon exhalation

   B. Performing abdominal crunches

   C. Performing a posterior pelvic tilt

   D. Pulling the abdominal wall in during a deep inhalation

5. The "neutral zone" is characterized by all the following except:

   A. The least symptomatic position

   B. The most stable position

   C. The most efficient position

   D. The close-packed position

Case 9

A 50-year-old female nurse sustained soft tissue injuries to her head and neck in a rear-end motor vehicle accident (MVA) while driving to work. The patient presents to your department 6 weeks post-MVA with complaints of headache, TMJ/facial pain and stiffness, and bilateral neck and shoulder pain. The patient has to work to support her two children, but each day is stressful because of the pain, impairment, and functional limitation. On the Pain Rating Index (PRI) of the McGill Pain Questionnaire, the patient had an overall score of 28, involving both sensory and affective aspects of pain.

1. The patient demonstrates 30 mm of mandibular depression and her jaw deflects to the right upon opening. An examination of lateral excursions reveals restriction of motion to the left side. What are the physical findings consistent with?

   A. An anterior disc displacement (ADD) without reduction on the right

   B. An ADD with reduction on the right

   C. Capsular hypomobility of the right TMJ

   D. A and C

2. The patient presents with marked forward head posture. With what is this finding often correlated?

   A. Reduction of the freeway space

   B. Inferior and posterior displacement of the mandible

   C. Decompression of the suboccipital region

   D. All of the above

3. Upon further questioning, the patient reveals that prior to the MVA her right TMJ would intermittently "click" and "pop" and that on one occasion it momentarily "locked." In light of this information, what do you expect the MRI to be positive for?

   A. Posterior disc displacement on the right

   B. Anterior disc displacement without reduction on the right

   C. An acoustic neuroma

   D. An impacted wisdom tooth

4. The patient also demonstrates an accentuated midthoracic kyphosis with protraction, elevation, and downward rotation of her scapulae. You suspect, but need to test for impairment, of which of the following?

   A. Flexion (T5 to T8)

   B. Extension (T5 to T8)

   C. Lower cervical spine flexion

   D. Glenohumeral internal rotation

5. The Alexander technique would assist this patient with the following:

   A. Restoring the "primary control" mechanism

   B. Releasing tension throughout the head, neck, and shoulder girdle

   C. Shortening the torso

   D. A and B

Case 10

A 70-year-old male college professor presents with a chief complaint of intermittent right calf pain and weakness exacerbated by running. When he runs less than 2 miles he is fine, but after that he is forced to stop and rest because the calf muscles become achy, tight, and weak.

The patient is otherwise healthy and is somewhat discouraged because he has been running competitively most of his adult life. The pain that forces him to stop running is given an intensity of 7 on a 0 through 10 scale (PI-NRS).

1. Based upon the patient's history, which of the following conditions is a possibility?
   A. Vascular intermittent claudication
   B. Neurogenic intermittent claudication
   C. A and B
   D. None of the above

2. The patient is taken to the track and asked to run until his right calf symptoms appear. Following a brief cool down, the patient is asked to stand still. The patient reports that his symptoms persist in standing, but following 3 minutes of sitting his symptoms begin to abate. What is the most likely diagnosis?
   A. Vascular intermittent claudication
   B. Neurogenic intermittent claudication
   C. A and B
   D. None of the above

3. What pathology is most consistent with this patient's symptomatology?
   A. Type II diabetes
   B. Herniated nucleus pulposus (HNP)
   C. Spinal stenosis
   D. Osteoarthritis of the right hip

4. Given that a positive crossed straight leg raise test (straight leg raising on the patient's well leg elicits pain in the leg with sciatica) has excellent "specificity" (0.90) but low "sensitivity" (0.25), what is this the clinical test of choice for?
   A. Rule-in nerve compression
   B. Rule-out nerve compression
   C. Identify the specific root level involved
   D. All of the above

5. What would placing this patient on a stationary bike and asking him to exercise for 20 minutes most likely result in?
   A. Right calf symptoms
   B. The absence of symptoms
   C. Low back pain
   D. None of the above

Case 11

A 26-year-old female physical therapy student presents with a chief complaint of numbness in her right arm and hand. An MRI of the cervical spine was unremarkable, as was electromyography. All blood work was normal. The patient's neurologist referred her for a physical therapy consult.

1. The patient may have which following condition?
   A. Cervical radiculopathy
   B. Thoracic inlet (outlet) syndrome (TOS)
   C. Carpal tunnel syndrome
   D. All of the above

2. The examination reveals that the Roos or Elevated Arm Stress Test (EAST) is positive on the right, whereas Spurling's test and Tinel's sign at the wrist are both negative. What is the most likely diagnosis?
   A. Cervical radiculopathy
   B. TOS
   C. Carpal tunnel syndrome
   D. None of the above

3. Disc herniation with resultant compression of the C6 nerve root most often occurs at which level?
   A. C4,5
   B. C5,6
   C. C6,7
   D. C7,T1

4. Elevation of the first rib may occur in response to hypertonicity of which of the following?
   A. Levator scapulae
   B. Posterior scalene
   C. Anterior scalene
   D. B and C

5. Direct fascial technique of which muscle is often beneficial in patients with TOS?

A. The quadratus lumborum

B. The rotator cuff

C. The temporalis

D. The pectoralis minor

Case 12

You were exposed to evidence-based practice in PT school, but your first job is in a department that is far from being evidence-based. For the most part, the idea of finding any evidence at all to support a given intervention is rarely discussed, let alone scouring the literature for the "best research evidence."

1. Your plan is to introduce the concept slowly and to start what?

A. Organizing a journal club

B. Speaking with the medical librarian about literature searches

C. Inviting guest speakers who are knowledgeable of the subject

D. All of the above

2. A few therapists in the department are threatened by this concept. They are convinced of the efficacy of their techniques, but are fearful of the changes that may be coming. What is your next step?

A. Tell them to "get with the program"

B. Find a new job

C. Stress the importance of clinical expertise in this paradigm

D. Leave the veterans alone and work with new graduates like yourself

3. The chief therapist realizes the financial liability of not being evidence-based. She wants to know what constitutes "best research evidence." What is your answer?

A. Expert opinion

B. Randomized controlled trials (RCTs)

C. Case studies

D. Retrospective cohort studies

4. One of the recalcitrant "veterans" wants to know whether a patient's input "counts for anything" in this new approach to patient care. What is your answer?

A. Yes

B. No

C. It depends on the patient's knowledge of evidence-based practice

D. They can't be trusted with such important decisions

5. One year has passed and progress has been made. However, one of the therapists is a proponent of therapy "X" for patients with chronic pain. He has undergone extensive training, but other than patient satisfaction he cannot produce sound scientific validation for the use of this intervention. What is your advice to him?

A. Design an acceptable outcome study given the department's resources

B. Submit a grant application for a randomized controlled trial on therapy "X"

C. A and B

D. "All things must come to an end"

Answers

Case 1

1. B) Although the patient's headaches appear related to bruxism, stress, and cervical/TMJ impairment, it is always wise to have headache patients worked up by a neurologist in order to rule out secondary headache. The patient may also be suffering from migraine. If that is the case, the patient may respond well to pharmacologic management.

2. C) The NTI-tss appliance has demonstrated efficacy for controlling the effects of bruxism as well as managing migraine and tension-type headache. It is the only appropriate dental intervention listed for this patient.

3. A) The fifth cranial nerve is the primary nociceptive afferent pathway involved with the mediation of head, neck, and TMJ/facial pain.

4. C) The most likely cause of TMJ clicking in a 25-year-old female is internal derangement. Of the possible types, an anterior disc displacement with reduction is the most prevalent.

5. D) The upper cervical spine can be the source of headaches and dizziness, and can contribute to a TMD through both sensory and motor excitation of the trigeminal nerve (ie, masticatory hypertonicity).

Case 2

1. A) Prior to the use of lumbar extension, McKenzie recommends correcting the lateral shift when present. Flexion exercises have not been shown to be effective for posterior derangements. Myofascial intervention of the quadratus lumborum is considered after the derangement is reduced and stable.

2. C) Whenever symptoms are not made worse by movement nor relieved by rest, the therapist should see a "red flag." The proper course of action is to have the physician rule out a nonmechanical disorder as soon as possible. According to Dr. Stanley Paris, "Physical therapists are experts in dysfunction; physicians are experts in disease."

3. C) Postural syndrome is the least likely option because this patient responded to mechanical interventions consistent with derangement and possibly dysfunction. Postural syndrome by definition may be symptomatic, but there is no limitation of motion nor deformity.

4. C) A right lateral shift adducts the left hip and thus places the left TFL under stretch. As a result, the left TFL is the most likely of the four choices to become irritated under tension and to be tender.

5. D) This is self-explanatory. See Chapter 17.

Case 3

1. B) Recall that forward head posture (FHP) = backward head + forward neck. The patient often appears to have an increased cervical lordosis, but upon radiographic inspection it can be seen that the he or she has a flattened cervical curve. There is evidence in the dental literature that mouth breathing plays a role in the development of FHP in children, which in turn affects the growth and development of the maxillofacial region (ie, retrognathia, malocclusion, TMD, etc). Rocabado has been instrumental in sharing this information with the orthopaedic physical therapy community. On the other hand, there are those who hypothesize that poor ergonomics and body mechanics cause the development of FHP as part of the aging process. Whether FHP works its way down from the head or up from the neck, the result is the same and the consequences are significant, as discussed in Chapter 8. It's no wonder that Alexander developed an entire approach to treatment based on the relationship that exists between the head, neck, and upper back.

2. C) Given that the patient's headaches are unilateral, posturally related, and associated with cervical motion loss, the best choice is cervicogenic headache. A history of a neck injury does not necessarily rule out migraine, but it is consistent with headache of cervical origin. Choices B and D are ruled out because of the long headache history.

3. B) Cervicogenic headache is thought to be more related to C2,3 impairment than any other segment in the neck including OA and AA.[1] B is the only choice that even comes close.

4. D) This is the clear peripheral nerve of choice for headache. As discussed in Chapter 8, greater occipital nerve compression can produce unilateral headache not unlike migraine. Its management, however, is quite different.

5. A) This interconnecting collection of sensory neurons, from the pars caudalis in the lower brainstem to at least the third level in the upper cervical spinal cord, provides the neuroanatomic means whereby the pain related to an upper cervical somatic impairment is able to be felt in the head and TMJ/facial region. It is primarily the ophthalmic division that forms this connection, which explains why cervicogenic headache is perceived most often in the temporoparietal and frontal region (V1) and not in the maxillary (V2) nor mandibular region (V3).

Case 4

1. A) Based on Fryette's first rule (type 1 spinal mechanics), the thoracic spine, from T5 through T11, will rotate to the right when it is first side bent left. Consequently, the ribs will be displaced posteriorly on the right as a result of the right vertebral rotation that occurs with this patient.

2. D) The other choices are all postural muscles, which according to Janda, tend to become facilitated, hypertonic, and tight.

3. B) As per the "arthrokinetic reflex,"[2] restricted midthoracic extension will inhibit the middle trapezius muscle. Consequently, joint manipulation should always precede muscle strengthening in the presence of weak phasic muscles.

4. D) The levator scapulae and latissimus dorsi muscles are both downward rotators of the scapulae and will restrict upward rotation of the scapulae when tight. As a result of limited scapular upward rotation, the suprahumeral tissues (ie, rotator cuff tendons, subdeltoid bursa, etc) are susceptible to compression at the coracoacromial arch during shoulder elevation, causing impingement to occur.

5. C) Of the choices given, this is the best one. It is thoracic spine hypomobility that often causes compensatory hypermobility in the cervical and lumbar spine, leading to pain in these areas. The astute therapist is always on the "look-out" for the AGR. The thoracic spine, like the hips, is a good place to look!

Case 5

1. C) Given the patient's history (ie, missed golf swing) and the physical signs of an iliosacral impairment on the right, it is reasonable to assume that the patient has sustained an anterior rotation subluxation of the right iliac bone. The only set of pelvic landmarks consistent with this diagnosis is choice C.

2. D) This is the muscle that is expected to become hypertonic and short in the presence of an anterior iliac rotation on the right.

3. D) By contracting its antagonistic muscles (ie, the gluteus maximus and hamstrings), the iliopsoas is relaxed through reciprocal inhibition. Once the contractile component of the lesioned complex is minimized, the ilium is free to resume its normal anatomic position on the sacrum. This is the neurophysiologic principle at work with muscle energy technique.

4. A) Large amplitude oscillations at the end of range.

5. B) This is the proper treatment sequence when dealing with tissue dysfunction. When managing a derangement, the sequence is quite different (ie, reduction, maintenance of the reduction, recovery of function, and prevention of recurrence).

Case 6

1. D) All of the above.

2. A) All, except enlargement of the right buttock, are typical of a McKenzie derangement six (ie, adverse sciatic tension, lateral lumbar shift, and centralization of symptoms with lumbar extension).

3. A) To ignore this potentially serious sign and proceed with "business as usual" is the wrong course of action. As the saying goes, "When in doubt, don't!"

4. C) The famous British orthopaedist, Dr. James Cyriax,[3] described the "sign of the buttock" as an indication of "major lesions in the buttock," including osteomyelitis of the upper femur, chronic septic sacroiliac arthritis, ischiorectal abscess, septic arthritis, rheumatic fever with bursitis, neoplasm at the upper femur, iliac neoplasm, and a fractured sacrum. It consists of buttock pain with trunk flexion, hip flexion, and straight leg raising. Passive rotations of the ipsilateral hip are painful, but there is no tissue resistance other than the patient's insistence that the movement be stopped (ie, an "empty end-feel"). Resisted hip movements are often painful, since they alter tensions in the buttock. Inspection of the affected buttock may reveal that it is larger than the other side; palpation may disclose a tumor. With the discovery of these findings, Cyriax recommends that the patient's temperature be taken, a rectal examination be performed, and a radiograph be ordered without delay.

5. B) Given that the tumor was compressing the sciatic nerve in the right buttock area, this patient closely resembled a discogenic patient with sciatic compression. Except for the large buttock and the fact that hip flexion with the knee flexed provoked right buttock pain, this patient would present very much like a patient with a McKenzie derangement six.

Case 7

1. C) Given symptoms of nerve root irritation in the left C7 dermatome (ie, "tingling" in the middle finger), the most likely disc derangement would be at the C6,7 level. Because the nerve roots in the cervical spine exit above the

pedicle of the corresponding vertebrae, a typical posterolateral cervical disc herniation impinges on the nerve root exiting at the level of the disc. For example, a disc herniation at the C4,5 level compresses the C5 nerve root.

2. B) A combined restriction in extension, rotation, and side bending to the left is referred to as an FRS right. The problem with an FRS right is that the left apophyseal joint is "stuck" in the "open" position and can't "close."

3. A) Since the triceps muscle is innervated by the efferent fibers of the left C7 nerve root, compression from a herniated disc at C6,7 can potentially lead to triceps weakness, atrophy, and hyporeflexia of the triceps jerk.

4. D) The correct answer would have been the flexors, right rotators, and right side benders. However, because the correct choice is not listed, the answer is D. Postisometric relaxation (PIR) is an extremely useful intervention in manual therapy. Because there is almost always an element of muscle hypertonicity in somatic impairment of the vertebral and peripheral joints, PIR should routinely be performed prior to mobilization of the noncontractile connective tissue capsule. There are several theories related to the neurophysiology of PIR. These include Golgi tendon organ reflex inhibition, Renshaw cell inhibition of the alpha motoneurons, presynaptic Ia inhibition, reduction in gamma motoneuron activity, and sensorimotor learning. In addition, it is conceivable that PIR achieves increased range of motion as a result of the fascial "stretch" produced by the contracting muscle belly. Postisometric relaxation is related to what Hammer[4] refers to as "postfacilitation stretch," which includes an isometric contraction of 7 seconds duration, followed by 12 seconds of stretching.

5. D) This is self-explanatory. See Chapter 8.

Case 8

1. B) As described by Panjabi,[5,6] clinical "instability" is the failure of the "spinal stabilization system" to restrict the neutral zone to the physiologic borders of a segment's range of motion. As discussed in the introduction to Chapter 20, the "spinal stabilization system" consists of three components, namely the passive, active, and neural control subsystems. In this case, our 17-year-old basketball player already shows signs of degenerative disc disease according to the MRI. According to Macnab,[7] the facet joints in this degenerative state subluxate into hyperextension and are held at the extreme of their limit or what Panjabi calls the elastic zone. Consequently, the extension strains of everyday living tend to push the joints past their physiologically permitted limits and thereby produce pain. In general, segmental "instability" is considered to be anything greater than 3.5 mm of horizontal translation (ie, along the Z-axis) on a standing lateral radiograph with the patient moving between flexion and extension.[8] It must be kept in mind, however, that the presence of "instability" must always be correlated with the patient's symptoms in the clinical decision making process.

2. B) Of all the choices, the only muscle that has been shown to control segmental motion of the spine is the multifidus. All the others (sacrospinalis, quadratus lumborum, and rectus abdominis) are postural muscles that tend towards hypertonicity and shortening, which do not provide physiologic stability to the lumbar spine.

3. D) The three muscles listed (ie, the transversus abdominis, pubococcygeus, and multifidus) are all core stabilizers. The fourth, which is not listed, is the respiratory diaphragm.

4. A) This is the correct way of eliciting a transversus abdominis contraction, but it is not the easy way. The easy but incorrect way is to "suck the belly in" with a deep inhalation or to perform a posterior pelvic tilt. However, neither have been shown to activate the transversus, and the patient must not be permitted to "cheat" by taking these measures.

5. D) It is the close-packed position of segmental hyperextension that causes this young athlete so much grief. The goal of "spinal stabilization training" is to activate the active and neural control subsystems so that the patient regains control of the neutral zone in hopes of recovering function and managing symptoms.

Case 9

1. D) Given the "capsular pattern" of the right TMJ, choices A and C are both possibilities. Based upon physical signs alone, we know that there is limited translation of the right mandibular condyle. However, at this point we don't know whether the capsule is inflamed or the disc is displaced without reduction. Stay tuned!

2. A) The only acceptable answer is A. Whereas head-neck extension increases the interocclusal or freeway space, forward head posture (FHP) has been shown to decrease it. It is theorized that the increase in temporalis activity, associated with occipital extension, plays a role in this response by displacing the mandible in a posterior and superior direction. The author submits that the forward translation of the occipital condyles on the atlas vertebra also plays a role by causing a vertical "drop" of the skull onto the mandible (ie, not only does FHP cause the mandible to be "pulled" upward, but it also causes the maxilla to "drop" down on the mandible, which in either case diminishes the freeway space between the upper and lower teeth).

3. B) The difference between question 1 and 3 is the patient's history. The additional information indicates the presence of a right sided TMJ internal derangement prior to her MVA. Consequently, we would expect the MRI to confirm a nonreducing anterior disc displacement (ie, a closed-lock).

4. B) The most likely restriction in light of an accentuated midthoracic kyphosis with scapular protraction, elevation, and downward rotation is thoracic extension. This can be tested with PAIVMs or PPIVMs as discussed in Chapter 4.

5. D) The Alexander technique accomplishes many things, but there are four core components. They are restoring "primary control" by allowing the neck to release so that the head can balance forward and up, which in turn facilitates a lengthening and widening of the torso, a lateral release of the shoulders away from the chest wall, and a release of the legs/hips away from the pelvis. Consequently, A and B are both good choices.

Case 10

1. C) Intermittent claudication (ie, limping or "lameness") has generally been attributed to an occlusive vascular disease of the legs. In the mid 1950's, however, Verbiest[9] also linked this clinical picture to narrowing of the spinal canal (ie, spinal stenosis) with resultant compression of the spinal nerve roots. Typically, the patient walks a certain distance until leg symptoms, such as pain, numbness, weakness, etc, force the patient to stop walking. Unlike vascular claudication, which requires only that the patient rests, neurogenic claudication requires that the patient decompress the impinged nerve roots by flexing his or her lumbar spine. Based on the history provided, our professor may have claudication of either a vascular or neurogenic nature. Stay tuned!

2. B) The crucial diagnostic distinction between a vascular and a neurologic disorder, in this instance, is found in the intervention that relieves the patient's symptoms. Because spinal flexion helped whereas rest alone did not, the right calf symptoms are therefore due to neurogenic claudication.

3. C) HNP is the only other choice that comes close. However, HNP is most prevalent in the 25 to 45 year old range, whereas stenosis is a more likely cause of nerve root compression at age 70 (this is because of the gradual loss of water content in the disc from approximately 90% in early adult life to 70% in the elderly). In addition, the peripheral symptoms associated with an HNP tend to worsen with spinal flexion rather than extension.

4. A) Given the excellent specificity (ie, the ability of a test to correctly identify patients without a disease ["negative in health"]) of the crossed straight leg raising test (0.90), it is more effective as a rule-in test for peripheral nerve compression, whereas ipsilateral straight leg raising (SLR) is more effective as a rule-out test, given its high degree (0.80) of sensitivity (ie, the proportion of persons with the disease who have a positive test "[positive in disease"]). In other words, because the crossed SLR is rarely positive in health (only 10% of the time), a positive test result almost always indicates impairment. Similarly, the absence of sciatica (or femoral nerve radicular pain) makes a clinically significant disc herniation very unlikely because, being such a sensitive finding (0.95), its absence becomes highly significant.[8]

5. B) Because the patient's lower limb circulatory status is not the problem, the "stationary bike test" should be normal. With intermittent neurogenic claudication secondary to spinal stenosis, the provoking factor is not ischemia, but rather activities that place the lumbar spine into an extended position. In fact, the flexion associated with riding a bicycle could prove to be therapeutic for patients suffering from spinal stenosis.

Case 11

1. D) Based on the history provided, all the choices listed are potential causes of the patient's chief complaint.

2. B) A positive Roos or Elevated Arm Stress Test (EAST) rules-in TOS. This, in conjunction with tests to rule-out the cervical spine (negative Spurling's test) and the carpal tunnel (negative Tinel's sign), makes the diagnosis more likely.

3. B) For the reason given in case 7, question 1, the answer is the C5,6 disc. This formula, however, changes at the thoracolumbar junction and below. Starting at T1 and throughout the remainder of the thoracolumbar spine, the nerve roots exit caudal to the pedicle of the corresponding vertebra. However, in the lower lumbar spine where most of the herniated discs occur, it is still the lower root level that is most often impinged (ie, an L4,5 disc herniation will compress the L5 nerve root). This is because the nerve root is not impinged at the level of the foramina where it exits, but posteriorly as it descends through the spinal canal. However, a large disc herniation and/or lateral recess stenosis may violate this rule and impinge the nerve root above (ie, L4 compression at the L4,5 level). According to Kramer,[10] herniated cervical discs occur most often at C5,6 (41%) followed by C6,7 (33%). Nerve root involvement by level is C5 = 4.1%, C6 = 36.1%, C7 = 34.6%, and C8 = 25.2%.

4. C) This is the only possible choice. The posterior scalene attaches to the second rib, where hypertonicity may cause a superiorly laterally flexed rib.

5. D) Of all the muscles listed, the pectoralis minor is the only one that has direct bearing on TOS. Because it is capable of impinging the neurovascular bundle (subclavian artery, vein, and lower trunk of the brachial plexus), direct fascial technique, for the purpose of releasing muscular tension and restrictions, is often quite effective in the management of TOS.

Case 12

1. D) A through C are all excellent ways of beginning the process. Before your department can be evidence-based, the therapists must learn how to access the literature. In addition, most clinicians require further postgraduate training in critiquing scientific papers. Guest speakers with expertise in research design can get the ball rolling.

2. C) Sackett et al[11] emphasize that EBM is the "integration of best research evidence with clinical expertise and patient values." Consequently, the anxious therapists in this department must realize that their clinical experience and expertise are not completely overlooked in this system. The goal of EBM is not to "throw the baby out with the bathwater," but rather to apply a systematic review process to all aspects of clinical physical therapy so that clinical practice guidelines can be established. The operative word here is "guideline" and not "mandate." If presented in this manner, EBM need not be feared but welcomed.

3. B) Of the five levels of potential evidence, Sackett et al[11] place the systematic review of high-quality RCTs at the top of the list (ie, level 1). Though not the only acceptable form of evidence, RCTs do qualify as the "best evidence" available.

4. A) Again, as per the definition of EBM mentioned above,[11] "patient values" do enter into the equation. It must always be remembered that above all else, the needs of the patient are paramount. Although EBM is an attempt to utilize interventions that are based upon the best evidence available, we as physical therapists are still treating human beings. Their needs, feelings, expectations, and welfare must always remain our top priority. If, for example, a patient "swears by ultrasound" and is convinced that it has helped in the past, this should then become part of the "evidence" in designing a treatment plan for this patient. It would be wrong, in the opinion of the author, to dismiss this patient's preference, unless there are known contraindications, simply because there was a lack of RCTs on this intervention. In other words, common sense sometimes needs to carry the day!

5. C) In the days of EBM it is no longer acceptable to say, "I know it works and that's all that matters." The retort is, "If it you know it works, then prove it"! In the long run, this therapist will benefit when his therapy "X" is shown to be effective. As someone has wisely said, "It's not science until it's published". The question is whether to refrain from providing a particular intervention when there are no acceptable studies one way or the other.[12] In this author's opinion, we must exercise extreme caution at this early stage in the development of EBM. The process must be given time and we must be patient!

References and Bibliography

References

1. Schoensee SK, Jensen G, Nicholson G, Gossman M, Katholi C. The effect of mobilization on cervical headaches. *J Orthop Sports Phys Ther*. 1995;21(4):184-196.

2. Wyke BD. Articular neurology and manipulative therapy. In: Glasgow EF, Twomey LT, Scull ER, Kleynhans AM, Idczak RMC, eds. *Aspects of Manipulative Therapy*. Melbourne: Churchill Livingstone; 1985.

3. Cyriax J. *Textbook of Orthopaedic Medicine, Vol. 1: Diagnosis of Soft Tissue Lesions*. London: Bailliere Tindall; 1978.

4. Hammer WI. *Functional Soft Tissue Examination and Treatment by Manual Methods: New Perspectives*. 2nd ed. Gaithersburg, Md: Aspen Publishers; 1999.

5. Panjabi M. The stabilizing system of the spine. Part I. Function, dysfunction, adaptation, and enhancement. *J Spinal Disorders*. 1989;5:383-389.

6. Panjabi M. The stabilizing system of the spine. Part II. Neutral zone and stability hypothesis. *J Spinal Disord Tech*. 1992;5:393-397.

7. Macnab I. *Backache*. Baltimore, Md: Williams & Wilkins; 1977.

8. Weinstein JN, Rydevik BL, Sonntag VKH, eds. *Essentials of the Spine*. New York, NY: Raven Press; 1995.

9. Verbiest H. A radicular syndrome from developmental narrowing of the lumbar spine vertebral canal. *J Bone Joint Surg (Br)*. 1954;36B:230-237.

10. Kramer J. *Intervertebral Disk Diseases: Causes, Diagnosis, Treatment and Prophylaxis*. 2nd ed. New York, NY: Thieme Medical Publishers; 1990.

11. Sackett DL. Straus SE, Richardson WS, et al. *Evidence-Based Medicine: How to Practice and Teach EBM*. 2nd ed. New York, NY: Churchill Livingstone; 2000.

12. Medeiros J. Knowledge-based practice. *Journal of Manual & Manipulative Therapy*. 2002;10(2):64-65.

Bibliography

Barry MJ. Evidence-based practice in pediatric physical therapy. *PT Magazine*. 2001;38-51.

Caplan D. *Back Trouble: A New Approach to Prevention and Recovery*. Gainesville, Fla: Triad Publishing; 1987.

Cibulka MT, Aslin K. How to use evidence-based practice to distinguish between three different patients with low back pain. *J Orthop Sports Phys Ther*. 2001;31(12):678-695.

Fairbank JCT, Pynsent PB. The Oswestry disability index. *Spine*. 2000;25(22):2940-2953.

Korr IM. Proprioceptors and somatic dysfunction. *JAOA*. 1975;74:638-650.

Lawlis GF, Cuencas R, Selby D, McCoy CE. The development of the Dallas Pain Questionnaire, an assessment of the impact of spinal pain on behavior. *Spine*. 1989;14:511-516.

Meadows JTS. *Orthopaedic Differential Diagnosis in Physical Therapy: A Case Study Approach*. New York, NY: McGraw-Hill; 1999.

Melzack R, Katz J. Pain measurement in persons in pain. In: Wall PD, Melzack R, eds. *Textbook of Pain*. 4th ed. Edinburgh: Churchill Livingstone; 1999.

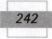

Moeti P, Marchetti G. Clinical outcome from mechanical intermittent cervical traction for the treatment of cervical radiculopathy: a case series. *J Orthop Sports Phys Ther.* 2001;31(4):207-213.

Savarese RG, ed. *OMT Review: A Comprehensive Review in Osteopathic Medicine.* 2nd ed. West Orange, NJ: Author; 1999.

Vernon H, Mior S. The neck disability index: a study of reliability and validity. *J Manipulative Physiol Ther.* 1991;14:411.

Index

Neuromuscular mobilization, pelvic, 191
Neuromusculoskeletal impairment, 51–52
Neuromusculoskeletal stabilization, 123–125
Neutral zone, 157
Newton's Third Law, 83
Nine-point Brighton scale for generalized hypermobility, 140
Northwick Park Neck Pain Questionnaire, 61
NTI-TSS device, 236
    for temporomandibular joint disorders, 113
Nuchal line, inferior, 67

Ober's test position, 186
Occipital cervical flexors, 89–90
Occipital distraction, inhibitive, 71–72
Occipital extension, 74
Occipital extensor stretch, 75, 76f
Occipital nerve, greater
    compression of, 237
    palpation of, 68
Occipital position
    evaluation of, 59
    in frontal plane, 59–60
Occipital protuberance, external, 67
Occipitoatlantal flexion mobilization, 75
One-legged stork test, 175–177
Onset, 12
Orbicularis oculi muscle, 111
Orthopaedic tests, lumbar spine, 140
Orthostatic posture, attaining, 14
Osler, Sir William, 15
Osteocentric position, 157
Osteopathic lesion, 11
Osteopathic manipulative therapy, 12
Oswestry Disability Index, Version 2.0, 230
Overturning, 7

Pain. *See also* Backache; Headache; Low back pain; Neck pain
    assessment of, 12
    cervical mobilization effects on, 221–222
    differential diagnosis of, 17f
    for cervical derangement, 86
    for herniated lumbar intervertebral disc with radiculopathy, 216–217
    in sagittal end-range spinal motion, 212–213
    management of
    neurogenic, 17f
    radiating, 12
    upper cervical, 91–94
    viscogenic, 17f
Palpation
    of lumbar spine, 139–140
    of pelvic/hip landmarks, 171–174
    of temporomandibular joint, 104f, 107–109

two-hand style of, 33–34
Paravertebral muscles, asymmetric, 132
Passive accessory intervertebral movements, 41
    evaluation of in scapulothoracic region, 27–29
Passive accessory rib mobility, 32
Passive mobilization, 213–214
Passive physiologic intervertebral movements, 41
    evaluation of in scapulothoracic region, 29–30
    of lumbar spine, 138–139
Pectoralis major/minor fascial technique, 35
Pelvic angle, 170f
Pelvic floor, 151
    contraction of, 156
    muscles of, 179
Pelvic floor fascial technique, 184
Pelvic floor syndrome, 183
Pelvic girdle
    connective tissue techniques and stretching procedures for, 183–190
    examination and evaluation of, 169–181
    manual therapy for, 191–198
    mechanical stability of, 169
    structural exam of, 170–175
    therapeutic and home exercises for, 199–203
Pelvic torsion test, 180–181
Pelvic/urogenital diaphragm release, 183
Pelvis
    angles in, 170
    asymmetry of, 169–175
    bony landmarks of, 170–175
    form/force closure of, 169
    normal angles of, 170f
    soft tissue structures of, 178–179
Peroneal nerve, common, mobilization of, 145
Phasic muscles, 13
    strengthening exercises for, 14, 89–90
Physical therapy
    for herniated lumbar intervertebral disc with radiculopathy, 216–217
    for neck pain, 220–221
Physical Therapy Forum, 162
Physiologic motion, 3
    barrier to, 7
Physiologic tripodism, loss of, 70
Piriformis fascial technique, 184–185
Piriformis muscle, 178
    self-stretch of, 199–200
    stretch of, 186
Plumb-line grid, 60
Posterior shear test, 180
Posteroanterior central spring test, 28–29
Postisometric relaxation, 36, 186, 189
    with thoracic manipulations, 48
Postural alignment, assessment of, 131–132
Postural balance, 14

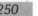

Build Your Library

Along with this title, we publish numerous products on a variety of topics. We are sure that you will find the below titles to be an essential addition to your library. Order your copies today or contact us for a copy of our latest catalog for additional product information.

SPINAL MANUAL THERAPY: AN INTRODUCTION TO SOFT TISSUE MOBILIZATION, SPINAL MANIPULATION, THERAPEUTIC AND HOME EXERCISES

Howard W. Makofsky, PT, DHSc, OCS

272 pp., Soft Cover, 2003, ISBN 1-55642-569-4, Order #45694, **$39.95**

Spinal Manual Therapy: An Introduction to Soft Tissue Mobilization, Spinal Manipulation, Therapeutic and Home Exercises is a systematic, easy-to-follow manual of clinical techniques for the spine, pelvis, and temporomandibular joint. It is the ideal resource for all those interested in grasping the basics of spinal manual therapy and transferring that knowledge into practice within a clinical environment.

THE MYOFASCIAL RELEASE MANUAL, THIRD EDITION

Carol Manheim, MS, MEd, PT, LPC

304 pp., Soft Cover, 2001, ISBN 1-55642-452-3, Order #44523, **$47.95**

The Myofascial Release Manual, Third Edition is an essential manual that includes answers to commonly asked questions and does an excellent job of illustrating hand placement for many of the muscles in the body. Carol J. Manheim, MS, MEd, PT, LPC, renowned in the area of Myofascial Release, has developed this new edition to be modeled after her own extensive background, teaching experiences, and lectures.

THE MANUAL OF TRIGGER POINT AND MYOFASCIAL THERAPY

Dimitrios Kostopoulos, PT, PhD and Konstantine Rizopoulos, PT, FABS

264 pp., Soft Cover, 2001, ISBN 1-55642-542-2, Order #45422, **$47.95**

The Manual of Trigger Point and Myofascial Therapy offers the reader a comprehensive therapeutic approach for the evaluation and treatment of Myofascial pain and musculoskeletal dysfunction. This user-friendly manual will serve as a quick reference for clinically relevant items that pertain to the identification and management of trigger points.

Contact us at

SLACK Incorporated, Professional Book Division
6900 Grove Road, Thorofare, NJ 08086
1-800-257-8290/1-856-848-1000, Fax: 1-856-853-5991
E-Mail: orders@slackinc.com or www.slackbooks.com

ORDER FORM

QUANTITY	TITLE	ORDER #	PRICE
	Spinal Manual Therapy	45694	$39.95
	Myofascial Release Manual, Third Edition	44523	$47.95
	Manual of Trigger Point and Myofascial Therapy	45422	$47.95
		Subtotal	$
		Applicable state and local tax will be added to your purchase	$
		Handling	$4.50
		Total	$

Name _____

Address: _____

City: _____ State: _____ Zip: _____

Phone: _____ Fax _____

Email: _____

• Check enclosed (Payable to SLACK Incorporated) _____

• Charge my: _____ [AMERICAN EXPRESS] _____ VISA _____ MasterCard

Account #: _____

Exp. date: _____ Signature _____

NOTE: Prices are subject to change without notice.
Shipping charges will apply.
Shipping and handling charges are non-refundable

CODE: 328